# Medical Terminology Systems

## A Body Systems Approach

D1370323

FIFTH EDITION

**Barbara A. Gylys,** MEd, CMA-A

Professor Emerita
College of Health and Human Services
Medical Assisting Technology
University of Toledo
Toledo, Ohio

**Mary Ellen Wedding,** MEd, MT(ASCP), CMA, AAPC

Professor of Health Professions
College of Health and Human Services
University of Toledo
Toledo, Ohio

# *Medical Terminology Systems*

## A Body Systems Approach

**F. A. DAVIS COMPANY** • Philadelphia

Medical terminology is presented in a clear and concise manner, using the classic word-building and body systems approach to learning.

# What's *Inside....*

The pages of Medical Terminology Systems: A Body Systems Approach, 5th Edition

## Chapter Outlines
to orient student to each chapter's content
(see page 107)

**CHAPTER OUTLINE**

Objectives
Key Terms
Anatomy and Physiology
  Mouth
  Teeth
  Tongue
  Hard and Soft Palates
  Pharynx, Esophagus, and
  Stomach
  Small Intestine
  Large Intestine
  Accessory Organs of Digestion
  Liver
  Pancreas
  Gallbladder
Medical Word Elements
  Combining Forms
  Mouth
  Esophagus, Pharynx, and
  Stomach
  Small Intestine
  Large Intestine
  Terminal End of Large Intestine
  Accessory Organs of Digestion

  Suffixes
  Prefixes
Pathology
  Ulcer
  Peptic Ulcer Disease
  Ulcerative Colitis
  Hernia
  Bowel Obstruction
  Hemorrhoids
  Liver Disorders
  Diverticulosis
  Oncology
Diagnostic, Symptomatic, and
  Related Terms
Diagnostic and Therapeutic
  Procedures
Pharmacology
Abbreviations
Learning Activities
Medical Record Activities
  GI evaluation
  Esophagogastroduodenoscopy with
  biopsy

**Key Terms**

This section introduces important digestive system terms and their definitions. Word analyses are also provided.

| Term | Definition |
|------|------------|
| **asymptomatic**<br>ā-simp-tō-MĂT-ĭk | Without symptoms |
| **defecation**<br>dĕf-ĕ-KĀ-shŭn | Elimination of feces from the gastrointestinal tract through the rectum |
| **duodenal bulb**<br>dū-ō-DĒ-năl BŬLB | Upper duodenal area just beyond the pylorus |
| **endoscope**<br>ĔN-dō-skōp<br>*endo-*: in, within<br>*-scope*: instrument for examining | Instrument consisting of a rigid or flexible fiberoptic tube and optical system for observing the inside of a hollow organ or cavity |
| **exocrine**<br>ĔKS-ō-krin<br>*exo-* : outside, outward<br>*-crine*: secrete | Pertaining to a gland that secretes outwardly through excretory ducts to the surface of an organ or tissue or into a vessel |

## Key Terms highlighted in the
beginning of each chapter
(see page 108)

| Abbreviation | Meaning |
|--------------|---------|
| COMMON | |
| ABC | aspiration biopsy cytology |
| alk phos | alkaline phosphatase |
| ALT | alanine aminotransferase (elevated in liver and heart disease); formerly *SGPT* |
| AST | |
| Ba | |
| BaE | |

| Abbreviation | Meaning |
|--------------|---------|
| COMMON | |
| **ABC** | aspiration biopsy cytology |
| **alk phos** | alkaline phosphatase |
| **ALT** | alanine aminotransferase (elevated in liver and heart disease); formerly *SGPT* |

## Abbreviations
for common terms
(see page 136)

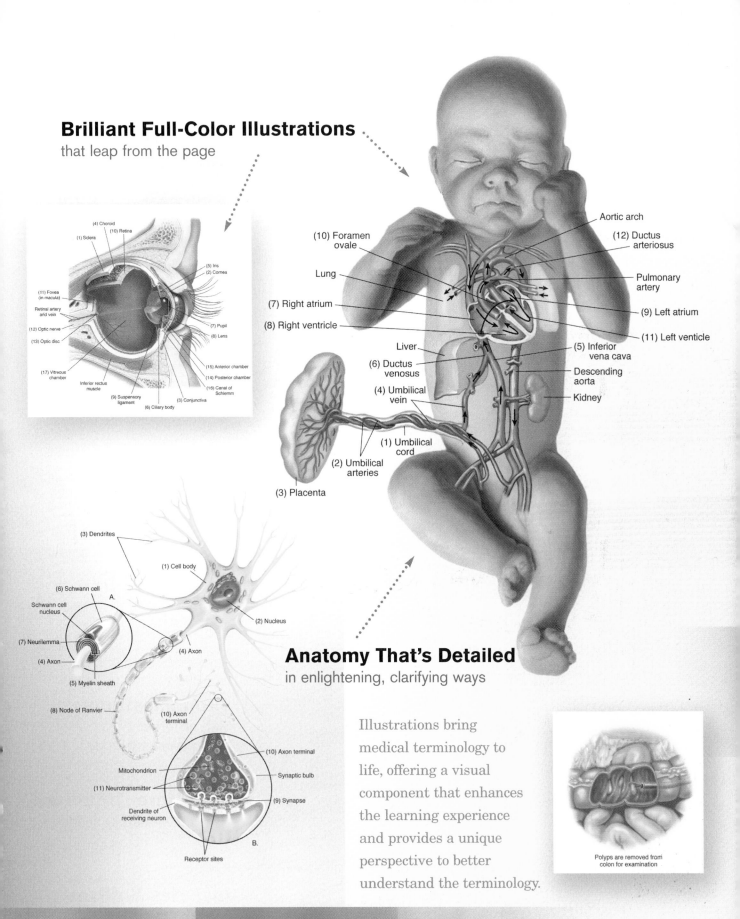

## Brilliant Full-Color Illustrations
that leap from the page

**Eye diagram labels:**
(4) Choroid
(10) Retina
(1) Sclera
(5) Iris
(2) Cornea
(11) Fovea (in macula)
Retinal artery and vein
(12) Optic nerve
(13) Optic disc
(7) Pupil
(8) Lens
(17) Vitreous chamber
(15) Anterior chamber
(14) Posterior chamber
(16) Canal of Schlemm
Inferior rectus muscle
(9) Suspensory ligament
(3) Conjunctiva
(6) Ciliary body

**Fetal circulation labels:**
(10) Foramen ovale
Aortic arch
(12) Ductus arteriosus
Lung
Pulmonary artery
(7) Right atrium
(9) Left atrium
(8) Right ventricle
(11) Left venticle
Liver
(5) Inferior vena cava
(6) Ductus venosus
Descending aorta
(4) Umbilical vein
Kidney
(1) Umbilical cord
(2) Umbilical arteries
(3) Placenta

**Neuron diagram labels:**
(3) Dendrites
(1) Cell body
(6) Schwann cell
Schwann cell nucleus
A.
(7) Neurilemma
(2) Nucleus
(4) Axon
(5) Myelin sheath
(4) Axon
(8) Node of Ranvier
(10) Axon terminal
Mitochondrion
(10) Axon terminal
Synaptic bulb
(11) Neurotransmitter
(9) Synapse
Dendrite of receiving neuron
B.
Receptor sites

## Anatomy That's Detailed
in enlightening, clarifying ways

Illustrations bring medical terminology to life, offering a visual component that enhances the learning experience and provides a unique perspective to better understand the terminology.

Polyps are removed from colon for examination

# ...A Unique Blend of Words and Art

**GI Evaluation**

**HISTORY OF PRESENT ILLNESS:** The patient's abdominal pain began 2 years ago when she first had intermittent, sharp epigastric pain. Each episode lasted 2 to 4 hours. Eventually, she was diagnosed as having cholecystitis with cholelithiasis and underwent cholecystectomy. Three to five large calcified stones were found.

Her postoperative course was uneventful until 4 months ago, when she began having continuous deep right-sided pain.

This pain followed a crescendo pattern and peaked several weeks ago, at a time when family stress was also at its climax. Since then, the pain has been following a decrescendo pattern. It does not cause any nausea or vomiting, does not trigger any urge to defecate, and was not alleviated by passage of flatus. Her PMH is significant only for tonsillectomy, appendectomy, and the cholecystectomy. Her PE findings indicate that there was no hepatomegaly or splenomegaly. The rectal examination confirmed normal sphincter tone and heme-negative stool.

**IMPRESSION:** Abdominal pain. R/O hepatomegaly and splenomegaly.

**PLAN:** Schedule a complete barium workup for possible obstruction.

**Analysis**

Review the medical record *GI Evaluation* to answer the following questions.

1. While referring to Figure 6–3, describe the location of the gallbladder in relation to the liver.

2. Why did the patient undergo the cholecystectomy?

3. List the patient's prior surgeries.

4. How does the patient's most recent postoperative episode of discomfort (pain) differ from the initial pain she described?

**Detailed Medical Records**
with each body system, that provide real-life examples
(see page 146)

**Procedure** | **Description**

**DIAGNOSTIC PROCEDURES**

**Endoscopic**

**endoscopy**
ĕn-DŎS-kō-pē

*endo-:* in, within
*-scopy:* visual examinination

**upper GI**

**lower GI**

Visual examination of a cavity or canal using a specialized lighted instrument called an *endoscope*
The organ, cavity, or canal being examined dictates the name of the endoscopic procedure. (See Figure 4–5.) A camera and video recorder are commonly used during the procedure to provide a permanent record.
Endoscopy of the esophagus (esophagoscopy), stomach (gastroscopy), and duodenum (duodenoscopy)
Endoscopy of the upper GI tract is performed to identify tumors, esophagitis, gastroesophageal varices, peptic ulcers, and the source of upper GI bleeding. It is also used to confirm the presence and extent of varices in the lower esophagus and stomach in patients with liver disease.
Endoscopy of the colon (colonoscopy), sigmoid colon (sigmoidoscopy), and rectum and anal canal (proctoscopy) (See Figure 6–9.)
Endoscopy of the lower GI tract is used to identify pathological conditions in the colon. It may also be used to remove polyps. When polyps are discovered in the colon, they are retrieved and tested for cancer.

**Fully Revised Table Format**
for better retention and quick learning
(see page 128)

| Element | Meaning | Word Analysis | *(Continued)* |
|---------|---------|---------------|-----|
| **gingiv/o** | gum(s) | gingiv/ectomy (jĭn-jĭ-VĔK-tō-mē): excision of diseased gingival tissue in surgical treatment of periodontal disease<br>*-ectomy:* excision, removal | |
| **sial/o** | saliva, salivary gland | sial/o/lith (sī-ĂL-ō-lĭth): calculus formed in a salivary gland or duct<br>*-lith:* stone, calculus | |
| Esophagus, Pharynx, and Stomach | | | |
| **esophag/o** | esophagus | esophag/o/scope (ē-SŎF-ă-gō-skōp): endoscope used to examine the esophagus<br>*-scope:* instrument for examining | |
| **pharyng/o** | pharynx (throat) | pharyng/o/tonsill/itis (fă-ŭng-gō-tŏn-sĭ-LĪ-tĭs): inflammation of the pharynx and tonsils<br>*tonsill:* tonsils<br>*-itis:* inflammation | |
| **gastr/o** | stomach | gastr/algia (găs-TRĂL-jē-ă): pain in the stomach from any cause; also called *stomachache*<br>*-algia:* pain | |
| **pylor/o** | pylorus | pylor/o/spasm (pī-LOR-ō-spăzm): involuntary contraction of the pyloric sphincter of the stomach, as in pyloric stenosis<br>*-spasm:* involuntary contraction, twitching | |
| Small Intestine | | | |
| **duoden/o** | duodenum (first part of small intestine) | duoden/o/scopy (dū-ŏd-ĕ-NŎS-kō-pē): visual examination of the duodenum<br>*-scopy:* visual examination | |
| **enter/o** | intestine (usually small intestine) | enter/o/pathy (ĕn-tĕr-ŎP-ă-thē): any intestinal disease<br>*-pathy:* disease | |

**Pronunciations**
with all terms
(see page 116)

**More Organized,**
user-friendly headings

**Includes Suffixes**
and their meanings

**Worksheets Containing Exercises and Activities** are featured in each chapter, to help track progress and to review for quizzes and tests (see pages 142-143)

Learning Activity 6–4

**Building surgical words**

*Build a surgical word that means:*

1. excision of gums (tissue) _____
2. partial or complete excision of the tongue _____
3. repair of the esophagus _____
4. removal of part or all of the stomach _____
5. forming an opening between the stomach _____
6. excision of (part of) the esophagus _____
7. forming an opening between the stomach and jejunum _____
8. surgical repair of the esophagus _____
9. fixation of the small intestine _____
10. suture of the bile duct _____
11. forming an opening into the colon _____
12. fixation of a movable liver (to the abdominal wall) _____
13. surgical repair of the anus or rectum _____
14. removal of the gallbladder _____
15. surgical repair of a bile duct _____

Check your answers in Appendix A. Review material that you did not answer correctly.

**CORRECT ANSWERS** _____ × 6.67 = _____ **% SCORE**

Learning Activity 6–5

**Matching pathological, diagnostic, symptomatic, and related terms**

*Match the following terms with the definitions in the numbered list.*

anorexia        dysphagia        hematemesis
cachexia        dyspnea          lesion
cirrhosis       fecalith         melena
dyspepsia       halitosis        obstipation

_____ vomiting blood
_____ difficulty swallowing or inability to swallow
1. _____ fecal concretion
2. _____ "bad" breath
3. _____ loss of appetite
4. _____ poor digestion
5. _____ degenerative liver disease
6. _____
7. _____

**Packaged with Interactive Medical Terminology 2.0** on CD-ROM. Designed to be used in tandem with the text, this interactive software helps students master medical terminology. IMT 2.0 includes:

- Nearly 1200 test items
- Choice of basic or advanced testing modes
- Interactive exercises such as crossword puzzles, word drag-and-drop, and word scrambles
- Comprehensive score reporting for each exercise

ARTHRODESIS
CARPAL
FRACTURE
HUMERUS
ISCHIAL
MUSCLE
OSTEOMALACIA
PATELLECTOMY
TENDON

One word Solved

Play

**Interactive Medical Terminology / Speci**

options ▼

- module menu
- exercise menu
- my progress
- games
- dictionary
- help

**Neurology:** Applied Activity

**Objectives:** To identify the word components related to the Nervous System.

Question 4 of 5

Drag and drop the word component(s) to its proper position.

Combining form:

mening/o        cerebr/o
encephal/o
medull/o

F. A. Davis Company
1915 Arch Street
Philadelphia, PA 19103
www.fadavis.com

Printed in the United States of America

Last digit indicates print number: 10 9 8 7 6 5 4 3 2 1

*Acquisitions Editor:* Andy McPhee
*Developmental Editor:* Brenna Mayer
*Art and Design Manager:* Joan Wendt

As new scientific information becomes available through basic and clinical research, recommended treatments and drug therapies undergo changes. The author(s) and publisher have done everything possible to make this book accurate, up to date, and in accord with accepted standards at the time of publication. The author(s), editors, and publisher are not responsible for errors or omissions or for consequences from application of the book, and make no warranty, expressed or implied, in regard to the contents of the book. Any practice described in this book should be applied by the reader in accordance with professional standards of care used in regard to the unique circumstances that may apply in each situation. The reader is advised always to check product information (package inserts) for changes and new information regarding dose and contraindications before administering any drug. Caution is especially urged when using new or infrequently ordered drugs.

**Library of Congress Cataloging-in-Publication Data**

0–8036–1249–X

**This book is dedicated with love**

■ ■ ■ ■ ■

to my best friend, colleague,
and husband, Julius A. Gylys

*and*

to my children,
Regina Maria
and Julius Anthony

*and*

to Andrew Masters,
Julia Masters, Caitlin Masters,
Anthony Mychal Bishop-Gylys,
and Matthew James Bishop-Gylys

**B.A.G.**


to my little ones,
Andrew Arthur Kurtz,
Katherine Louise Kurtz,
Daniel Keith Wedding, II,
Carol Ann Estelle Wedding,
Jonathan Michael Kurtz,
Donald Keith Wedding, III,
and Emily Michelle Wedding

**M.E.W.**

# Acknowledgments

The authors would like to acknowledge the valuable contributions of F. A. Davis's editorial and production team who were responsible for this project:

- **Andy McPhee, Acquisitions Editor,** who provided the overall design and layout for the fifth edition. His vision of the work helped focus the authors at the onset of the project and his guidance throughout this endeavor provided cohesiveness.
- **Susan Rhyner, Manager of Creative Development,** whose expertise and care are evident in the quality of support staff she selected for the fifth edition. We are especially grateful for her continued support and help whenever it was needed.
- **Margaret Biblis, Publisher,** Health Professions and Medicine, whose untiring "behind-the-scenes" efforts are evident in the quality of the finished product.
- **Brenna Mayer, Developmental Editor,** whose careful and conscientious edits and suggestions for the manuscript are evident throughout the entire work. Her untiring assistance and support during this project are deeply appreciated and the authors extend their sincerest gratitude.
- **Anne Rains, Artist,** who developed high-quality illustrations throughout the textbook. Her ability to capture in line and color the words and concepts envisioned by the authors is outstanding. The authors wish to acknowledge her artistic talents and thank her for being a part of this project.

In addition, we wish to acknowledge the many, exceptionally dedicated publishing partners that helped in this publication:

- Robert Butler, Production Manager
- Mimi McGinnis, Managing Editor
- Joan Wendt, Design Manager
- Jack Brandt, Illustrations Specialist
- Kirk Pedrick, Senior Developmental Editor, Electronic Publishing
- Ralph Zickgraf, Manager, Electronic Publishing
- Melissa Reed, Assistant Editor of Development
- Kimberly Harris, Administrative Assistant.

We also extend our sincerest appreciation to Neil Kelly, Director of Sales, and his staff of sales representatives whose continued efforts have undoubtedly contributed to the success of this textbook.

# Reviewers

We sincerely thank the clinical reviewers who read and edited the manuscript and provided detailed evaluations and ideas for improving the text and illustrations:

**Ann M. Barrow, MSN, RN**
Coordinator of College Relations
College of Nursing
Villanova University
Villanova, Pennsylvania

**Katie Barton, LPN, BA, NMCA**
Medical Assistant Coordinator
Kerr Business College
Augusta, Georgia

**Lisa Morris Bonsall, RN, MSN, CRNP**
Independent Clinical Consultant
West Chester, Pennsylvania

**John Clouse, MSR, RT(R)**
Associate Professor
Department of Radiography
Owensboro Community College
Owensboro, Kentucky

**Michael W. Cook, MA, RRT, RCP**
Professor
Department of Respiratory Therapy
Mountain Empire Community College
Big Stone Gap, Virginia

**Patti A. Fayash, CMA, CCS**
Evening Adult CE Instructor
Schuykill Technology Center
Frackville, Pennsylvania
Coder
Medical Records Department
Hazleton Healthcare Alliance,
    Broad Street Campus
Hazleton, Pennsylvania

**Collette Bishop Hendler, RN, BS, CCRN**
Clinical Leader, Intensive Care Unit
Abington Memorial Hospital
Abington, Pennsylvania

**Sue Hunt, MA, RN, CMA**
Professor and Coordinator
Department of Medical Assisting
Middlesex Community College
Lowell, Massachusetts

**Carol Masker**
Instructor, Medical Terminology
Morris County School of Technology
Denville, New Jersey

**Kay A. Nave, CMA/MRT**
Program Director, Medical Assisting Program
Medical Department
Hagerstown Business College
Hagerstown, Maryland

**Michelle Shipley, MS, RHIA, CCS**
Director and Assistant Professor
Health Information Technology
Washburn University
Topeka, Kansas

In addition, we wish to acknowledge the following individuals who edited portions of the manuscript:

**Suzanne Wambold, PhD, RN, RDCS, FASE**
Director of the Cardiovascular
    Technology Program
University of Toledo
Toledo, Ohio

**Craig Patrick Black, PhD, RRT-NPS**
Respiratory Care Program
University of Toledo
Toledo, Ohio

**Suzanne Spacek, MEd, RRT-NPS, CPFT**
Director, Respiratory Care Program
University of Toledo
Toledo, Ohio

**Judith A. Ruple, PhD, RN, NREMT-P**
Director of the Emergency Medical
    Health Services Program
University of Toledo
Toledo, Ohio

Lastly, we feel it is only appropriate to acknowledge our deepest gratitude to Robert H. Craven, Jr., President, for his continued support of our publication efforts on this, the 125th anniversary of F. A. Davis Company, a family-owned business. In 1981 (25 years ago), Mr. Craven, through Mr. Robert Martone, Publisher, awarded these two authors an initial contract for the *Body Systems* textbook. We thank Mr. Craven and Mr. Martone for giving us the opportunity to become authors for one of the most successful and prestigious medical textbook publishing companies.

# Preface

The fifth edition of *Medical Terminology Systems: A Body Systems Approach* lives up to its well-established track record of presenting medical word building principles based on a competency-based curricula. *Systems* is designed with the educational foundation of a textbook-workbook format that complements traditional lecture and classroom teaching methods. The purpose of the book is to help students learn medical terminology so they can effectively communicate with other members of the healthcare team. A variety of pedagogical features will help them develop a strong foundation in medical terminology and broaden their medical vocabulary. Although the study of medical terminology demands hard work and discipline, various self-paced activities offer interest and variety to the learning process.

All of the changes in the fifth edition are structured to make learning easier and improve retention of medical terms. Perhaps the most striking changes to this edition are the all-new, visually impressive, full-color illustrations. The artwork is specifically designed to present accurate and aesthetically pleasing representations of anatomical structures, disease conditions, and medical procedures. At the same time, the illustrations enhance course content in new and interesting ways, provide a clearer perspective for the reader, and promote long-lasting learning.

Another new feature of the fifth edition is the omission of possessive forms of all eponyms, (such as *Bowman capsule, Cushing syndrome,* and *Parkinson disease*). Medical dictionaries as well as the American Association for Medical Transcription and the American Medical Association support these changes. The fifth edition also contains updated, comprehensive lists of medical abbreviations and their meanings, including a "do not use" abbreviations list mandated by the Joint Commission on Accreditation of Healthcare Organizations.

Each chapter incorporates the most current technological changes in medicine. Educators and practitioners in various healthcare disciplines have provided excellent suggestions for this edition, and many of those suggestions have been integrated into the text to augment its educational effectiveness. Pharmacology information has been significantly expanded and now includes commonly used drugs, their generic and trade names, and their modes of action.

The popular, basic features of the previous edition remain intact but have been expanded and enhanced. Here's a breakdown of those features:

- **Chapter 1** explains the techniques of medical word building using basic word elements.
- **Chapter 2** categorizes major surgical, diagnostic, symptomatic, and grammatical suffixes.
- **Chapter 3** presents major prefixes of position, number and measurement, direction, and other parameters.
- **Chapter 4** introduces anatomical, physiological, and pathological terms. Combining forms denoting cellular and body structure, body position and direction, regions of the body, and additional combining forms related to body structure, diagnostic methods, and pathology are also presented. General diagnostic and therapeutic terms are described and provide a solid foundation for specific terms addressed in the body system chapters that follow.

- **Chapters 5 to 15** are organized according to specific body systems and may be taught in any sequence. These chapters include key terms; anatomy and physiology; combining forms, suffixes, and prefixes; pathology; diagnostic, symptomatic, and related terms; diagnostic and therapeutic procedures; pharmacology; abbreviations; learning activities; and medical record activities. All activities allow self-assessment and evaluation of competency.
- **Appendix A: Answer Key** contains answers to each learning activity to validate competency and provide immediate feedback for student assessment.
- **Appendix B: Abbreviations** includes an updated, comprehensive list of medical abbreviations and their meanings.
- **Appendix C: Glossary of Medical Word Elements** contains an alphabetical list of medical word elements and their meanings.
- **Appendix D: Index of Genetic Disorders** lists genetic disorders presented in the textbook.
- **Appendix E: Index of Diagnostic Imaging Procedures** lists radiographic and other diagnostic imaging procedures presented in the textbook.
- **Appendix F: Index of Pharmacology** lists medications presented in the textbook.
- **Appendix G: Index of Oncological Terms** lists terms related to oncology presented in the textbook.

## Instructor's Resource Disk

The Instructor's Resource Disk (IRD) features many new and some familiar teaching aids created to make your teaching job easier and more effective. The supplemental teaching aids it provides can be used in various classroom settings—traditional classroom, distance learning, or independent studies. The IRD consists of an Activity Pack, three PowerPoint presentations, and a computerized test bank in Brownstone, a powerful test-generation program.

## Activity Pack

**The Activity Pack\*** contains a wealth of information and resources for you, including:

- *Question Bank.* The questions and answers in this popular section are taken from the *Brownstone Computerized Test Bank* found elsewhere on the IRD. These multiple-choice and true/false questions are only a small sample of the more than 1,100 test items available in the Brownstone test bank. Questions are available for each body-system chapter. The multiple-choice and true/false questions mirror the testing format used on many allied health national board examinations.
- *Suggested Course Outlines.* Course outlines are provided to help you plan the best method of covering the material presented in the textbook.
- *Student and Instructor Directed Activities.* These comprehensive teaching aids are newly developed for this edition. They provide an assortment of exercises for each body-system chapter that offers variety and interest to the course material. You can select from the various activities and determine if they are to be used as required content or supplemental material, and whether the activities are to be undertaken individually or as a group project. If group projects are selected, a Peer Evaluation Form is available.
- *Community and Internet Resources.* This section provides updated and expanded resources that offer a rich supply of technical journals, community organizations, and Internet resources to supplement classroom, Internet, and directed activities.

---

\*The *Activity Pack* is available in hard copy on request for those who adopt the textbook.

- *Supplemental Medical Record Activities.* In addition to updating the medical record activities from the previous edition, we've added supplemental activities for each of the body system chapters. As in the textbook, these medical record activities use common clinical scenarios to show how medical terminology is used in the clinical area to document patient care. Activities for terminology, pronunciation, and medical record analysis are provided for each medical record, along with an answer key. In addition, each medical record focuses on a specific medical specialty. These records can be used for group activities, oral reports, medical coding activities, or individual assignments. The medical records are designed to reinforce and enhance the terminology presented in the textbook.
- *Crossword Puzzles.* These fun, educational activities are included for each body system chapter. They are designed to reinforce material covered in the chapter and can be used individually or in a group activity. They can also be used as a way of providing extra credit or "just for fun." An answer key is included for each puzzle.
- *Pronunciations and Answer Keys.* We've included in this edition a special answer key for the medical record research activities in the textbook. This key should prove to be a helpful addition when you discuss the material or correct assignments.
- *Master Transparencies.* The transparency pages offer large, clear, black-and-white anatomical illustrations perfect for making overhead transparencies and are provided for each body system.

## PowerPoint Presentations

This edition of *Systems* contains not one but *three* PowerPoint presentations for your use. One, called *Lecture Notes,* provides an outline-based presentation for each body-system chapter. It consists of a chapter overview, the main functions of the body system, and selected pathology, vocabulary, and procedures for each. Full-color illustrations from the book are included. A second presentation, called *Illustrations,* contains most illustrations from the text, with one illustration per slide. The third presentation, called *Med TERMinator,* is an interactive presentation in which terms from a chapter drop into view each time you click the mouse. You can ask students to say the term aloud, define the term, or provide other feedback before moving to the next term.

## Electronic Test Bank

As in the previous edition, this edition offers a powerful Brownstone test bank that allows you to create custom-generated or randomly-selected tests in a printable format from more than 1,100 multiple-choice test items. The program requires Windows 95, Windows 98, or Windows NT and is available for Macintosh on request.

## Audio CD-ROM

Depending on which *Systems* version you ordered, you may find an **audio CD-ROM** in the textbook. The CD is designed to strengthen your students' ability to spell, pronounce, and understand the meaning of selected medical terms using exercises for each body system chapter. These exercises provide continuous reinforcement of correct pronunciation and usage of medical terms.

The audio CD can also be used for students in beginning transcription courses. Medical secretarial and medical transcription students can use the CD to learn beginning transcription skills by typing each word as it is pronounced. After the words are typed, spelling can be corrected by referring to either the textbook or a medical dictionary.

## Interactive Medical Terminology 2.0

Interactive Medical Terminology 2.0 (IMT), a powerful interactive CD-ROM program, comes with the text, depending on which version you've chosen. IMT is a competency-based, self-paced, multimedia program that includes graphics, audio, and a dictionary culled from *Taber's Cyclopedic Medical Dictionary*. Help menus provide navigational support. The software comes with numerous interactive learning activities, including:

- word-building and word-breakdown activities
- drag-and-drop anatomical exercises
- word-search puzzles
- word scrambles
- crossword puzzles.

The exercises throughout are designed at a 90% competency level, providing immediate feedback on student competency. Students can also print their progress as they go along. The CD-ROM is especially valuable as a distance-learning tool because it provides evidence of student drill and practice in various learning activities.

## Taber's Cyclopedic Medical Dictionary

The world-famous *Taber's Cyclopedic Medical Dictionary* is the recommended companion reference for this book. Virtually all terms in the new edition of *Systems* may be found in *Taber's*. In addition, *Taber's* contains etymologies for nearly all main entries presented in this textbook. We hope you enjoy this new edition as much as we enjoyed preparing it. We think you will find that it is the best edition ever.

Barbara A. Gylys
Mary Ellen Wedding

# Contents at a Glance

# Appendices

# Contents

## C h a p t e r   5
## Integumentary System   75

## Chapter 6
## Digestive System    107

**C h a p t e r   9**

## Blood, Lymph, and Immune Systems   225

## Chapter 12
## Female Reproductive System    345

# Chapter 13
# Endocrine System  387

# Appendices

# Chapter

# 1

# Basic Elements of a Medical Word

## CHAPTER OUTLINE

## OBJECTIVES

*Upon completion of this chapter, you will be able to:*

- Identify the four basic word elements used to form medical words.
- Divide medical words into their component parts.
- Use the guidelines to define and build medical words.
- Locate the pronunciation guidelines and interpret pronunciation marks.

## Medical Word Elements

The language of medicine is a specialized vocabulary used by health-care practitioners. Many medical word elements in current use had their origin as early as the 1st century B.C., when Hippocrates practiced medicine. With technological and scientific advancements in medicine, many new terms have evolved to reflect these innovations. For example, radiographic terms, such as magnetic resonance imaging (MRI) and ultrasound (US), are now used to describe current diagnostic procedures.

A medical word consists of some or all of the following elements: word root, combining form, suffix, and prefix. How you combine these elements, and whether all or some of them are present in a medical word, determines the meaning of a word. The purpose of this chapter is to help you learn to identify these elements and use them to build medical terms.

## Word Roots

A **word root** is the core of a medical term and contains the fundamental meaning of the word. It is the foundation on which other elements are added to develop a complete term. Most word roots are derived from Greek or Latin. Because of this twofold origin, two different roots may have the same meaning. For example, the Greek word *derm* and the Latin word *cutane* both refer to the skin. As a general rule, Greek word roots are used to build words that describe a disease, condition, treatment, or diagnosis; Latin word roots are used to build words that describe anatomic structures. Consequently, the Greek root *derm* is used primarily in terms that describe a disease, condition, treatment, or diagnosis of the skin; the Latin root *cutane* is used primarily to describe an anatomic structure. Most medical terms contain at least one word root. (See Table 1–1.)

## Table 1–1    EXAMPLES OF WORD ROOTS

This table lists examples of word roots as well as their phonetic pronunciations. Begin learning the pronunciations as you review the information below.

| Greek or Latin Word | Word Root | Meaning | Word Analysis |
|---|---|---|---|
| **dermatos (Gr\*)** | derm | skin | dermat/itis (dĕr-mă-TĪ-tĭs): inflammation of the skin<br>*A term that describes a skin disease* |
| **nephros (Gr)** | nephr | kidney | nephr/oma (nĕ-FRŌ-mă): tumor of the kidney<br>*A term that describes a kidney disease* |
| **stoma (Gr)** | stomat | mouth | stomat/o/pathy (stō-mă-TŎP-ă-thē): any disease of the mouth<br>*A term that describes a mouth disease* |
| **cutis (L)** | cutane | skin | sub/cutane/ous (sŭb-kū-TĀ-nē-ŭs): beneath the skin<br>*A term that describes the anatomic tissue layer beneath the skin* |
| **oris (L)** | or | mouth | or/al (OR-ăl): pertaining to the mouth<br>*A term that describes an anatomic structure* |
| **renes (L)** | ren | kidney | ren/al (RĒ-năl): pertains to the kidney<br>*A term that describes an anatomic structure* |

\*It is not important to know the origin of a medical word. This information is only provided to illustrate that there may be two different word roots for a single term.

## Combining Forms

A combining form is a word root to which a vowel (usually an *o*) is added. The vowel has no meaning of its own, but enables two elements to be connected. Like the word root, the combining form is the basic foundation on which other elements are added to build a complete word. In this text, a combining form will be listed as *word root/vowel* (such as *gastr/o*), as illustrated in Table 1–2.

| Table 1–2 | EXAMPLES OF COMBINING FORMS |
|---|---|

This table illustrates how word roots and vowels create combining forms. Learning combining forms rather than word roots makes pronunciation a little easier because of the terminal vowel. For example, in the table below, the word roots *gastr* and *nephr* are difficult to pronounce, whereas their combining forms *gastr/o* and *nephr/o* are easier to pronounce.

| Word Root | + | Vowel | = | Combining Form | Meaning |
|---|---|---|---|---|---|
| erythr/ | + | *o* | = | erythr/o | red |
| gastr/ | + | *o* | = | gastr/o | stomach |
| hepat/ | + | *o* | = | hepat/o | liver |
| immun/ | + | *o* | = | immun/o | immune, immunity, safe |
| nephr/ | + | *o* | = | nephr/o | kidney |
| oste/ | + | *o* | = | oste/o | bone |

It is time to review word roots and combining forms by completing Learning Activities 1–1 and 1–2.

## Suffixes

A **suffix** is a word element placed at the end of a word or word root that changes the meaning of the word. In the terms tonsill/*itis*, and tonsill/*ectomy*, the suffixes are *-itis* (inflammation) and *-ectomy* (excision, removal). Changing the suffix changes the meaning of the word. In medical terminology, a suffix usually indicates a procedure, condition, disease, or part of speech. Many suffixes are derived from Greek or Latin words. (See Table 1–3.)

## Prefixes

A prefix is a word element attached to the beginning of a word or word root. Adding or changing a prefix changes the meaning of the word. The prefix usually indicates a number, time, position, direction, or negation. Many of the same prefixes found in medical terminology are also found in the English language. (See Table 1–4.)

## Table 1-3   EXAMPLES OF SUFFIXES

This table lists examples of suffixes as well as their phonetic pronunciations. Begin learning the pronunciations as you review the information below.

| Combining Form | + | Suffix | = | Medical Word | Meaning |
|---|---|---|---|---|---|
| **gastr/o**<br>(stomach) | + | *-itis*<br>(inflammation) | = | gastritis<br>găs-TRĪ-tĭs | inflammation of the stomach |
| | + | *-megaly*<br>(enlargement) | = | gastromegaly<br>găs-trō-MĔG-ă-lē | enlargement of the stomach |
| | + | *-oma*<br>(tumor) | = | gastroma<br>găs-TRŌ-mă | tumor of the stomach |
| **hepat/o**<br>(liver) | + | *-itis*<br>(inflammation) | = | hepatitis<br>hĕp-ă-TĪ-tĭs | inflammation of the liver |
| | + | *-megaly*<br>(enlargement) | = | hepatomegaly<br>hĕp-ă-tō-MĔG-ă-lē | enlargement of the liver |
| | + | *-oma*<br>(tumor) | = | hepatoma<br>hĕp-ă-TŌ-mă | tumor of the liver |

## Table 1-4   EXAMPLES OF PREFIXES

This table lists examples of prefixes as well as their phonetic pronunciations. Begin learning the pronunciations as you review the information below.

| Prefix | + | Word Root | + | Suffix | = | Medical Word | Meaning |
|---|---|---|---|---|---|---|---|
| **a-**<br>(without) | + | *mast*<br>(breast) | + | *-ia*<br>(condition) | = | amastia<br>ă-MĂS-tē-ă | without a breast |
| **hyper-**<br>(excessive, above normal) | + | *therm*<br>(heat) | + | *-ia*<br>(condition) | = | hyperthermia<br>hī-pĕr-THĔR-mē-ă | condition of excessive heat |
| **intra-**<br>(in, within) | + | *muscul*<br>(muscle) | + | *-ar*<br>(relating to) | = | intramuscular<br>ĭn-tră-MŬS-kū-lăr | within the muscle |
| **macro-**<br>(large) | + | *card*<br>(heart) | + | *-ia*<br>(condition) | = | macrocardia<br>măk-rō-KĂR-dē-ă | condition of a large heart |
| **micro-**<br>(small) | + | *card*<br>(heart) | + | *-ia*<br>(condition) | = | microcardia<br>mī-krō-KĂR-dē-ă | condition of a small heart |

 **It is time to review suffixes and prefixes by completing Learning Activity 1–3.**

 ## Basic Rules

Defining and building medical words are crucial skills in mastering medical terminology. Following the basic rules for each will help you master these skills.

## Defining Medical Words

Here are the three basic rules for defining medical words using the example term *gastroenteritis*.

### Rule #1

Define the **suffix,** or last part of the word. In this case, *-itis,* which means *inflammation.*

### Rule #2

Define the first part of the word (which may be a **word root, combining form,** or **prefix**). In this case, the combining form *gastr/o* means *stomach.*

### Rule #3

Define the middle parts of the word. In this case, *enter/* means *intestine.*
When you analyze *gastroenteritis* following the three previous rules, the meaning is revealed as:

1. inflammation (of)
2. stomach (and)
3. intestine

Thus, the definition of *gastroenteritis* is "inflammation (of) stomach (and) intestine." Table 1–5 further illustrates this process.

**Table 1–5      DEFINING GASTROENTERITIS**

This table illustrates the three rules of defining a medical word using the example *gastroenteritis.*

| Combining Form | Middle | Suffix |
|---|---|---|
| **gastr/o** | **enter/** | **-itis** |
| stomach | intestine | inflammation |
| (rule 2) | (rule 3) | (rule 1) |

## Building Medical Words

There are three basic rules for building medical words.

### Rule #1

A word root links a suffix that begins with a vowel.

| Word Root | + | Suffix | = | Medical Word | Meaning |
|---|---|---|---|---|---|
| **hepat/**<br>liver | + | **-itis**<br>inflammation | = | hepatitis<br>hĕp-ă-TĪ-tĭs | inflammation of the liver |

### Rule #2

A combining form (root + *o*) links a suffix that begins with a consonant.

| Combining Form | + | Suffix | = | Medical Word | Meaning |
|---|---|---|---|---|---|
| **hepat/o**<br>liver | + | **-cyte**<br>cell | = | hepatocyte<br>HĔP-ă-tō-sīt | liver cell |

### Rule #3

Use a combining form to link a root to another root to form a compound word. This rule holds true even if the next root begins with a vowel, as in *osteoarthritis*. Keep in mind that the rules for linking multiple roots to each other are slightly different from the rules for linking roots and combining forms to suffixes.

| Combining Form | + | Word Root | + | Suffix | = | Medical Word | Meaning |
|---|---|---|---|---|---|---|---|
| **oste/o**<br>bone | + | **chondr/**<br>cartilage | + | **-itis**<br>inflammation | = | osteochondritis<br>ŏs-tē-ō-kŏn-<br>DRĪ-tĭs | inflammation<br>of bone and<br>cartilage |
| **oste/o**<br>bone | + | **arthr/**<br>joint | + | **-itis**<br>inflammation | = | osteoarthritis<br>ŏs-tē-ō-ăr-<br>THRĪ-tĭs | inflammation<br>of bone and<br>joint |

 It is time to review word building rules by completing Learning Activity 1–4.

 ## Pronunciation Guidelines

Although the pronunciation of medical words usually follows the same rules that govern the pronunciation of English words, some medical words may be difficult to pronounce when first encountered. Therefore, selected terms in this book include phonetic pronunciation. In addition, pronunciation guidelines can be found on the inside front cover of this book. Use it whenever you need help with pronunciation of medical words. Locate and study these guidelines before proceeding with Learning Activity 1–5.

 It is time to review pronunciation guidelines by completing Learning Activity 1–5.

# LEARNING ACTIVITIES

The following activities provide a review of the basic medical word elements introduced in this chapter. Complete each activity and review your answers to evaluate your understanding of this chapter.

## Learning Activity 1–1

### Understanding medical word elements

*Fill in the following blanks to complete the sentences correctly.*

1. The four elements used to form words are _____.

2. A root is the main part or foundation of a word. In the words *teacher, teaches,* and *teaching*, the root is _____.

*Identify the following statements as true or false. If false, rewrite the statement correctly on the line provided.*

3. A combining vowel is usually an *e*.                         True        False

   _____

4. A word root links a suffix that begins with a consonant.    True        False

   _____

5. A combining form links multiple roots to each other.        True        False

   _____

6. A combining form links a suffix that begins with a consonant.  True     False

   _____

7. To define a medical word, first define the prefix.          True        False

   _____

8. A word root links a suffix that begins with a vowel.        True        False

   _____

*Underline the word root in each of following combining forms.*

9. splen/o (spleen)
10. hyster/o (uterus)
11. enter/o (intestine)
12. neur/o (nerve)
13. ot/o (ear)
14. dermat/o (skin)
15. hydr/o (water)

Check your answers in Appendix A. Review material that you did not answer correctly.

**CORRECT ANSWERS** _____ × 6.67 = _____ **% SCORE**

Learning Activity 1–2

## Identifying word roots and combining forms

*Underline the word roots in the following terms.*

| Medical Word | Meaning |
|---|---|
| 1. nephritis | inflammation of the kidneys |
| 2. arthrodesis | surgical fixation of a joint |
| 3. phlebotomy | incision of a vein |
| 4. dentist | specialist in teeth |
| 5. gastrectomy | excision of the stomach |
| 6. chondritis | inflammation of cartilage |
| 7. hepatoma | tumor of the liver |
| 8. cardiologist | specialist in the heart |
| 9. gastria | condition of the stomach |
| 10. osteoma | tumor of the bone |

*Underline the following elements that are combining forms.*

| | |
|---|---|
| 11. nephr | kidney |
| 12. cardi/o | heart |
| 13. arthr | joint |
| 14. oste/o/arth | bone, joint |
| 15. cholangi/o | bile vessel |

✓ Check your answers in Appendix A. Review material that you did not answer correctly.

**CORRECT ANSWERS** _____ × **6.67** = _____ **% SCORE**

Learning Activity 1–3

## Identifying suffixes and prefixes

*Pronounce the following medical terms. Then analyze each term and write the element from each that is a suffix in the right-hand column. The first suffix is completed for you.*

| Term | Suffix |
|------|--------|
| 1. **thoracotomy** <br> thō-răk-ŎT-ō-mē | *-tomy* |
| 2. **gastroscope** <br> GĂS-trō-skōp | |
| 3. **tonsillitis** <br> tŏn-sĭl-Ī-tĭs | |
| 4. **gastritis** <br> găs-TRĪ-tĭs | |
| 5. **tonsillectomy** <br> tŏn-sĭl-ĔK-tō-mē | |

*Pronounce the following medical terms. Then analyze each term and write the element from each that is a prefix in the right-hand column. The first prefix is completed for you.*

| Term | Prefix |
|------|--------|
| 6. **microcardia** <br> mī-krō-KĂR-dē-ă | *micro-* |
| 7. **hyperthermia** <br> hī-pĕr-THĔR-mē-ă | |
| 8. **macroglossia** <br> măk-rō-GLŎS-ē-ă | |
| 9. **intramuscular** <br> ĭn-tră-MŬS-kū-lăr | |
| 10. **amastia** <br> ă-MĂS-tē-ă | |

 Check your answers in Appendix A. Review material that you did not answer correctly.

**CORRECT ANSWERS** _____ × 10 = _____ **% SCORE**

Learning  Activity  1–4

## Defining and building medical words

The three basic steps for defining medical words are:

1.  Define the last part of the word, or **suffix.**
2.  Define the first part of the word, or **prefix, word root,** or **combining form.**
3.  Define the **middle** of the word.

*Use the previous steps to define the following words. If you are not certain of a definition, refer to Appendix C, Part 1, of this textbook, which provides an alphabetical list of word elements and their definitions.*

| Term | Definition |
| --- | --- |
| 1.  **gastritis**<br>gǎs-TRĪ-tǐs | |
| 2.  **nephritis**<br>něf-RĪ-tǐs | |
| 3.  **gastrectomy**<br>gǎs-TRĔK-tō-mē | |
| 4.  **osteoma**<br>ŏs-tē-Ō-mǎ | |
| 5.  **hepatoma**<br>hěp-ǎ-TŌ-mǎ | |
| 6.  **hepatitis**<br>hěp-ǎ-TĪ-tǐs | |

*Refer to the section "Building Medical Words" on page 5 to complete this activity. Write the number for the rule that applies to each listed term as well as a short summary of the rule. Use the abbreviation WR to designate word root, CF to designate combining form. The first one is completed for you.*

| Term | Rule | Summary of the Rule |
| --- | --- | --- |
| 7.  **arthr/itis**<br>ǎr-THRĪ-tǐs | 1 | *A WR links a suffix that begins with a vowel.* |
| 8.  **scler/osis**<br>sklě-RŌ-sǐs | | |
| 9.  **arthr/o/centesis**<br>ǎr-thrō-sěn-TĒ-sǐs | | |
| 10.  **colon/o/scope**<br>kō-LŎN-ō-skōp | | |
| 11.  **chondr/itis**<br>kŏn-DRĪ-tǐs | | |

| Term | Rule | Summary of the Rule |
|------|------|---------------------|
| **12. chondr/oma**<br>kŏn-DRŌ-mă | ___ | _____ |
| **13. oste/o/chondr/itis**<br>ŏs-tē-ō-kŏn-DRĪ-tĭs | ___ | _____ |
| **14. muscul/ar**<br>MŬS-kū-lăr | ___ | _____ |
| **15. oste/o/arthr/itis**<br>ŏs-tē-ō-ăr-THRĪ-tĭs | ___ | _____ |

 Check your answers in Appendix A. Review material that you did not answer correctly.

**CORRECT ANSWERS** _____ × 10 = _____ **% SCORE**

## Learning Activity 1–5

## Understanding pronunciations

*Review the pronunciation guidelines (located inside the front cover of this book) and then underline the correct answer in each of the following statements.*

1. The diacritical mark ‾ is called a (breve, macron).

2. The diacritical mark ˘ is called a (breve, macron).

3. The ‾ indicates the (short, long) sounds of vowels.

4. The ˘ indicates the (short, long) sounds of vowels.

5. The combination *ch* is sometimes pronounced like *(k, chiy)*. Examples are *ch*olesterol, *ch*olemia.

6. When *pn* is at the beginning of a word, it is pronounced only with the sound of *(p, n)*. Examples are *pn*eumonia, *pn*eumotoxin.

7. When *pn* is in middle of a word, the *p* *(is, is not)* pronounced. Examples are ortho*pn*ea, hyper*pn*ea.

8. When *i* is at the end of a word, it is pronounced like *(eye, ee)*. Examples are bronch*i*, fung*i*, nucle*i*.

9. For *ae* and *oe*, only the (first, second) vowel is pronounced. Examples are burs*ae*, pleur*ae*.

10. When *e* and *es* form the final letter or letters of a word, they are commonly pronounced as (combined, separate) syllables. Examples are syncop*e*, systol*e*, nar*es*.

 Check your answers in Appendix A. Review material that you did not answer correctly.

**CORRECT ANSWERS** _____ × 10 = _____ **% SCORE**

# Chapter

# Suffixes

## OBJECTIVES

*Upon completion of this chapter, you will be able to:*

- Define and provide examples of surgical, diagnostic, pathological, and related suffixes.
- Determine the use of a combining form and word root when linking these elements to a suffix.
- Identify adjective, noun, and diminutive suffixes.
- Locate and apply guidelines for pluralizing terms.
- Demonstrate your knowledge of the chapter by completing the learning activities.

## Suffix Linking

In medical words, a suffix is added to the end of a root or combining form to change its meaning. For example, the combining form *gastr/o* means stomach. The suffix *-megaly* means enlargement, and *-itis* means inflammation. *Gastr/o/megaly* is an enlargement of the stomach; *gastr/itis* is an inflammation of the stomach. Whenever you change the suffix, you change the meaning of the word. Suffixes are also used to denote singular and plural forms of a word as well as a part of speech. The following tables provide additional examples to reinforce the rules you learned in Chapter 1. (See Tables 2–1 and 2–2.)

### Table 2–1    WORD ROOTS AND COMBINING FORMS WITH SUFFIXES

This table lists examples of word roots used to link a suffix that begins with a vowel. It also lists combining forms (root + o) used to link a suffix that begins with a consonant.

| Element | + | Suffix | = | Medical Word | Meaning |
|---|---|---|---|---|---|
| **Word Roots** | | | | | |
| **gastr** (stomach) | + | *-itis* (inflammation) | = | gastritis găs-TRĪ-tĭs | inflammation of the stomach |
| **hemat** (blood) | + | *-emesis* (vomiting) | = | hematemesis hĕm-ăt-ĔM-ē-sĭs | vomiting of blood |
| **arthr** (joint) | + | *-itis* (inflammation) | = | arthritis ăr-THRĪ-tĭs | inflammation of a joint |
| **Combining Forms** | | | | | |
| **gastr/o** (stomach) | + | *-dynia* (pain) | = | gastrodynia găs-trō-DĬN-ē-ă | pain in the stomach |
| **hemat/o** (blood) | + | *-logy* (study of) | = | hematology hĕm-ă-TŎL-ō-jē | study of blood |
| **arthr/o** (joint) | + | *-centesis* (surgical puncture) | = | arthrocentesis ăr-thrō-sĕn-TĒ-sĭs | surgical puncture of a joint |

### Table 2–2    COMPOUND WORDS WITH SUFFIXES

This table lists examples of a combining form used to link a root to another root to form a compound word. This rule holds true even if the next root begins with a vowel, as in *osteoarthritis*. Recall that the rules for linking multiple roots to each other are slightly different from the rules for linking roots and combining forms to suffixes.

| Combining Form | + | Word Root | + | Suffix | = | Medical Word | Meaning |
|---|---|---|---|---|---|---|---|
| **gastr/o** (stomach) | + | *enter* (intestine) | + | *-itis* (inflammation) | = | gastroenteritis găs-trō-ĕn-tĕr-Ī-tĭs | inflammation of stomach and intestine |

## Table 2-2    COMPOUND WORDS WITH SUFFIXES

| Combining Form | + | Word Root | + | Suffix | = | Medical Word | Meaning |
|---|---|---|---|---|---|---|---|
| **oste/o**<br>(bone) | + | *arthr*<br>(joint) | + | *-itis*<br>(inflammation) | = | osteoarthritis<br>ŏs-tē-ō-ăr-THRĪ-tĭs | inflammation of bone and joint |
| **encephal/o**<br>(brain) | + | *mening*<br>(meninges) | + | *-itis*<br>(inflammation) | = | encephalomeningitis<br>ĕn-sĕf-ă-lō-mĕn-in-JĪ-tĭs | inflammation of brain and meninges |

## Suffix Types

An effective strategy in mastering medical terminology is to learn the major types of suffixes, such as surgical, diagnostic, pathological, and related suffixes, as well as grammatical and singular and plural suffixes.

### Surgical, Diagnostic, Pathological, and Related Suffixes

Surgical suffixes describe a type of invasive procedure performed on a body part. (See Table 2–3.) Diagnostic suffixes denote a procedure or test performed to identify the cause and nature of an illness. (See Table 2–4.) Pathological suffixes describe an abnormal condition or disease. (See Table 2–4.)

## Table 2-3    COMMON SURGICAL SUFFIXES

This table lists commonly used surgical suffixes along with their meanings and word analyses.

| Suffix | Meaning | Word Analysis |
|---|---|---|
| **-centesis** | surgical puncture | arthr/o/centesis (ăr-thrō-sĕn-TĒ-sĭs): puncture of a joint space with a needle to remove accumulated fluid from a joint<br>    *arthr/o:* joint |
| **-clasis** | to break; surgical fracture | oste/o/clasis (ŏs-tē-ŎK-lă-sĭs): surgical fracture of a bone in order to correct a deformity<br>    *oste/o:* bone |
| **-desis** | binding, fixation (of a bone or joint) | arthr/o/desis (ăr-thrō-DĒ-sĭs): binding together of a joint<br>    *arthr/o:* joint |
| **-ectomy** | excision, removal | append/ectomy (ăp-ĕn-DĔK-tō-mē): excision of the appendix<br>    *append:* appendix |
| **-lysis** | separation; destruction; loosening | thromb/o/lysis (thrŏm-BŎL-ĭ-sĭs): dissolution of a blood clot<br>    *thromb/o:* blood clot<br>*Drug therapy is usually used to dissolve a blood clot.* |

*(Continued)*

| Table 2-3 | COMMON SURGICAL SUFFIXES *(Continued)* |
|---|---|

| Suffix | Meaning | Word Analysis |
|---|---|---|
| **-pexy** | fixation (of an organ) | mast/o/pexy (MĂS-tō-pĕks-ē): surgical fixation of the breast(s)<br>   *mast/o:* breast<br>*Mastopexy, an elective surgery, is performed to affix sagging breasts in a more elevated position, often improving their shape.* |
| **-plasty** | surgical repair | rhin/o/plasty (RĪ-nō-plăs-tē): surgical repair in which the structure of the nose is changed<br>   *rhin/o:* nose |
| **-rrhaphy** | suture | my/o/rrhaphy (mī-OR-ă-fē): suture of a muscle<br>   *my/o:* muscle |
| **-stomy** | forming an opening (mouth) | trache/o/stomy (trā-kē-ŎS-tō-mē): artificial opening through the neck into the trachea into which a breathing tube is inserted<br>   *trache/o:* trachea (windpipe)<br>*A tracheostomy is usually performed to bypass an obstructed upper airway.* |
| **-tome** | instrument to cut | oste/o/tome (ŎS-tē-ō-tōm): surgical instrument for cutting through bone<br>   *oste/o:* bone |
| **-tomy** | incision | trache/o/tomy (trā-kē-ŎT-ō-mē): incision through the neck into the trachea<br>   *trache/o:* trachea (windpipe)<br>*Tracheotomy is performed to gain access to an airway below a blockage.* |
| **-tripsy** | crushing | lith/o/tripsy (LĬTH-ō-trĭp-sē): crushing of a stone<br>   *lith/o:* stone, calculus |

**It is time to review surgical suffixes by completing Learning Activities 2–1, 2–2, and 2–3.**

| Table 2-4 | COMMON DIAGNOSTIC, PATHOLOGICAL, AND RELATED SUFFIXES |
|---|---|

This table lists commonly used diagnostic, pathological, and related suffixes along with their meanings and word analyses.

| Suffix | Meaning | Word Analysis |
|---|---|---|
| **Diagnostic** | | |
| **-gram** | record, writing | electr/o/cardi/o/gram (ē-lĕk-trō-KĂR-dē-ō-grăm): graphic recording of the electrical activity of the heart<br>   *electr/o:* electricity<br>   *cardi/o:* heart<br>*An electrocardiogram allows diagnosis of specific cardiac abnormalities.* |

| Table 2–4 | COMMON DIAGNOSTIC, PATHOLOGICAL, AND RELATED SUFFIXES | |
|---|---|---|

| Suffix | Meaning | Word Analysis |
|---|---|---|
| **Diagnostic** | | |
| **-graph** | instrument for recording | cardi/o/graph (KĂR-dē-ŏ-grăf): instrument used to record electrical activity of the heart<br>*cardi/o:* heart |
| **-graphy** | process of recording | angi/o/graphy (ăn-jē-ŎG-ră-fē): radiographic image of blood vessels after injection of a contrast medium<br>*angi/o:* vessel (usually blood or lymph) |
| **-meter** | instrument for measuring | pelv/i/meter* (pěl-VĬM-ě-těr): instrument for measuring the pelvis<br>*pelv/i:* pelvis |
| **-metry** | act of measuring | pelv/i/metry (pěl-VĬM-ě-trē): act or process of determining the dimension of the pelvis<br>*pelv/i:* pelvis |
| **-scope** | instrument for examining | endo/scope (ĔN-dō-skōp): flexible or rigid instrument consisting of a tube and optical system for observing the inside of a hollow organ or cavity<br>*endo-:* in, within |
| **-scopy** | visual examination | endo/scopy (ěn-DŎS-kō-pē): visual examination of a cavity or canal using a specialized lighted instrument called an *endoscope*<br>*endo-:* in, within |
| **Pathological and Related** | | |
| **-algia** | pain | neur/algia (nū-RĂL-jē-ă): pain occurring along the path of a nerve<br>*neur:* nerve |
| **-dynia** | | ot/o/dynia (ō-tō-DĬN-ē-ă): pain in the ear; earache<br>*ot/o:* ear |
| **-cele** | hernia, swelling | hepat/o/cele (hě-PĂT-ō-sēl): hernia of the liver<br>*hepat/o:* liver |
| **-ectasis** | dilation, expansion | bronchi/ectasis (brŏng-kē-ĔK-tă-sĭs): abnormal dilation of one or more bronchi<br>*bronchi:* bronchus (plural, bronchi)<br>*Bronchiectasis is associated with various lung conditions and is commonly accompanied by chronic infection.* |
| **-edema** | swelling | lymph/edema (lĭmf-ě-DĒ-mă): swelling and accumulation of tissue fluid<br>*lymph:* lymph<br>*Lymphedema may be caused by a blockage of the lymph vessels.* |
| **-emesis** | vomiting | hyper/emesis (hī-pěr-ĔM-ě-sĭs): excessive vomiting<br>*hyper-:* excessive, above normal |
| **-emia** | blood condition | an/emia (ă-NĒ-mē-ă): blood condition caused by iron deficiency or decrease in red blood cells<br>*an-:* without, not |

*(Continued)*

| Table 2–4 | COMMON DIAGNOSTIC, PATHOLOGICAL, AND RELATED SUFFIXES *(Continued)* |
|---|---|

| Suffix | Meaning | Word Analysis |
|---|---|---|
| **Pathological and Related** | | |
| **-gen** | forming, producing, origin | carcin/o/gen (kăr-SĬN-ō-jĕn): substance or agent that causes the development or increases the incidence of cancer<br>*carcin/o:* cancer |
| **-genesis** | | carcin/o/genesis (kăr-sĭ-nō-JĔN-ĕ-sĭs): the process of initiating and promoting cancer<br>*carcin/o:* cancer<br>*Carcinogenesis is the transformation of normal cells into cancer cells, commonly as a result of chemical, viral, or radioactive damage to genes.* |
| **-iasis** | abnormal condition (produced by something specific) | chol/e/lith/iasis* (kō-lē-lĭ-THĬ-ă-sĭs): presence or formation of gallstones in the gallbladder or common bile duct<br>*chol/e:* bile, gall<br>*lith:* stone, calculus |
| **-itis** | inflammation | gastr/itis (găs-TRĬ-tĭs): inflammation of the stomach<br>*gastr:* stomach |
| **-lith** | stone, calculus | chol/e/lith* (KŌ-lē-lĭth): gallstone<br>*chlo/e:* bile, gall |
| **-malacia** | softening | chondr/o/malacia (kŏn-drō-măl-Ā-shē-ă): softening of the articular cartilage, usually involving the patella<br>*chondr/o:* cartilage |
| **-megaly** | enlargement | cardi/o/megaly (kăr-dē-ō-MĔG-ă-lē): enlargement of the heart<br>*cardi/o:* heart |
| **-oma** | tumor | neur/oma (nū-RŌ-mă): tumor composed of nerve cells or swelling of a nerve that usually results from compression<br>*neur:* nerve |
| **-osis** | abnormal condition; increase (used primarily with blood cells) | cyan/osis (sī-ă-NŌ-sĭs): dark blue or purple discoloration of the skin and mucous membrane<br>*cyan:* blue<br>*Cyanosis indicates a deficiency of oxygen in the blood.* |
| **-pathy** | disease | my/o/pathy (mī-ŎP-ă-thē): any disease of muscle<br>*my/o:* muscle |
| **-penia** | decrease, deficiency | erythr/o/penia (ĕ-rĭth-rō-PĒ-nē-ă): abnormal decrease in red blood cells<br>*erythr/o:* red |
| **-phagia** | eating, swallowing | dys/phagia (dĭs-FĀ-jē-ă): inability or difficulty in swallowing<br>*dys-:* bad; painful; difficult |
| **-phasia** | speech | a/phasia (ă-FĀ-zē-ă): absence or impairment of speech<br>*a-:* without, not |
| **-phobia** | fear | hem/o/phobia (hē-mō-FŌ-bē-ă): fear of blood<br>*hem/o:* blood |

| Table 2-4 | COMMON DIAGNOSTIC, PATHOLOGICAL, AND RELATED SUFFIXES | |
|---|---|---|

| Suffix | Meaning | Word Analysis |
|---|---|---|
| **Pathological and Related** | | |
| **-plasia** | formation, growth | dys/plasia (dĭs-PLĀ-zē-ă): abnormal development of cells, tissues, or organs<br>*dys-*: bad; painful; difficult<br>*Dysplasia is a general term for abnormal formation of an anatomic structure.* |
| **-plasm** | | neo/plasm (NĒ-ō-plăzm): a new and abnormal formation of tissue, such as a tumor or growth<br>*neo-*: new |
| **-plegia** | paralysis | hemi/plegia (hĕm-ē-PLĒ-jē-ă): paralysis of one side of the body<br>*hemi-*: one half<br>*Hemiplegia affects the right or left side of the body and is caused by a brain injury or stroke.* |
| **-rrhage** | bursting (of) | hem/o/rrhage (HĔM-ĕ-rĭj): loss of a large amount of blood within a short period, either externally or internally<br>*hem/o*: blood |
| **-rrhagia** | | men/o/rrhagia (mĕn-ō-RĀ-jē-ă): profuse discharge of blood during menstruation<br>*men/o*: menses, menstruation |
| **-rrhea** | discharge, flow | dia/rrhea (dī-ă-RĒ-ă): abnormally frequent discharge or flow of fluid fecal matter from the bowel<br>*dia-*: through, across |
| **-rrhexis** | rupture | arteri/o/rrhexis (ăr-tē-rē-ō-RĔK-sĭs): rupture of an artery<br>*arteri/o*: artery |
| **-spasm** | involuntary contraction, twitching | blephar/o/spasm (BLĔF-ă-rō-spăsm): twitching of the eyelid<br>*blephar/o*: eyelid |
| **-stenosis** | narrowing, stricture | arteri/o/stenosis (ăr-tē-rē-ō-stĕ-NŌ-sĭs): abnormal narrowing of an artery<br>*arteri/o*: artery |
| **-toxic** | poison | hepat/o/toxic (HĔP-ă-tō-tŏk-sĭk): toxic to the liver<br>*hepat/o*: liver |
| **-trophy** | nourishment, development | dys/trophy (DĬS-trō-fē): abnormal condition caused by defective nutrition or metabolism<br>*dys-*: bad; painful; difficult |

*The *i* in *pelv/i/meter* and the *e* in *chol/e/lithiasis* and *chol/e/lith* are exceptions to the rule of using the connecting vowel *o*.

 **It is time to review diagnostic, pathological, and related suffixes by completing Learning Activities 2–4 and 2–5.**

## Grammatical Suffixes

Grammatical suffixes may be attached to word roots to form a part of speech, such as adjectives and nouns, or a singular or plural form of a medical word. They are also used to denote a diminutive form of a word that designates a smaller version of the object indicated by the root. Many of these suffixes are the same as those used in the English language. (See Table 2–5.)

### Table 2–5   ADJECTIVE, NOUN, AND DIMINUTIVE SUFFIXES

This table lists adjective, noun, and diminutive suffixes along with their meanings and word analyses.

| Suffix | Meaning | Word Analysis |
|---|---|---|
| **Adjective** | | |
| -ac | pertaining to, relating to | cardi/ac (KĂR-dē-ăk): pertaining to the heart<br>    *cardi:* heart |
| -al | | neur/al (NŪ-răl): pertaining to a nerve<br>    *neur:* nerve |
| -ar | | muscul/ar (MŬS-kū-lăr): pertaining to muscle<br>    *muscul:* muscle |
| -ary | | pulmon/ary (PŬL-mō-nĕr-ē): pertaining to the lungs<br>    *pulmon:* lung |
| -eal | | esophag/eal (ē-sŏf-ă-JĒ-ăl): pertaining to the esophagus<br>    *esophag:* esophagus |
| -ic | | thorac/ic (thō-RĂS-ĭk): pertaining to the chest<br>    *thorac:* chest |
| -ical* | | path/o/log/ical (păth-ō-LŎJ-ĭ-kăl): pertaining to the study of disease<br>    *path/o:* disease<br>    *log:* study of |
| -ile | | pen/ile (PĒ-nĭl): pertaining to the penis<br>    *pen:* penis |
| -ior | | poster/ior (pŏs-TĒ-rē-or): pertaining to the back of the body<br>    *poster:* back (of body), behind, posterior |
| -ous** | | cutane/ous (kū-TĀ-nē-ŭs): pertaining to the skin<br>    *cutane:* skin |
| -tic | | acous/tic (ă-KOOS-tĭk): pertaining to hearing<br>    *acous:* hearing |
| **Noun** | | |
| -esis | condition | di/ur/esis (dī-ū-RĒ-sĭs): abnormal secretion of large amounts of urine<br>    *di-:* double<br>    *ur:* urine |
| -ia | | pneumon/ia (nū-MŌ-nē-ă): infection of the lung usually caused by bacteria, viruses, or diseases<br>    *pneumon:* air; lung |
| -ism | | hyper/thyroid/ism (hī-pĕr-THĪ-royd-ĭzm): condition characterized by overactivity of the thyroid gland<br>    *hyper-:* excessive, above normal<br>    *thyroid:* thyroid gland |

## Table 2–5    ADJECTIVE, NOUN, AND DIMINUTIVE SUFFIXES

| Suffix | Meaning | Word Analysis |
|---|---|---|
| **Noun** | | |
| **-iatry** | medicine; treatment | pod/iatry (pō-DĪ-ă-trē): specialty concerned with treatment and prevention of conditions of the human foot<br>*pod:* foot |
| **-ician** | specialist | obstetr/ician (ŏb-stĕ-TRĬSH-ăn): physician who specializes in the branch of medicine concerned with pregnancy and childbirth<br>*obstetr:* midwife |
| **-ist** | | hemat/o/log/ist (hē-mă-TŎL-ō-jĭst): physician who specializes in the treatment of disorders of blood and blood-forming tissues<br>*hemat/o:* blood<br>*log:* study of |
| **-y** | condition; process | neur/o/path/y (nū-RŎP-ă-thē): disease of the nerves<br>*r/o:* nerve<br>*path:* disease |
| **Diminutive** | | |
| **-icle** | small, minute | ventr/icle (VĔN-trĭk-l): small cavity, as of the brain or heart<br>*ventr:* belly, belly side |
| **-ole** | | arteri/ole (ăr-TĒ-rē-ōl): the smallest of the arteries; minute artery<br>*arteri:* artery<br><br>*Arteries narrow to form arterioles (small arteries), which branch into capillaries (the smallest blood vessels).* |
| **-ule** | | ven/ule (VĔN-ūl): small vein continuous with a capillary<br>*ven:* vein |

*The suffix *-ical* is a combination of *-ic* and *-al*. **The suffix *-ous* also means *composed of* or *producing*.

 **It is time to review grammatical suffixes by completing Learning Activity 2–6.**

## Plural Suffixes

Because many medical words have Greek or Latin origins, there are a few unusual rules you need to learn to change a singular word into its plural form. Once you begin learning them, you will find that they are easy to apply. You will also find that some English endings have also been adopted for commonly used medical terms. When a word changes from a singular to a plural form, the suffix of the word is the part that changes. A summary of the rules for changing a singular word into its plural form is located on the inside back cover of this textbook. Use it to complete Learning Activity 2–7 and whenever you need help forming plural words.

 **It is time to review the rules for forming plural words by completing Learning Activity 2–7.**

# LEARNING ACTIVITIES

The following activities provide review of the suffixes introduced in this chapter. Complete each activity and review your answers to evaluate your understanding of the chapter.

## Learning Activity 2–1

## Completing and building surgical words

*Use the meanings in the right column to complete the surgical words in the left column. The first one is completed for you. Note: The word roots are underlined in the left column.*

| Incomplete Word | Meaning |
|---|---|
| 1. episi /o/ _t o m y_ | incision of the perineum |
| 2. col_ _ _ _ _ _ | excision (of all or part)* of the colon |
| 3. arthr/o/ _ _ _ _ _ _ _ _ | surgical puncture of a joint (to remove fluid) |
| 4. splen_ _ _ _ _ _ | excision of the spleen |
| 5. col/o/ _ _ _ _ _ | forming an opening (mouth) into the colon |
| 6. oste/o/ _ _ _ _ | instrument to cut bone |
| 7. tympan/o/ _ _ _ _ _ | incision of the tympanic membrane |
| 8. trache/o/ _ _ _ _ _ _ | forming an opening (mouth) into the trachea |
| 9. mast_ _ _ _ _ _ | excision of a breast |
| 10. lith/o/ _ _ _ _ | incision to remove a stone or calculus |
| 11. hemorrhoid_ _ _ _ _ _ | excision of hemorrhoids |

*Information in parentheses is used to clarify the meaning of the word but not to build the medical term.

**Build a surgical word that means:**

12. forming an opening (mouth) into the colon: _____

13. excision of the colon: _____

14. instrument to cut bone: _____

15. surgical puncture of a joint: _____

16. incision to remove a stone: _____

17. excision of a breast: _____

18. incision of the tympanic membrane: _____

19. forming an opening (mouth) into the trachea: _____

20. excision of the spleen: _____

**CORRECT ANSWERS** _____ × 5 = _____ % SCORE

✓ Check your answers in Appendix A. Review any material that you did not answer correctly.

*Note:* If you are not satisfied with your level of comprehension in Learning Activity 2–1, review it and try the exercise again.

# Learning Activity 2–2

## Completing and building more surgical words

*Use the meanings in the right column to complete the surgical words in the left column.*

| Incomplete Word | Meaning |
|---|---|
| 1. arthr/o/ _ _ _ _ _ | fixation or binding of a joint |
| 2. rhin/o/ _ _ _ _ _ _ | surgical repair of the nose |
| 3. ten/o/ _ _ _ _ _ _ | surgical repair of tendons |
| 4. my/o/ _ _ _ _ _ _ _ | suture of muscle |
| 5. mast/o/ _ _ _ _ | fixation of a (pendulous)* breast |
| 6. cyst/o/ _ _ _ _ _ _ _ | suture of the bladder |
| 7. oste/o/ _ _ _ _ _ _ | surgical fracture of a bone |
| 8. lith/o/ _ _ _ _ _ _ | crushing of a stone |
| 9. enter/o/ _ _ _ _ _ | separating intestinal (adhesions) |
| 10. neur/o/ _ _ _ _ _ _ | crushing a nerve |

*Information in parentheses is used to clarify the meaning of the word but not to build the medical term.

### Build a surgical word that means:

11. surgical repair of the nose: _____

12. fixation of a joint: _____

13. suture of muscle: _____

14. fixation of a (pendulous) breast: _____

15. suture of the bladder: _____

16. repair of tendons: _____

17. surgical fracture of a bone: _____

18. crushing stones: _____

19. separating intestinal (adhesions): _____

20. crushing a nerve: _____

✓ Check your answers in Appendix A. Review any material that you did not answer correctly.

**CORRECT ANSWERS** _____ × 5 = _____ % SCORE

Learning Activity 2–3

## Selecting a surgical suffix

*Use the suffixes in this list to build surgical words in the right column that reflect the meanings in the left column.*

| | | | |
|---|---|---|---|
| -centesis | -ectomy | -plasty | -tome |
| -clasis | -lysis | -rrhaphy | -tomy |
| -desis | -pexy | -stomy | -tripsy |

1. crushing of a stone:                          lith/o/ _____
2. puncture of a joint (to remove fluid)*:       arthr/o/ _____
3. excision of the spleen:                       splen/ _____
4. forming an opening (mouth) into the colon:    col/o/ _____
5. instrument to cut skin:                       derma/ _____
6. forming an opening (mouth) into the trachea:  trache/o/ _____
7. incision to remove a stone or calculus:       lith/ _____ / _____
8. excision of a breast:                         mast/ _____
9. excision of hemorrhoids:                       hemorrhoid/ _____
10. incision of the trachea:                      trache/ _____ / _____
11. fixation of a breast:                         mast/ _____ / _____
12. excision of the colon:                        col/ _____
13. suture of the stomach (wall):                 gastr/ _____ / _____
14. fixation of the uterus:                        hyster/ _____ / _____
15. surgical repair of the nose:                  rhin/ _____ / _____
16. fixation or binding of a joint:               arthr/ _____ / _____
17. to break or surgically fracture a bone:       oste/ _____ / _____
18. loosening of nerve (tissue):                  neur/ _____ / _____
19. suture of muscle:                              my/o/ _____
20. incision of the tympanic membrane:            tympan/ _____ / _____

*Information in parentheses is used to clarify the meaning of the word but not to build the medical term.

✓ Check your answers in Appendix A. Review any material that you did not answer correctly.

**CORRECT ANSWERS** _____ × 5 = _____ **% SCORE**

## Learning Activity 2-4

## Selecting diagnostic, pathological, and related suffixes

*Use the suffixes in this list to build diagnostic, pathological, and related words in the right column that reflect the meanings in the left column.*

| | | |
|---|---|---|
| -algia | -malacia | -phagia |
| -cele | -megaly | -phasia |
| -ectasis | -metry | -plegia |
| -emia | -oma | -rrhage |
| -genesis | -osis | -rrhea |
| -graph | -pathy | -rrhexis |
| -iasis | -penia | -spasm |

1. tumor of the liver:                                    hepat/ _____
2. pain (along the course) of a nerve:                    neur/ _____
3. dilation of a bronchus:                                bronchi/ _____
4. producing or forming cancer:                           carcin/o/ _____
5. abnormal condition of the skin:                        dermat/ _____
6. enlarged kidney:                                       nephr/o/ _____
7. discharge or flow from the ear:                        ot/ ____ / _____
8. rupture of the uterus:                                 hyster/ ____ / _____
9. spasm or twitching of the eyelid:                      blephar/ ____ / _____
10. herniation of the bladder:                            cyst/ ____ / _____
11. bursting forth (of) blood:                            hem/o/ _____
12. abnormal condition of a stone or calculus:            lith/ _____
13. paralysis affecting one side (of the body):           hemi/ _____
14. diseases of muscle (tissue):                          my/ ____ / _____
15. difficult or painful eating:                          dys/ _____
16. softening of the bones:                               oste/ ____ / _____
17. without, or absence of, speech:                       a/ _____
18. white blood condition:                                leuk/ _____
19. deficiency in red (blood) cells:                      erythr/ ____ / _____
20. measuring the pelvis:                                 pelv/i/ _____

✓ Check your answers in Appendix A. Review any material that you did not answer correctly.

**CORRECT ANSWERS** _____ × 5 = _____ **% SCORE**

Learning Activity 2–5

## Building pathological and related words

*Use the meanings in the right column to complete the pathological and related words in the left column.*

| **Incomplete Word** | **Meaning** |
|---|---|
| 1. bronchi _ _ _ _ _ _ _ | dilation of a bronchus |
| 2. chole _ _ _ _ | gallstone |
| 3. carcin/o/ _ _ _ _ _ _ _ | forming or producing cancer |
| 4. oste/_ / _ _ _ _ _ _ _ | softening of bone |
| 5. hepat/_ / _ _ _ _ _ _ | enlargement of the liver |
| 6. cholelith _ _ _ _ _ | abnormal condition of gallstones |
| 7. hepat/_ / _ _ _ _ | herniation of the liver |
| 8. neur/o/ _ _ _ _ _ | disease of the nerves |
| 9. dermat _ _ _ _ | abnormal condition of the skin |
| 10. hemi _ _ _ _ _ _ | paralysis of one half of the body |
| 11. dys _ _ _ _ _ _ | difficult swallowing |
| 12. a _ _ _ _ _ _ | without speech or absence of speech |
| 13. cephal _ _ _ _ _ | pain in the head; headache |
| 14. blephar/_ / _ _ _ _ _ | twitching of the eyelid |
| 15. hyper _ _ _ _ _ _ | excessive formation (of an organ or tissue) |

✓ Check your answers in Appendix A. Review any material that you did not answer correctly.

**CORRECT ANSWERS** _____ × 6.67 = _____ **% SCORE**

Learning Activity 2–6

## Selecting adjective, noun, and diminutive suffixes

*Use the adjective suffixes in the following list to create a medical word. The first one is completed for you. Note: When in doubt about the validity of a word, refer to a medical dictionary.*

| -ac | -ary | -ic | -tic |
|-----|------|-----|------|
| -al | -eal | -ous | -tix |

| Element | Medical Term | Meaning |
|---------|-------------|---------|
| 1. thorac/ | *thoracic* | pertaining to the chest |
| 2. gastr/ | _____ | pertaining to the stomach |
| 3. bacteri/ | _____ | pertaining to bacteria |
| 4. aqua/ | _____ | pertaining to water |
| 5. axill/ | _____ | pertaining to the armpit |
| 6. cardi/ | _____ | pertaining to the heart |
| 7. spin/ | _____ | pertaining to the spine |
| 8. membran/ | _____ | pertaining to a membrane |

**Use the noun suffixes in the following list to create a medical word.**

| -er | -ism |
|-----|------|
| -ia | -ist |
| -is | -y |

| Element | Medical Term | Meaning |
|---------|-------------|---------|
| 9. intern/ | _____ | specialist in internal medicine |
| 10. leuk/em/ | _____ | condition of "white" blood |
| 11. sigmoid/o/scop/ | _____ | visual examination of the sigmoid colon |
| 12. alcohol/ | _____ | condition of (excessive) alcohol |
| 13. senil/ | _____ | condition associated with aging |
| 14. allerg/ | _____ | specialist in treating allergic disorders |
| 15. man/ | _____ | condition of madness |

**Use the diminutive suffixes in the following list to create a medical word.**

| -icle | -ole | -ule |
|-------|------|------|

| Element | Medical Term | Meaning |
|---------|-------------|---------|
| 16. arteri/ | _____ | minute artery |
| 17. ventr/ | _____ | small cavity |
| 18. ven/ | _____ | small vein |

Check your answers in Appendix A. Review any material that you did not answer correctly.

**CORRECT ANSWERS** _____ × 5.6 = _____ **% SCORE**

Learning Activity 2–7

## Forming plural words

*Review the guidelines for plural suffixes (located inside the back cover of this book). Then write the plural form for each of the following singular terms and briefly state the rule that applies. The first one is completed for you.*

| Singular | Plural | Rule |
|---|---|---|
| 1. diagnosis | *diagnoses* | *Drop the is and add es.* |
| 2. fornix | | |
| 3. vertebra | | |
| 4. keratosis | | |
| 5. bronchus | | |
| 6. spermatozoon | | |
| 7. septum | | |
| 8. coccus | | |
| 9. ganglion | | |
| 10. prognosis | | |
| 11. thrombus | | |
| 12. appendix | | |
| 13. bacterium | | |
| 14. testis | | |
| 15. nevus | | |

✓ Check your answers in Appendix A. Review any material that you did not answer correctly.

**CORRECT ANSWERS** _____ × **6.67** = _____ **% SCORE**

# Chapter

# 3

# Prefixes

## CHAPTER OUTLINE

Objectives

Prefix Linking

Prefix Types
  *Prefixes of Position, Number and
    Measurement, and Direction*
  *Other Prefixes*

Learning Activities

## OBJECTIVES

*Upon completion of this chapter, you will be able to:*

■ Explain the use of prefixes in medical terminology.

■ Explain how a prefix changes the meaning of a medical word.

■ Identify prefixes of position, number and measurement, and direction.

■ Demonstrate your knowledge of this chapter by completing the learning activities.

## Prefix Linking

Most medical words contain a root, or combining form, and a suffix. Some of them also contain prefixes. A prefix is a word element located at the beginning of a word. Substituting one prefix for another alters the meaning of the word. For example, in the term *macro/cyte*, *macro-* is a prefix meaning *large*; *-cyte* is a suffix meaning cell. A *macrocyte* is a large cell. By changing the prefix *macro-* to *micro-* (small), the meaning of the word changes. A *microcyte* is a small cell. See Table 3–1 for three other examples of how a prefix can change the meaning of a word.

## Table 3–1    CHANGING PREFIXES AND MEANINGS

In this table, each word has the same root, *nat* (birth). By substituting different prefixes, a new word with a different meaning is formed.

| Prefix | + | Word Root | + | Suffix | = | Medical Word | Meaning |
|---|---|---|---|---|---|---|---|
| **pre-** (before) | + | *nat* (birth) | + | *-al* (pertaining to, relating to) | = | prenatal prē-NĀ-tăl | pertaining to (the period) before birth |
| **peri-** (around) | + | *nat* (birth) | + | *-al* (pertaining to, relating to) | = | perinatal pĕr-ĭ-NĀ-tăl | pertaining to (the period) around birth |
| **post-** (after) | + | *nat* (birth) | + | *-al* (pertaining to, relating to) | = | postnatal pōst-NĀ-tăl | pertaining to (the period) after birth |

## Prefix Types

Learning the major types of prefixes, such as prefixes of position, number and measurement, and direction, as well as some others, will help you master medical terminology.

### Prefixes of Position, Number and Measurement, and Direction

Prefixes are used in medical terms to denote position, number and measurement, and direction. Prefixes of position describe a place or location. (See Table 3–2.) Prefixes of number and measurement describe an amount, size, or degree of involvement. (See Table 3–3.) Prefixes of direction indicate a pathway or route. (See Table 3–4.)

## Table 3–2    PREFIXES OF POSITION

This table lists commonly used prefixes of position along with their meanings and word analyses.

| Prefix | Meaning | Word Analysis |
|---|---|---|
| **epi-** | above, upon | epi/derm/is (ĕp-ĭ-DĔR-mĭs): outermost layer of the skin *derm*: skin *-is*: noun ending |

| Table 3-2 | PREFIXES OF POSITION |

| Prefix | Meaning | Word Analysis |
|---|---|---|
| **hypo-** | under, below, deficient | hypo/derm/ic (hī-pō-DĔR-mĭk): under or inserted under the skin, as in a hypodermic injection<br>*derm:* skin<br>*-ic:* pertaining to, relating to |
| **infra-** | under, below | infra/cost/al (ĭn-fră-KŎS-tăl): below the ribs<br>*cost:* ribs<br>*-al:* pertaining to, relating to |
| **sub-** | | sub/nas/al (sŭb-NĀ-săl): under the nose<br>*nas:* nose<br>*-al:* pertaining to, relating to |
| **inter-** | between | inter/cost/al (ĭn-tĕr-KŎS-tăl): between the ribs<br>*cost:* ribs<br>*-al:* pertaining to, relating to |
| **post-** | after, behind | post/nat/al (pōst-NĀ-tăl): pertaining to the period after birth<br>*nat:* birth |
| **pre-** | before, in front of | pre/nat/al (prē-NĀ-tăl): pertaining to the period before birth<br>*nat:* birth<br>*-al:* pertaining to, relating to |
| **pro-** | | pro/gnosis (prŏg-NŌ-sĭs): prediction of the course and end of a disease, and the estimated chance of recovery<br>*-gnosis:* knowing |
| **retro-** | backward, behind | retro/version (rĕt-rō-VĔR-shŭn): tipping backward of an organ (such as the uterus) from its normal position<br>*-version:* turning |

| Table 3-3 | PREFIXES OF NUMBER AND MEASUREMENT |

This table lists commonly used prefixes of number and measurement along with their meanings and word analyses.

| Prefix | Meaning | Word Analysis |
|---|---|---|
| **bi-** | two | bi/later/al (bī-LĂT-ĕr-ăl): pertaining to, affecting, or relating to two sides<br>*later:* side, to one side<br>*-al:* pertaining to, relating to |
| **dipl-** | double | dipl/opia (dĭp-LŌ-pē-ă): double vision<br>*-opia:* vision |
| **diplo-** | | diplo/bacteri/al (dĭp-lō-băk-TĒ-rē-ăl): bacterial cells linked together in pairs<br>*bacteri:* bacteria<br>*-al:* pertaining to, relating to |
| **hemi-** | one half | hemi/plegia (hĕm-ē-PLĒ-jē-ă): paralysis of one side of the body<br>*-plegia:* paralysis |

*(Continued)*

## Table 3–3   PREFIXES OF NUMBER AND MEASUREMENT *(Continued)*

| Prefix | Meaning | Word Analysis |
|---|---|---|
| **hyper-** | excessive, above normal | hyper/calc/emia (hī-pĕr-kăl-SĒ-mē-ă): excessive concentration of calcium in the blood<br>   *calc:* calcium<br>   *-emia:* blood condition |
| **macro-** | large | macro/cyte (MĂK-rō-sīt): abnormally large erythrocyte, such as those found in pernicious anemia<br>   *-cyte:* cell<br>*An erythrocyte is a red blood cell.* |
| **micro-** | small | micro/scope (MĪ-krō-skōp): optical instrument that greatly magnifies minute objects<br>   *-scope:* instrument for examining |
| **mono-** | one | mono/chromat/ism (mŏn-ō-KRŌ-mă-tĭzm): complete color blindness in which all colors are perceived as shades of gray<br>   *chromat:* color<br>   *-ism:* condition |
| **uni-** | | uni/nucle/ar (ū-nĭ-NŪ-klē-ăr): having only one nucleus<br>   *nucle:* nucleus<br>   *-ar:* pertaining to, relating to |
| **multi-** | many, much | multi/gravida (mŭl-tĭ-GRĂV-ĭ-dă): woman who has been pregnant more than once<br>   *-gravida:* pregnant woman |
| **poly-** | | poly/phobia (pŏl-ē-FŌ-bē-ă): abnormal fear of many things<br>   *-phobia:* fear |
| **primi-** | first | primi/gravida (prī-mĭ-GRĂV-ĭ-dă): woman during her first pregnancy<br>   *-gravida:* pregnant woman |
| **quadri-** | four | quadri/plegia (kwŏd-rĭ-PLĒ-jē-ă): paralysis of all four limbs<br>   *-plegia:* paralysis |
| **tri-** | three | tri/plegia (trī-PLĒ-jē-ă): hemiplegia with paralysis of one limb on the other side of the body<br>   *-plegia:* paralysis |

## Table 3–4   PREFIXES OF DIRECTION

This table lists commonly used prefixes of direction as well as their meanings and word analyses.

| Prefix | Meaning | Word Analysis |
|---|---|---|
| **ab-** | from, away from | ab/duction (ăb-DŬK-shŭn): movement of a limb away from the body (See Figure 10–2.)<br>   *-duction:* act of leading, bringing, conducting |
| **ad-** | toward | ad/duction (ă-DŬK-shŭn): movement of a limb toward the axis of the body (See Figure 10–2.)<br>   *-duction:* act of leading, bringing, conducting |

*(Continued)*

| Table 3-4 | PREFIXES OF DIRECTION |
|---|---|

| Prefix | Meaning | Word Analysis |
|---|---|---|
| **circum-** | around | circum/duction (sĕr-kŭm-DŬK-shŭn): movement of a part, such as an extremity, in a circular direction<br>   *-duction:* act of leading, bringing, conducting |
| **peri-** | | peri/odont/al (pĕr-ē-ō-DŎN-tăl): located around a tooth<br>   *odont:* teeth<br>   *-al:* pertaining to, relating to |
| **dia-** | through, across | dia/rrhea (dī-ă-RĒ-ă): abnormally frequent discharge or flow of fluid fecal matter from the bowel<br>   *-rrhea:* discharge, flow |
| **trans-** | | trans/vagin/al (trăns-VĂJ-ĭn-ăl): across or through the vagina<br>   *vagin:* vagina<br>   *-al:* pertaining to, relating to |
| **ecto-** | outside, outward | ecto/gen/ous (ĕk-TŎJ-ĕ-nŭs): originating outside the body or structure<br>   *gen:* forming, producing, origin<br>   *-ous:* pertaining to, relating to |
| **exo-** | | exo/tropia (ĕks-ō-TRŌ-pē-ă): abnormal turning outward of one or both eyes<br>   *-tropia:* turning |
| **extra-** | | extra/crani/al (ĕks-tră-KRĀ-nē-ăl): outside the skull<br>   *crani:* cranium (skull)<br>   *-al:* pertaining to, relating to |
| **endo-** | in, within | endo/crine (ĔN-dō-krĭn): secreting internally<br>   *-crine:* secrete<br>*Endocrine refers to a gland that secretes directly into the bloodstream.* |
| **intra-** | | intra/muscul/ar (ĭn-tră-MŬS-kū-lăr): within the muscle<br>   *muscul:* muscle<br>   *-ar:* pertaining to, relating to |
| **para-*** | near, beside; beyond | para/nas/al (păr-ă-NĀ-săl): beside the nose<br>   *nas:* nose<br>   *-al:* pertaining to, relating to |
| **super-** | upper, above | super/ior (soo-PĒ-rē-or): toward the head or upper portion of a structure<br>   *-ior:* pertaining to, relating to |
| **supra-** | above; excessive; superior | supra/pelv/ic (soo-pră-PĔL-vĭk): located above the pelvis<br>   *pelv:* pelvis<br>   *-ic:* pertaining to, relating to |
| **ultra-** | excess, beyond | ultra/son/ic (ūl-tră-SŎN-ĭk): pertaining to sound frequencies too high to be perceived by the human ear<br>   *son:* sound<br>   *-ic:* pertaining to, relating to |

*\*Para-* may also be used as a suffix meaning *to bear (offspring).*

## Other Prefixes

Many other prefixes may also be used to change the meaning of a word. See Table 3–5 for a list of some other common prefixes.

### Table 3–5    OTHER PREFIXES

This table lists other commonly used prefixes along with their meanings and word analyses.

| Prefix | Meaning | Word Analysis |
|---|---|---|
| **a-*** | without, not | a/mast/ia (ă-MĂS-tē-ă): without a breast<br>  *mast:* breast<br>  *-ia:* condition<br>*Amastia may be the result of a congenital defect, an endocrine disorder, or mastectomy.* |
| **an-**** | | an/esthesia (ăn-ĕs-THĒ-zē-ă): partial or complete loss of sensation with or without loss of consciousness<br>  *-esthesia:* feeling |
| **anti-** | against | anti/bacteri/al (ăn-tĭ-băk-TĒ-rē-ăl): pertaining to agents that destroy or stop the growth of bacteria<br>  *bacteri:* bacteria<br>  *-al:* pertaining to, relating to |
| **contra-** | | contra/ception (kon-tră-SEP-shŭn): prevention of conception or impregnation<br>  *-ception:* conceiving |
| **brady-** | slow | brady/cardia (brăd-ē-KĂR-dē-ă): slow heart rate<br>  *-cardia:* heart |
| **dys-** | bad; painful; difficult | dys/tocia (dĭs-TŌ-sē-ă): difficult childbirth<br>  *-tocia:* childbirth, labor |
| **eu-** | good, normal | eu/pnea (ūp-NĒ-ă): normal breathing<br>  *-pnea:* breathing |
| **hetero-** | different | hetero/graft (HĔT-ĕ-rō-grăft): transplant of tissue from one species to a different species; *also called xenograft*<br>  *-graft:* transplantation |
| **homo-** | same | homo/graft (HŌ-mō-grăft): transplant of tissue between the same species; also called *allograft*<br>  *-graft:* transplantation |
| **homeo-** | | homeo/plasia (hō-mē-ō-PLĀ-zē-ă): formation of new tissue similar to that already existing in a part<br>  *-plasia:* formation, growth |
| **mal-** | bad | mal/nutrition (măl-nū-TRĬ-shŭn): any disorder of nutrition |
| **pan-** | all | pan/arthr/itis (păn-ăr-THRĪ-tĭs): abnormal condition characterized by the inflammation of many joints of the body<br>  *arthr:* joint<br>  *-itis:* inflammation |
| **pseudo-** | false | pseudo/cyesis (soo-dō-sī-Ē-sĭs): condition in which a woman believes she is pregnant when she is not<br>  *-cyesis:* pregnancy |

## Table 3–5     OTHER PREFIXES

| Prefix | Meaning | Word Analysis |
|---|---|---|
| **syn-\*\*\*** | union, together, joined | syn/dactyl/ism (sĭn-DĂK-tĭl-ĭzm): congenital anomaly characterized by the fusion of the fingers or toes<br>*dactyl:* fingers; toes<br>*-ism:* condition |
| **tachy-** | rapid | tachy/pnea (tăk-ĭp-NĒ-ă): abnormally rapid rate of breathing<br>*-pnea:* breathing |

*The prefix *a-* is usually used before a consonant. ** The prefix *an-* is usually used before a vowel. *** The prefix *syn-* appears as *sym-* before *b, p, ph,* or *m*.

**It is time to review prefixes by completing Learning Activities 3–1, 3–2, and 3–3.**

# LEARNING ACTIVITIES

The following activities provide review of the prefixes introduced in this chapter. Complete each activity and review your answers to evaluate your understanding of the chapter.

## Learning Activity 3–1

### Identifying and defining prefixes

*Place a slash after each of the following prefixes and then define the prefix. The first one is completed for you.*

| Word | Definition of Prefix |
|---|---|
| 1. inter/dental | *between* |
| 2. hypodermic | |
| 3. epidermis | |
| 4. retroversion | |
| 5. sublingual | |
| 6. transvaginal | |
| 7. infracostal | |
| 8. postnatal | |
| 9. quadriplegia | |
| 10. hypercalcemia | |
| 11. primigravida | |
| 12. microscope | |

13.  t r i p l e g i a                    _____
14.  p o l y d i p s i a                  _____
15.  a b d u c t i o n                    _____
16.  a n e s t h e s i a                  _____
17.  m a c r o c y t e                    _____
18.  i n t r a m u s c u l a r            _____
19.  s u p r a p e l v i c                _____
20.  d i a r r h e a                      _____
21.  c i r c u m d u c t i o n            _____
22.  a d d u c t i o n                    _____
23.  p e r i o d o n t a l                _____
24.  b r a d y c a r d i a                _____
25.  t a c h y p n e a                    _____
26.  d y s t o c i a                      _____
27.  e u p n e a                          _____
28.  h e t e r o g r a f t                _____
29.  m a l n u t r i t i o n              _____
30.  p s e u d o c y e s i s              _____

✓ Check your answers in Appendix A. Review any material that you did not answer correctly.

**CORRECT ANSWERS** _____ × **3.34** = _____ **% SCORE**

## Learning Activity 3–2

## Matching prefixes of position, number and measurement, and direction

*Match the following terms with the definitions in the numbered list.*

*diarrhea*          *macrocyte*          *pseudocyesis*
*ectogenous*        *periodontal*        *quadriplegia*
*hemiplegia*        *polyphobia*         *retroversion*
*hypodermic*        *postoperative*      *subnasal*
*intercostal*       *prenatal*           *suprarenal*

1.  _____ tipping back of an organ
2.  _____ pertaining to under the skin
3.  _____ before birth
4.  _____ pertaining to under the nose
5.  _____ after surgery
6.  _____ pertaining to between the ribs
7.  _____ false pregnancy
8.  _____ pertaining to around the teeth

9. _____ flow through (watery bowel movement)

10. _____ pertaining to an origin outside (the body or structure)

11. _____ above the kidney

12. _____ paralysis of one half (of the body)

13. _____ paralysis of four (limbs)

14. _____ abnormally large (blood cell)

15. _____ many fears

 Check your answers in Appendix A. Review any material that you did not answer correctly.

**CORRECT ANSWERS** _____ × 6.67 = _____ % SCORE

## Learning Activity 3–3

## Matching other prefixes

*Match the following terms with the definitions in the numbered list.*

| | | |
|---|---|---|
| *amastia* | *dyspepsia* | *homosexual* |
| *anesthesia* | *dystocia* | *malnutrition* |
| *antibacterial* | *eupnea* | *panarthritis* |
| *bradycardia* | *heterosexual* | *syndactylism* |
| *contraception* | *homograft* | *tachycardia* |

1. _____ difficult digestion

2. _____ pertaining to a different (opposite) sex

3. _____ inflammation of many joints of the body

4. _____ against bacteria

5. _____ slow heartbeat

6. _____ poor or bad nutrition

7. _____ without a breast

8. _____ without sensation

9. _____ good or normal breathing

10. _____ condition of fusion of fingers and toes

11. _____ rapid heartbeat

12. _____ against conception

13. _____ pertaining to the same sex

14. _____ difficult childbirth

15. _____ transplant (of tissue between the) same (species)

Check your answers in Appendix A. Review any material that you did not answer correctly.

**CORRECT ANSWERS** _____ × 6.67 = _____ % SCORE

# Chapter

# 4

# Body Structure

### OBJECTIVES

*Upon completion of this chapter, you will be able to:*

- Understand and identify levels of organization and anatomical planes of the body.
- Identify the cavities, quadrants, and regions of the body.

- Understand the terms related to direction, position, and planes of the body.
- Recognize, pronounce, spell, and build words related to body structure and identify common abbreviations.
- Describe diagnostic and therapeutic procedures and other terms associated with body structure.
- Demonstrate your knowledge of this chapter by completing the learning and medical record activities.

 **Key Terms**

This section introduces important body structure terms and their definitions. Word analyses are also provided.

| Term | Definition |
|---|---|
| **cytoplasm**<br>SĪ-tō-plăzm<br><br>*cyt/o:* cell<br>*-plasm:* formation, growth | Gel-like substance that surrounds the nucleus of a cell but is contained within the cell membrane<br><br>*The cytoplasm contains structures, called organelles, which carry out the essential functions of the cell.* |
| **deoxyribonucleic acid (DNA)**<br>dē-ok-sē-rī-bō-<br>noo-KLĒ-ĭk ĂS-ĭd | Molecule that holds genetic information and makes an exact copy of itself whenever the cell divides |
| **diagnosis**<br>dī-ăg-NŌ-sĭs<br><br>*dia-:* through, across<br>*-gnosis:* knowing | Identification of a disease or condition by scientific evaluation of physical signs, symptoms, history, laboratory and clinical test results, and radiographic procedures |
| **endoscope**<br>ĔN-dō-skōp<br><br>*endo-:* in, within<br>*-scope:* instrument for examining | Instrument consisting of a rigid or flexible fiberoptic tube and optical system for observing the inside of a hollow organ or cavity<br><br>*Most endoscopes consist of an elongated probe fitted with a light and camera.* |
| **etiology**<br>ē-tē-ŎL-ō-jē<br><br>*eti/o:* cause<br>*-logy:* study of | Study of the causes of disease |
| **fluoroscope**<br>FLOO-or-ō-skōp<br><br>*fluor/o:* luminous, fluorescent<br>*-scope:* instrument for examining | Instrument, consisting of an x-ray machine and a fluorescent screen, used to view the internal organs of the body<br><br>*The patient stands between the x-ray machine and the fluorescent screen, and as radiation passes through the body it produces an image. Although the regular x-ray film shows more detail, fluoroscopy is preferable when live images and movement of internal organs are required.* |

| Term | Definition |
|------|-----------|
| **idiopathic**<br>ĭd-ē-ō-PĂTH-ĭk<br><br>*idi/o:* unknown, peculiar<br>*path:* disease<br>*-ic:* pertaining to, relating to | Pertaining to conditions without clear pathogenesis, or disease without recognizable cause, as of spontaneous origin |
| **metabolism**<br>mĕ-TĂB-ō-lĭzm | Chemical changes that take place in a cell or an organism and produce energy and basic materials needed for all life processes |
| **prognosis**<br>prŏg-NŌ-sĭs<br><br>*pro-:* before, in front of<br>*-gnosis:* knowing | Prediction of the course and end of a disease and the estimated chance of recovery |
| **sign**<br>SĪN | Any objective evidence or manifestation of an illness or a disordered function of the body |
| **symptom**<br>SĬM-tŭm | Any change in the body or its functions as perceived by the patient |

 ## Introduction

This chapter provides the basic foundation for understanding the body system chapters that follow. It presents the basic structural and functional organization of the body—from the cellular level to the organism level. It also introduces terms used to describe planes of the body, body cavities, divisions of the spinal column, and quadrants and regions of the abdominal cavity. Such terms are an essential part of medical terminology and are relevant to all body systems. Pathology is also covered, as well as the terminology associated with the disease process. Finally, this chapter presents and describes terms associated with diagnostic and therapeutic procedures.

 ## Levels of Organization

The body is composed of several levels of structure and function. Each of these levels incorporates the previous level, and contributes to the structure and function of the entire organism. The levels of organization from simplest to most complex are:

- cell
- tissue
- organ
- system
- organism

### Cell

The study of the body at the cellular level is called *cytology*. The cell is the structural and functional unit of life. Body cells perform all activities associated with life, including obtaining nourishment, eliminating waste, and reproducing. Cells are composed of:

- cell membrane
- cytoplasm
- nucleus

## Cell Membrane and Cytoplasm

The cell membrane acts as a barrier that encloses the entire cell. It regulates the transport of a multitude of substances to and from the cell. Within the cell membrane is a gelatinous matrix of proteins, salts, water, dissolved gases, and nutrients called **cytoplasm.** Embedded in cytoplasm are various structures called *organelles* that provide specialized functions for the cell.

## Nucleus

The nucleus is responsible for metabolism, growth, and reproduction. It also carries the genetic blueprint of the organism. This blueprint is contained in a complex molecule called **deoxyribonucleic acid (DNA)** that is organized into chromatin. When the cell is ready to divide, chromatin forms chromosomes upon which approximately 31,000 genes are located. Each gene determines a unique human characteristic. Genes transmit biological information from one generation to the next and include such diverse traits as hair color, body structure, and metabolic activity. In the human, all cells except sperm cells and egg cells contain 23 pairs, or 46 chromosomes.

## Tissue

The study of tissues is called *histology.* Groups of cells that perform a specialized activity are called *tissues.* Between the cells that make up tissues are varying amounts and types of nonliving, intercellular substances that provide pathways for cellular interaction. More than 200 cell types compose four major tissues of the body:

- *Epithelial tissue* covers surfaces of organs; lines cavities and canals; forms tubes, ducts, and secreting portions of glands; and makes up the epidermis of the skin. It is composed of cells arranged in a continuous sheet consisting of one or several layers.
- *Connective tissue* supports and connects other tissues and organs and is made up of diverse cell types, including fibroblasts, fat cells, and blood.
- *Muscle tissue* provides the contractile tissue of the body, which is responsible for movement.
- *Nervous tissue* transmits electrical impulses.

## Organ

Organs are body structures composed of at least two or more tissue types that perform specialized functions. For example, the stomach is composed of muscle tissue, epithelial tissue, and nervous tissue. Muscle and connective tissue forms the wall of the stomach. Epithelial and connective tissue covers the internal and external surfaces of the stomach. Nervous tissue penetrates both the muscular wall and its epithelial lining to provide stimulation for the release of digestive juices and contraction of muscles in the stomach wall for digestion.

## System

A body system is composed of varying numbers of organs and accessory structures that have similar or interrelated functions. For example, some of the organs of the gastrointestinal system include the esophagus, stomach, and small intestine. Some of its accessory structures include the liver, gallbladder, and pancreas. The purpose of this system is to digest food, extract nutrients from it, and eliminate waste products. Other body systems include the reproductive, respiratory, urinary, and cardiovascular systems.

## Organism

The highest level of organization is the organism. An organism is a complete living entity capable of independent existence. All complex organisms, including humans, are composed of several body systems that work together to sustain life.

## Anatomical Position

The *anatomical position* is a body posture used as a reference when describing anatomical parts in relation to each other. In this position, the body is erect and the eyes are looking forward. The upper limbs hang to the sides, with the palms facing forward; the lower limbs are parallel, with the toes pointing straight ahead. Regardless how the body being examined or described is positioned—standing or reclining, facing forward or backward—or how the limbs are actually placed, the positions and relationships of a structure are always described as if the body were in the anatomical position. (See Figure 4–1.)

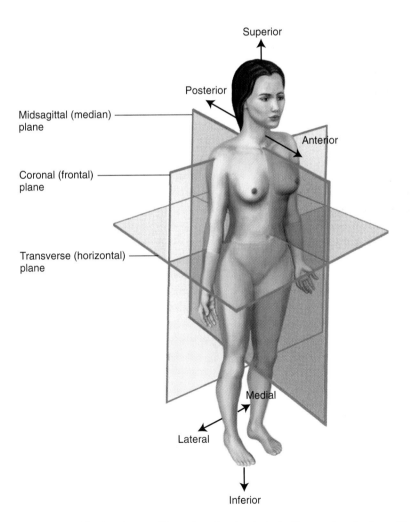

**Figure 4–1**   Body planes. Note that the body is in the anatomical position.

## Planes of the Body

To identify various sections of the body, anatomists use an imaginary flat surface called a *plane*. Prior to the development of modern imaging techniques, conventional x-ray images were taken only on a single plane, and many body abnormalities were difficult, if not impossible, to visualize. Current imaging procedures, such as magnetic resonance imaging (MRI) and computed tomography (CT), produce three-dimensional images on more than one plane. Thus, structural abnormalities and body masses that were previously not observable with a standard x-ray taken on a single plane are currently detected using scanning devices that produce images taken in several body planes.

The most commonly used planes are midsagittal, coronal, and transverse. (See Table 4–1.) The section is named for the plane along which it is cut. Thus, a cut along a transverse plane produces a transverse, or horizontal, section. The anatomical divisions of these body planes are illustrated in Figure 4–1. Various imaging procedures are presented in this chapter and developed more extensively in the body systems chapters.

| Table 4–1 | PLANES OF THE BODY |
| --- | --- |

This table lists planes of the body as well as the anatomical division for each.

| Plane | Anatomical Division |
| --- | --- |
| Midsagittal (median) | Right and left halves |
| Coronal (frontal) | Anterior (ventral) and posterior (dorsal) aspects |
| Transverse (horizontal) | Superior (upper) and inferior (lower) aspects |

## Body Cavities

The body has two major cavities: the dorsal cavity (posterior) and the ventral cavity (anterior). (See Table 4–2.) Each of these cavities has further subdivisions, as shown in Figure 4–2.

**Table 4-2    BODY CAVITIES**

This table lists the body cavities and some of the major organs found within them. The thoracic cavity is separated from the abdominopelvic cavity by a muscular wall called the *diaphragm*.

| Cavity | Major Organ(s) in the Cavity |
| --- | --- |
| **Dorsal** | |
| Cranial | Brain |
| Spinal | Spinal cord |
| **Ventral** | |
| Thoracic | Heart, lungs, and associated structures |
| Abdominopelvic | Digestive, excretory, and reproductive organs and structures |

**Figure 4–2**  Body cavities.

## Abdominopelvic Divisions

The abdominopelvic area of the body is located beneath the diaphragm. It contains the organs of digestion (abdominal area) and the organs of reproduction and excretion (pelvic area). Two anatomical methods are used to divide this area of the body for medical purposes:

- quadrants
- regions.

### Quadrants

The quadrants are four divisions of the lower torso demarcated for the purpose of topographical location. They provide a means of defining specific sites for descriptive and diagnostic purposes. (See Table 4–3.) The divisions of quadrants are used in clinical examinations and medical reports. Pain, lesions, abrasions, punctures, and burns are frequently described as located in a specific quadrant. Incision sites are also identified by using body quadrants as the method of location. An imaginary cross passing through the navel identifies the four quadrants. (See Figure 4–3A.)

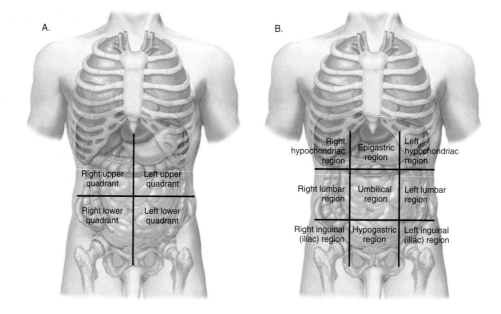

**Figure 4–3** (A) Four quadrants of the abdomen. (B) Nine regions of the abdomen.

## Table 4–3    BODY QUADRANTS

This table lists the quadrants of the body along with their corresponding abbreviations and identifies their major structures.

| Quadrant | Abbreviation | Major Structures |
| --- | --- | --- |
| Right upper | RUQ | Right lobe of liver, gallbladder, part of pancreas, part of the small and large intestines |
| Left upper | LUQ | Left lobe of liver, stomach, spleen, part of pancreas, part of small and large intestines |
| Right lower | RLQ | Part of the small and large intestines, appendix, right ovary, right fallopian tube, right ureter |
| Left lower | LLQ | Part of the small and large intestines, left ovary, left fallopian tube, left ureter |

## Regions

Whereas the quadrants of the body are used primarily to identify topographical sites, the abdominopelvic regions are used primarily to identify the location of underlying body structures and visceral organs. (See Table 4–4.) For example, the stomach is located in the left hypochondriac and epigastric region and the appendix is located in the hypogastric region. (See Figure 4–3B.)

## Table 4–4    ABDOMINOPELVIC REGIONS

This table lists the names of the abdominopelvic regions and where they are located.

| Region | Location |
| --- | --- |
| Left hypochondriac | Upper left region beneath the ribs |
| Epigastric | Region above the stomach |
| Right hypochondriac | Upper right region beneath the ribs |
| Left lumbar | Left middle lateral region |
| Umbilical | Region of the navel |
| Right lumbar | Right middle lateral region |
| Left inguinal (iliac) | Left lower lateral region |
| Hypogastric | Lower middle region beneath the navel |
| Right inguinal (iliac) | Right lower lateral region |

**It is time to review the planes of the body and quadrants and regions of the abdominopelvic area by completing Learning Activities 4–1 and 4–2.**

## Spine

The spine is divided into sections corresponding to the vertebrae located in the spinal column. (For a more complete discussion, refer to Chapter 10, Musculoskeletal System.) These divisions are:

- cervical (neck)
- thoracic (chest)
- lumbar (loin)
- sacral (lower back)
- coccyx (tailbone).

## Directional Terms

Directional terms are used to indicate the position of a structure in relation to another structure. For example, the kidneys are superior to the urinary bladder. The directional phrase *superior to* denotes *above*. This example indicates that the kidneys are located above the urinary bladder. (See Table 4–5.)

### Table 4–5    DIRECTIONAL TERMS

This table lists directional terms along with their definitions. In this list, opposing terms are presented consecutively to aid memorization.

| Term | Definition |
|---|---|
| Abduction | Movement away from the median plane of the body or one of its parts |
| Adduction | Movement toward the median plane of the body |
| Medial | Pertaining to the midline of the body or structure |
| Lateral | Pertaining to a side |
| Superior (cephalad) | Toward the head or upper portion of a structure |
| Inferior (caudal) | Away from the head, or toward the tail or lower part of a structure |
| Proximal | Nearer to the center (trunk of the body) or to the point of attachment to the body |
| Distal body | Further from the center (trunk of the body) or from the point of attachment to the |
| Anterior (ventral) | Near the front of the body |
| Posterior (dorsal) | Near the back of the body |

**Table 4–5     DIRECTIONAL TERMS**

| Term | Definition |
|------|------------|
| Parietal | Pertaining to the outer wall of the body cavity |
| Visceral | Pertaining to the viscera, or internal organs, especially the abdominal organs |
| Prone | Lying horizontal with the face downward, or indicating the hand with palms turned downward |
| Supine | Lying on the back with the face upward, or indicating the position of the hand or foot with the palm or foot facing upward |
| Inversion | Turning inward or inside out |
| Eversion | Turning outward |
| Palmar | Pertaining to the palm of the hand |
| Plantar | Pertaining to the sole of the foot |
| Superficial | Toward the surface of the body |
| Deep | Away from the surface of the body (internal) |

It is time to review body cavity, spine, and directional terms by completing Learning Activity 4–3.

## Medical Word Elements

This section introduces combining forms, suffixes, and prefixes related to body structure. Word analyses are also provided.

| Element | Meaning | Word Analysis |
|---------|---------|---------------|
| **COMBINING FORMS** | | |
| **Cellular Structure** | | |
| **cyt/o** | cell | cyt/o/logist (sī-TŎL-ō-jĭst): specialist in the study of the formation, structure, and function of cells<br><br>-*logist:* specialist in the study of |

*(Continued)*

| Element | Meaning | Word Analysis | *(Continued)* |
|---|---|---|---|
| **hist/o** | tissue | hist/o/logy (hĭs-TŎL-ō-jē): study of the microscopic structures of tissues<br>*-logy:* study of | |
| **nucle/o** | nucleus | nucle/ar (NŪ-klē-ăr): pertaining to the nucleus<br>*-ar:* pertaining to, relating to | |
| **kary/o** | | kary/o/lysis (kăr-ē-ŎL-ĭ-sĭs): destruction of the nucleus resulting in cell death<br>*-lysis:* separation; destruction; loosening | |

**Position and Direction**

| Element | Meaning | Word Analysis | |
|---|---|---|---|
| **anter/o** | anterior, front | anter/ior (ăn-TĬR-ē-or): pertaining to the front of the body, organ, or structure<br>*-ior:* pertaining to, relating to | |
| **caud/o** | tail | caud/ad (KAW-dăd): toward the tail; in a posterior direction<br>*-ad:* toward | |
| **crani/o** | cranium (skull) | crani/al (KRĀ-nē-ăl): pertaining to the cranium<br>*-al:* pertaining to, relating to | |
| **dist/o** | far, farthest | dist/al (DĬS-tăl): pertaining to a point further from the center (trunk of the body) or from the point of attachment to the body<br>*-al:* pertaining to, relating to | |
| **dors/o** | back (of body) | dors/al (DOR-săl): pertaining to the back of the body<br>*-al:* pertaining to, relating to | |
| **infer/o** | lower, below | infer/ior (ĭn-FĒ-rē-or): pertaining to the undersurface of a structure; underneath; beneath<br>*-ior:* pertaining to, relating to | |
| **later/o** | side | later/al (LĂT-ĕr-ăl): pertaining to a side<br>*-al:* pertaining to, relating to | |
| **medi/o** | middle | medi/ad (MĒ-dē-ăd): toward the middle or center<br>*-ad:* toward | |
| **poster/o** | back (of body), behind, posterior | poster/ior (pŏs-TĒ-rē-or): pertaining to the back of the body<br>*-ior:* pertaining to, relating to | |

| Element | Meaning | Word Analysis |
|---|---|---|
| **proxim/o** | near, nearest | proxim/al (PRŎK-sĭm-ăl): nearer to the center (trunk of the body) or to the point of attachment to the body<br>*-al:* pertaining to, relating to |
| **ventr/o** | belly, belly side | ventr/al (VĔN-trăl): pertaining to the belly side or front of the body<br>*-al:* pertaining to, relating to |

## Regions of the Body

| Element | Meaning | Word Analysis |
|---|---|---|
| **abdomin/o** | abdomen | abdomin/al (ăb-DŎM-ĭ-năl): pertaining to the abdomen<br>*-al:* pertaining to, relating to |
| **cervic/o** | neck; cervix uteri (neck of uterus) | cervic/al (SĔR-vĭ-kăl): pertaining to the neck<br>*-al:* pertaining to, relating to |
| **crani/o** | cranium (skull) | crani/al (KRĀ-nē-ăl): pertaining to the cranium<br>*-al:* pertaining to, relating to |
| **gastr/o** | stomach | hypo/gastr/ic (hī-pō-GĂS-trĭk): pertaining to beneath or below the stomach<br>*hypo-:* under, below<br>*-ic:* pertaining to, relating to |
| **ili/o** | ilium (lateral, flaring portion of hip bone) | ili/al (ĬL-ē-ăl): pertaining to the ilium<br>*-al:* pertaining to, relating to |
| **inguin/o** | groin | inguin/al (ĬNG-gwĭ-năl): pertaining to the groin, the depression located between the thigh and trunk<br>*-al:* pertaining to, relating to |
| **lumb/o** | loins, lower back | lumb/ar (LŬM-băr): pertaining to the loins, the lower back<br>*-ar:* pertaining to, relating to |
| **umbilic/o** | navel | umbilic/al (ŭm-BĬL-ĭ-kăl): pertaining to the navel region<br>*-al:* pertaining to, relating to |
| **pelv/i**<br><br>**pelv/o** | pelvis | pelv/i/meter* (pĕl-VĬM-ĕ-tĕr): instrument for measuring the pelvis<br>*-meter:* instrument for measuring<br>pelv/ic (PĔL-vĭk): pertaining to the pelvis<br>*-ic:* pertaining to, relating to |

*(Continued)*

| Element | Meaning | Word Analysis | (Continued) |
|---|---|---|---|
| **spin/o** | spine | spin/al (SPĪ-năl): pertaining to the spine<br><br>*-al:* pertaining to, relating to | |
| **thorac/o** | chest | thorac/ic (thō-RĂS-ĭk): pertaining to the chest<br><br>*-ic:* pertaining to, relating to | |
| **Color** | | | |
| **albin/o** | white | albin/ism (ĂL-bĭn-ĭzm): partial or total lack of pigment in skin, hair, and eyes<br><br>*-ism:* condition | |
| **leuk/o** | | leuk/o/cyte (LOO-kō-sīt): white blood cell<br><br>*-cyte:* cell | |
| **chlor/o** | green | chlor/opia (klō-RŌ-pē-ă): disorder in which viewed objects appear green<br><br>*-opia:* vision<br><br>*Chloropia is associated with a toxic reaction to digitalis.* | |
| **chrom/o** | color | hetero/chrom/ic (hĕt-ĕr-ō-KRŌ-mĭk): having different colors, especially of the iris or sections of the iris of both eyes<br><br>*hetero-:* different<br>*-ic:* pertaining to, relating to | |
| **cirrh/o** | yellow | cirrh/osis (sĭr-RŌ-sĭs): abnormal yellowing, especially of the skin and mucous membranes<br><br>*-osis:* abnormal condition; increase (used primarily with blood cells)<br><br>*Cirrhosis of the liver is usually associated with alcoholism or chronic hepatitis.* | |
| **jaund/o** | | jaund/ice (JAWN-dĭs): yellow discoloration of the skin, mucous membrane, and sclera of the eye<br><br>*-ice:* noun ending<br><br>*Jaundice is caused by an abnormal increase of bilirubin (a yellow compound formed when red blood cells are destroyed) in the blood.* | |
| **xanth/o** | | xanth/o/cyte (ZĂN-thō-sīt): cell containing yellow pigment<br><br>*-cyte:* cell | |
| **cyan/o** | blue | cyan/o/tic (sī-ăn-ŎT-ĭk): pertaining to blueness, especially of the skin and mucous membranes<br><br>*-tic:* pertaining to, relating to | |
| **erythr/o** | red | erythr/o/cyte (ĕ-RĬTH-rō-sīt): red blood cell<br><br>*-cyte:* cell | |

| Element | Meaning | Word Analysis |
|---------|---------|---------------|
| **melan/o** | black | melan/oma (měl-ă-NŌ-mă): malignant tumor of melanocytes<br><br>*-oma:* tumor<br><br>*Melanocytes are found in the lower epidermis and are responsible for skin pigmentation.* |
| **poli/o** | gray; gray matter (of brain or spinal cord) | polio/myel/itis (pōl-ē-ō-mī-ĕl-Ī-tǐs): inflammation of the gray matter of the spinal cord<br><br>*myel:* bone marrow; spinal cord<br>*-itis:* inflammation |
| **Other** | | |
| **acr/o** | extremity | acro/o/cyan/osis (ăk-rō-sī-ă-NŌ-sǐs): pertaining to blueness of the extremities<br><br>*cyan:* blue<br>*-osis:* abnormal condition; increase (used primarily with blood cells) |
| **eti/o** | cause | eti/o/logy (ē-tē-ŎL-ō-jē): study of the causes of disease<br><br>*-logy:* study of |
| **fasci/o** | band, fascia (fibrous membrane supporting and separating muscles) | fasci/itis (făs-ē-Ī-tǐs): inflammation of any fascia, the fibrous membrane that supports and separates muscles<br><br>*-itis:* inflammation |
| **idi/o** | unknown, peculiar | idi/o/path/ic (ĭd-ē-ō-PĂTH-ĭk): pertaining to conditions without clear pathogenesis, or disease without recognizable cause, as of spontaneous origin<br><br>*path:* disease<br>*-ic:* pertaining to, relating to |
| **morph/o** | form, shape, structure | morph/o/logy (mor-FŎL-ō-jē): study of form, shape, and structure, especially of cells<br><br>*-logy:* study of |
| **path/o** | disease | path/o/logist (pă-THŎL-ō-jǐst): physician specializing in examining tissues, cells, and body fluids for evidence of disease<br><br>*-logist:* specialist in the study of |
| **radi/o** | radiation, x-ray; radius (lower arm bone on thumb side) | radi/o/logist (rā-dē-ŎL-ŏ-jǐst): physician specializing in imaging techniques for diagnosis and treatment of disease<br><br>*-logist:* specialist in the study of |

*(Continued)*

| Element | Meaning | Word Analysis | (Continued) |
|---------|---------|---------------|-------------|
| **somat/o** | body | somat/ic (sō-MĂT-ĭk): pertaining to the body<br>*-ic:* pertaining to, relating to | |
| **son/o** | sound | son/o/graphy (sō-NŎG-ră-fē): process of recording an image or photograph of an organ or tissue using ultrasound (inaudible sound); also called *ultrasonography*<br>*-graphy:* process of recording<br>*Sonography is a noninvasive imaging technique that does not use x-rays and is painless.* | |
| **viscer/o** | internal organs | viscer/al (VĬS-ĕr-ăl): pertaining to the viscera, or internal organs, in the abdominal cavity<br>*-al:* pertaining to, relating to | |
| **xer/o** | dry | xer/osis (zē-RŌ-sĭs): abnormal dryness of the skin, mucous membranes, or conjunctiva<br>*-osis:* abnormal condition; increase (used primarily with blood cells) | |

**SUFFIXES**

| Element | Meaning | Word Analysis | |
|---------|---------|---------------|-|
| **-logy** | study of | hemat/o/logy (hē-mă-TŎL-ō-jē): study of blood and its components<br>*hemat/o:* blood | |
| **-logist** | specialist in the study of | dermat/o/logist (dĕr-mă-TŎL-ō-jĭst): physician specializing in disorders of the skin<br>*dermat/o:* skin | |
| **-genesis** | forming, producing, origin | path/o/genesis (păth-ō-JĔN-ĕ-sĭs): source or cause of an illness or abnormal condition<br>*path/o:* disease | |
| **-gnosis** | knowing | pro/gnosis (prŏg-NŌ-sĭs): prediction of the course and end of a disease, and the estimated chance of recovery<br>*pro-:* before, in front of | |
| **-gram** | record, writing | arteri/o/gram (ăr-TĒ-rē-ō-grăm): record of an artery after injection of a radiopaque contrast medium<br>*arteri/o:* artery | |
| **-graph** | instrument for recording | radi/o/graph (RĀ-dē-ō-grăf): film on which an image is produced through exposure to x-rays<br>*radi/o:* radiation, x-rays; radius (lower arm bone on thumb side) | |

| Element | Meaning | Word Analysis |
|---------|---------|---------------|
| **-graphy** | process of recording | arthr/o/graphy (ăr-THRŎG-ră-fē): process of obtaining an image of a joint after injection of a radiopaque contrast medium<br><br>*arthr/o:* joint |
| **-meter** | instrument for measuring | therm/o/meter (thĕr-MŎM-ĕ-tĕr): instrument used for measuring heat<br><br>*therm/o:* heat |
| **-metry** | act of measuring | ventricul/o/metry (vĕn-trĭk-ū-LŎM-ĕ-trē): measurement of the intraventricular cerebral pressure<br><br>*ventricul/o:* ventricle (of heart or brain) |
| **-pathy** | disease | gastr/o/pathy (găs-TRŎP-ă-thē): any disease of the stomach<br><br>*gastr/o:* stomach |

PREFIXES

| Element | Meaning | Word Analysis |
|---------|---------|---------------|
| **ab-** | from, away from | ab/duction (ăb-DŬK-shŭn): movement of a limb away from the body<br><br>*-duction:* act of leading, bringing, conducting |
| **ad-** | toward | ad/duction (ă-DŬK-shŭn): movement of a limb toward the axis of the body<br><br>*-duction:* act of leading, bringing, conducting |
| **infra-** | below, under | infra/cost/al (ĭn-fră-KŎS-tăl): pertaining to the area below the ribs<br><br>*cost:* ribs<br>*-al:* pertaining to, relating to |
| **hetero-** | different | hetero/morph/ous (hĕt-ĕr-ō-MOR-fŭs): deviating from a normal type or shape<br><br>*morph:* form, shape, structure<br>*-ous:* pertaining to, relating to |
| **homeo-** | same, alike | homeo/stasis (hō-mē-ō-STĀ-sĭs): relative equilibrium in the internal environment of the body<br><br>*-stasis:* standing still |
| **peri-** | around | peri/cardi/al (pĕr-ĭ-KĂR-dē-ăl): pertaining to the area around the heart<br><br>*cardi:* heart<br>*-al:* pertaining to, relating to |

*(Continued)*

| Element | Meaning | Word Analysis | (Continued) |
|---------|---------|---------------|-------------|
| **super-** | upper, above | super/ior (soo-PĒ-rē-or): pertaining to the head or upper portion of a structure<br><br>*-ior:* pertaining to, relating to | |
| **trans-** | across, through | trans/abdomin/al (trăns-ăb-DŎM-ĭ-năl): across the abdomen<br><br>*abdomin:* abdomen<br>*-al:* pertaining to, relating to | |
| **ultra-** | excess, beyond | ultra/son/ic (ŭl-tră-SŎN-ĭk): pertaining to sound frequencies too high to be perceived by the human ear<br><br>*son:* sound<br>*-ic:* pertaining to, relating to | |

*The *i* in *pelv/i/meter* is an exception to the rule of using the connecting vowel *o*.

**It is time to review medical word elements by completing Learning Activity 4–4.**

## Pathology

All body cells require oxygen and nutrients for survival. They also need a stable internal environment that provides a narrow range of temperature, water, acidity, and salt concentration. This stable internal environment is called *homeostasis*. When homeostasis is significantly interrupted and cells, tissues, organs, or systems are unable to meet the challenges of everyday life, the condition is called *disease*. From a clinical point of view, disease is a *pathological* or *morbid* condition that presents a group of signs, symptoms, and clinical findings. *Signs* are objective indicators that are observable by others. A palpable mass and tissue redness are examples of signs. A *symptom* is subjective and is experienced only by the patient. Dizziness, pain, and malaise are examples of symptoms. Clinical findings are results of diagnostic and other tests performed on the patient.

*Etiology* is the study of the cause or origin of a disease or disorder. Here are some possible causes of disease with examples:

- metabolic (diabetes)
- infectious (measles, mumps)
- congenital (cleft lip)
- hereditary (hemophilia)
- environmental (burns, trauma)
- neoplastic (cancer).

Establishing the cause and nature of a disease is referred to as **diagnosis.** Determining a diagnosis helps in the selection of a treatment. A **prognosis** is the prediction of the course of a disease and its probable outcome. Any disease whose cause is unknown is said to be **idiopathic.** A variety of diagnostic procedures are used to identify a specific disease and determine its extent or involvement. Diagnostic tests can be uncomplicated, such as listening to chest sounds with a stethoscope, or complex, such as a biopsy. Many of the diagnostic tests listed in this text can be categorized as surgical, clinical, endoscopic, laboratory, and radiologic. Some of these tests include more than one testing modality.

 ## Diagnostic, Symptomatic, and Related Terms

This section introduces diagnostic, symptomatic, and related terms and their meanings. Word analyses for selected terms are also provided.

| Term | Definition |
| --- | --- |
| **adhesion** <br> ăd-HĒ-zhŭn | Abnormal fibrous band that holds normally separated tissues together, usually occurring within a body cavity |
| **analyte** <br> ĂN-ă-lit | Substance being analyzed or tested, generally by means of a chemical |
| **contrast medium** <br> KŎN-trăst MĒD-ē-ŭm | In radiology, a substance that is injected into the body, introduced via catheter, or swallowed to facilitate radiographic imaging of internal structures that otherwise are difficult to visualize on x-ray films |
| **dehiscence** <br> dē-HĬS-ĕns | Bursting open of a wound, especially a surgical abdominal wound |
| **febrile** <br> FĒ-brĭl | Feverish; pertaining to a fever |
| **homeostasis** <br> hō-mē-ō-STĀ-sĭs <br><br> *homeo-:* same, alike <br> *-stasis:* standing still | Relative constancy or equilibrium in the internal environment of the body, which is maintained by the ever-changing processes of feedback and regulation in response to external or internal changes <br><br> *In homeostasis, such properties as temperature, acidity, and the concentrations of nutrients and wastes remain constant.* |
| **inflammation** <br> ĭn-flă-MĀ-shŭn | Body defense against injury, infection, or allergy marked by redness, swelling, heat, pain and, sometimes, loss of function <br><br> *Inflammation is one mechanism used by the body to protect against invasion by foreign organisms and to repair injured tissue.* |

*(Continued)*

| Term | Definition | (Continued) |
|------|-----------|-------------|
| **morbid**<br>MOR-bĭd | Diseased; pertaining to a disease | |
| **nuclear medicine**<br>NŪ-klē-ăr | Branch of medicine concerned with the use of radioactive substances for diagnosis, treatment, and research | |
| **radiology**<br>rā-dē-ŎL-ō-jē<br><br>   *radi/o:* radiation, x-ray; radius (lower arm bone on thumb side)<br>   *-logy:* study of | Medical discipline concerned with the use of electromagnetic radiation, ultrasound, and imaging techniques for diagnosis and treatment of disease and injury (See Figure 4–4.) | |
|   **diagnostic**<br>  di-ăg-NŎS-tĭk<br><br>    *dia-:* through, across<br>    *gnos:* knowing<br>    *-tic:* pertaining to, relating to | Medical imaging using external sources of radiation to evaluate body structures and functions of organs | |
|   **interventional**<br>  ĭn-tĕr-VĔN-shŭn-ăl | Use of imaging techniques in the nonsurgical treatment of various disorders, such as balloon angioplasty and cardiac catheterization | |
|   **therapeutic**<br>  thĕr-ă-PŪ-tĭk<br><br>    *therapeut:* treatment<br>    *-ic:* pertaining to, relating to | Use of ionizing radiation in the treatment of malignant tumors; also called *radiation oncology* | |
| **radionuclides**<br>rā-dē-ō-NŪ-klid | Substances that emit radiation spontaneously; also called *tracers*<br>*The quantity and duration of radioactive material used in these tests are safe for humans and should not have harmful effect.* | |
| **radiopharmaceutical**<br>rā-dē-ō-fărm-ă-SŪ-tĭ-kăl | Radionuclide attached to a protein, sugar, or other substance that travels to the organ or area of the body that will be scanned | |
| **scan**<br>SKĂN | Term used to describe a computerized image by modality (such as computed tomography, magnetic resonance, and nuclear) or by structure (such as thyroid and bone) | |
| **sepsis**<br>SĔP-sĭs | Pathological state, usually febrile, resulting from the presence of microorganisms or their products in the bloodstream | |
| **suppurative**<br>SŬP-ū-rā-tĭv | Producing or associated with generation of pus | |

(A)  Radiographic film.

(B)  Ultrasonography.

(C)  Nuclear scan.

(D)  CT scan.

(E)  MRI scan.

(F)  PET scan of brain.

**Figure 4–4**   Medical imaging.

 **Diagnostic and Therapeutic Procedures**

This section introduces procedures used to diagnose and treat a variety of disorders. Specific examples of these procedures are found in the body systems chapters. Descriptions are provided as well as pronunciations and word analyses for selected terms.

| Procedure | Description |
| --- | --- |
| **DIAGNOSTIC PROCEDURES** | |
| Endoscopic | |
| **endoscopy**<br>ĕn-DŎS-kō-pē<br><br>  *endo-:* in, within<br>  *-scopy:* visual examination | Visual examination of a cavity or canal using a specialized lighted instrument called an *endoscope*<br><br>*Endoscopy is used for biopsy, surgery, aspirating fluids, and coagulating bleeding areas. The organ, cavity, or canal being examined dictates the name of the endoscopic procedure. (See Figure 4–5.) A camera and video recorder are commonly used during the procedure to provide a permanent record.* |

*(Continued)*

| Procedure | Description | (Continued) |
|---|---|---|
| **laparoscopy**<br>lăp-ăr-ŎS-kō-pē<br><br>*lapar/o:* abdomen<br>*-scopy:* visual examination | Visual examination of the organs of the pelvis and abdomen through very small incisions in the abdominal wall | |
| **thoracoscopy**<br>thor-ă-KŎS-kŏ-pē<br><br>*thorac/o:* chest<br>*-scopy:* visual examination | Examination of the lungs, pleura, and pleural space with a scope inserted through a small incision between the ribs<br><br>*Thoracoscopy is an endoscopic procedure usually performed for lung biopsy, repairing perforations in the lungs, and diagnosing pleural disease.* | |

### Laboratory

| | | |
|---|---|---|
| **complete blood count** | Common blood test that enumerates red blood cells, white blood cells, and platelets; measures hemoglobin (the oxygen-carrying molecule in red blood cells); estimates red cell volume; and sorts white blood cells into five subtypes with their percentages | |
| **urinalysis**<br>ū-rĭ-NĂL-ĭ-sĭs | Common urine test that evaluates the physical, chemical, and microscopic properties of urine | |

**Figure 4–5**  Endoscopy (gastroscopy).

| Procedure | Description |
|---|---|
| **Radiographic** | |
| **computed tomography (CT) scan**<br>kŏm-PŪ-tĕd tō-MŎG-ră-fē<br><br>*tom/o:* to cut<br>*-graphy:* process of recording | Imaging technique achieved by rotating an x-ray emitter around the area to be scanned and measuring the intensity of transmitted rays from different angles; formerly called *computerized axial tomography*<br><br>*In a CT scan, the computer generates a detailed cross-sectional image that appears as a slice. (See Figure 4–4D.) Tumor masses, bone displacement, and accumulations of fluid may be detected. During a period of two held breaths, as many as 50 continuous tomographic images can be produced in a single-slice mode. This technique may be used with or without a contrast medium.* |
| **Doppler**<br>DŎP-lĕr | Ultrasound technique used to detect and measure blood-flow velocity and direction through the cardiac chambers, valves, and peripheral vessels by reflecting sound waves off of moving blood cells<br><br>*Doppler is used to identify irregularities in blood flow through the heart and its valves as well as peripheral vascular problems, such as blood clots, venous insufficiency, and arterial blockage.* |
| **fluoroscopy**<br>floo-or-ŎS-kō-pē<br><br>*fluor/o:* luminous, fluorescent<br>*-scopy:* visual examination | Radiographic technique in which x-rays are directed through the body to a fluorescent screen that displays continuous imaging of the motion of internal structures and immediate serial images<br><br>*Fluoroscopy is used to view the motion of organs, such as the digestive tract and heart, and joints or for intervascular placement of catheters or other devices.* |
| **magnetic resonance imaging (MRI)**<br>măg-NĔT-ĭc RĔZ-ĕn-ăns ĬM-ĭj-ĭng | Noninvasive imaging technique that uses radio waves and a strong magnetic field rather than an x-ray beam to produce multiplanar cross-sectional images (See Figure 4–4E.)<br><br>*MRI is the method of choice for diagnosing a growing number of diseases because it provides superior soft tissue contrast, allows multiple plane views, and avoids the hazards of ionizing radiation. MRI commonly proves superior to CT scan for most central nervous system images, particularly those of the brainstem and spinal cord as well as the musculoskeletal and pelvic area. The procedure usually does not require a contrast medium.* |
| **nuclear scan**<br>NŪ-klē-ăr | Diagnostic technique that uses a radioactive material (radiopharmaceutical) introduced into the body (inhaled, ingested, or injected) and a scanning device to determine size, shape, location, and function of various organs and structures (See Figure 4–4C.)<br><br>*A nuclear scan is the reverse of a conventional radiograph. Rather than being directed into the body, radiation comes from inside the body and is then detected by the scanning device to produce an image.* |

*(Continued)*

| Procedure | Description | (Continued) |
|---|---|---|
| **positron emission tomography (PET)**<br>PŎZ-ĭ-trŏn  ē-MĬSH-ŭn tō-MŎG-ră-fē | Scan using computed tomography to record the positrons (positive charged particles) emitted from a radiopharmaceutical, producing a cross-sectional image of metabolic activity in body tissues to determine the presence of disease (See Figure 4–4F.)<br>*PET is especially useful in scanning the brain and nervous system to diagnose disorders that involve abnormal tissue metabolism, such as schizophrenia, brain tumors, epilepsy, stroke, and Alzheimer disease as well as cardiac and pulmonary disorders.* | |
| **radiography**<br>rā-dē-ŎG-ră-fē<br><br>*radi/o:* radiation, x-ray, radius (lower arm bone on thumb side)<br>*-graphy:* process of recording | Image produced when an x-ray is passed through the body or area and captured on a film; also called *x-ray* (See Figure 4–4A.)<br>*On the radiograph, dense material, such as bone, appears white, and softer material, such as the stomach and liver, appears in shades of gray.* | |
| **single photon emission computed tomography (SPECT)**<br>SĬNG-gŭl  FŌ-tŏn ē-MĬ-shŭn tō-MŎG-ră-fē | Noninvasive imaging technique that provides clear, three-dimensional pictures of a major organ by injecting a radionuclide and detecting the emitted radiation using a special device called a gamma camera<br>*A healthy organ absorbs the radionuclide at a specific rate. Overabsorption (hot spot) or underabsorption (cold spot) may be an indication of pathology.* | |
| **tomography**<br>tō-MŎG-ră-fē<br><br>*tom/o:* to cut<br>*-graphy:* process of recording | Radiographic technique that produces an image representing a detailed cross-section or "slice" of an area, tissue, or organ at a predetermined depth<br>*Types of tomography include computed tomography (CT), positron emission tomography (PET), and single photon emission computed tomography (SPECT).* | |
| **ultrasonography (US)**<br>ŭl-tră-sŏn-ŎG-ră-fē<br><br>*ultra-:* excess, beyond<br>*son/o:* sound<br>*-graphy:* process of recording | Image produced by high-frequency sound waves (ultrasound) and displaying the reflected "echoes" on a monitor; also called *ultrasound, sonography, echo,* and *echogram* (See Figure 4–4B.)<br>*Ultrasound, unlike most other imaging methods, can create real-time moving images to view organs and functions of organs in motion. A computer analyzes the reflected echos and converts them into an image on a video monitor. Because this procedure does not use ionizing radiation (x-ray) it is used for visualizing fetuses as well as the neck, abdomen, pelvis, brain, and heart.* | |

| Procedure | Description |
|---|---|
| **Surgical** | |
| **biopsy**<br>BĪ-ŏp-sē | Representative tissue sample removed from a body site for microscopic examination, usually to establish a diagnosis |
| **needle** | Removal of a small tissue sample for examination using a hollow needle, usually attached to a syringe |
| **punch** | Removal of a small core of tissue using a hollow instrument (punch)<br>*An anesthetic and suturing are usually required for a punch biopsy, and minimal scarring is expected.* |
| **shave** | Removal of tissue using a surgical blade to shave elevated lesions |
| **frozen section** | Ultra-thin slice of tissue cut from a frozen specimen for immediate pathological examination<br>*Frozen section is used for rapid diagnosis of malignancy, while the patient awaits surgery.* |

## THERAPEUTIC PROCEDURES

| | |
|---|---|
| **Surgical** | |
| **ablation**<br>ăb-LĀ-shŭn | Removal of a part, pathway, or function by surgery, chemical destruction, electrocautery, freezing, or radiofrequency (RF) |
| **anastomosis**<br>ă-năs-tō-MŌ-sĭs | Surgical joining of two ducts, vessels, or bowel segments to allow flow from one to another (See Figure 4–6.) |

*(Continued)*

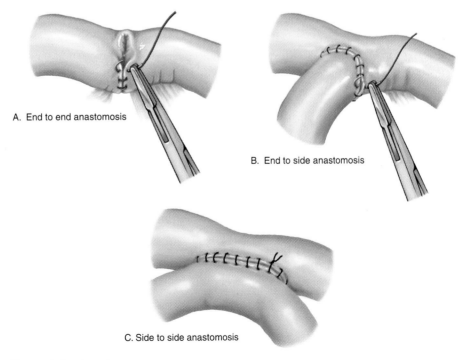

A. End to end anastomosis

B. End to side anastomosis

C. Side to side anastomosis

**Figure 4–6**    Anastomoses.

| Procedure | Description | (Continued) |
|---|---|---|
| **cauterize** KAW-tĕr-īz | Destroy tissue by electricity, freezing, heat, or corrosive chemicals | |
| **curettage** kū-rĕ-TAZH | Scraping of a body cavity with a spoon-shaped instrument called a *curette* (curet) | |
| **incision and drainage (I&D)** ĭn-SĬZH-ŭn, DRĀN-ĭj | Incision made to allow the free flow or withdrawal of fluids from a wound or cavity | |
| **laser surgery** LĀ-zĕr SŬR-jĕr-ē | Surgical technique employing a device that emits intense heat and power at close range to cut, burn, vaporize, or destroy tissues | |
| **radical dissection** RĂD-ĭ-kăl dī-SĔK-shŭn | Surgical removal of tissue in an extensive area surrounding the surgical site in an attempt to excise all tissue that may be malignant to decrease the chance of recurrence (such as radical mastectomy) | |
| **resection** rē-SĔK-shŭn | Partial excision of a bone, organ, or other structure | |

**It is time to review diagnostic and therapeutic terms and procedures by completing Learning Activity 4–5.**

# Abbreviations

This section introduces body structure abbreviations and their meanings.

| Abbreviation | Meaning |
|---|---|
| **ant** | anterior |
| **AP** | anteroposterior |
| **Bx, bx** | biopsy |
| **CT** | computed tomography |
| **CT scan, CAT scan** | computed (axial) tomography scan |

| Abbreviation | Meaning |
|---|---|
| DSA | digital subtraction angiography |
| Dx | diagnosis |
| LAT, lat | lateral |
| LLQ | left lower quadrant |
| LUQ | left upper quadrant |
| MRI | magnetic resonance imaging |
| PA | posteroanterior; pernicious anemia |
| PET | positron emission tomography |
| post | posterior |
| RLQ | right lower quadrant |
| RUQ | right upper quadrant |
| sono | sonogram |
| SPECT | single photon emission computed tomography |
| Sx | symptom |
| Tx | treatment |
| U&L, U/L | upper and lower |
| US | ultrasound |

# LEARNING ACTIVITIES

The following activities provide review of the body structure terms introduced in this chapter. Complete each activity and review your answers to evaluate your understanding of the chapter.

## Learning Activity 4–1

### Identifying body planes

*Label the following illustration using the terms below.*

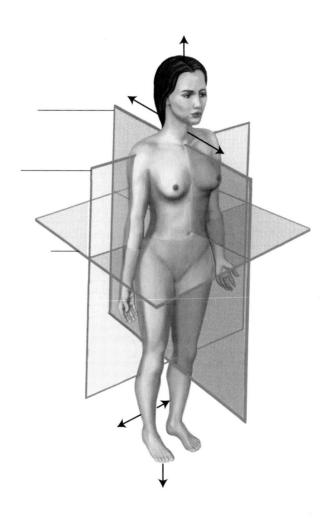

| | | |
|---|---|---|
| *anterior* | *lateral* | *posterior* |
| *coronal (frontal) plane* | *medial* | *superior* |
| *inferior* | *midsagittal (median) plane* | *transverse (horizontal) plane* |

 Check your answers by referring to Figure 4–1 on page 43. Review material that you did not answer correctly.

## Learning Activity 4-2

### Identifying abdominopelvic divisions

*Label the quadrants on Figure A and regions on Figure B using the terms below.*

A.

B.

| | | |
|---|---|---|
| epigastric region | left lumbar region | right lower quadrant |
| hypogastric region | left upper quadrant | right lumbar region |
| left hypochondriac region | right hypochondriac region | right upper quadrant |
| left iliac region | right iliac region | umbilical region |
| left lower quadrant | | |

Check your answers by referring to Figure 4-3A and 4-3B on page 46. Review material that you did not answer correctly.

Learning Activity 4–3

## Matching body cavity, spine, and directional terms

*Match each term on the left with its meaning on the right.*

1. _____ abdominopelvic
2. _____ adduction
3. _____ cervical

4. _____ coccyx
5. _____ deep
6. _____ eversion
7. _____ inferior (caudal)
8. _____ inversion

9. _____ lumbar
10. _____ plantar
11. _____ posterior (dorsal)
12. _____ prone

13. _____ proximal
14. _____ superficial
15. _____ thoracic

a. pertaining to the sole of the foot
b. tailbone
c. ventral cavity that contains heart, lungs, and associated structures
d. toward the surface of the body
e. lying horizontal with face downward
f. turning outward
g. nearer to the center (trunk of the body)
h. ventral cavity that contains digestive, reproductive, and excretory structures
i. turning inward or inside out
j. part of the spine known as the neck
k. movement toward the median plane
l. away from the head; toward the tail or lower part of a structure
m. away from the surface of the body; internal
n. part of the spine known as the loin
o. near the back of the body

 Check your answers in Appendix A. Review any material that you did not answer correctly.

**CORRECT ANSWERS** _____ × 6.67 = _____ **% SCORE**

Learning Activity 4–4

## Matching word elements

*Match the following word elements with the definitions in the numbered list.*

| **Combining Forms** | | **Suffixes** | **Prefixes** |
|---|---|---|---|
| *caud/o* | *dist/o* | *-genesis* | *ad-* |
| *dors/o* | *eti/o* | *-gnosis* | *infra-* |
| *hist/o* | *idi/o* | *-graphy* | *ultra-* |
| *jaund/o* | *kary/o* | | |
| *leuk/o* | *morph/o* | | |
| *poli/o* | *somat/o* | | |
| *viscer/o* | *xer/o* | | |

1. _____ nucleus
2. _____ far, farthest
3. _____ process of recording
4. _____ knowing
5. _____ white
6. _____ internal organs
7. _____ yellow
8. _____ tissue
9. _____ forming, producing, origin
10. _____ below, under
11. _____ excess, beyond
12. _____ tail
13. _____ back (of body)
14. _____ gray
15. _____ cause
16. _____ form, shape, structure
17. _____ dry
18. _____ unknown, peculiar
19. _____ toward
20. _____ body

✓ Check your answers in Appendix A. Review any material that you did not answer correctly.

**CORRECT ANSWERS** _____ × 5 = _____ **% SCORE**

## Learning Activity 4–5

## Matching diagnostic and therapeutic terms and procedures

*Match the following terms with the definitions in the numbered list.*

| | | |
|---|---|---|
| *ablation* | *fluoroscopy* | *radionuclide* |
| *cauterize* | *morbid* | *resection* |
| *Doppler* | *nuclear scan* | *suppurative* |
| *endoscopy* | *punch biopsy* | *thoracoscopy* |
| *febrile* | *radiology* | *ultrasonography* |

1. _____ medical specialty concerned with the use of electromagnetic radiation, ultrasound, and imaging techniques

2. _____ measurement of blood flow in a vessel by reflecting sound waves off moving blood cells

3. _____ image produced by using high-frequency sound waves and displaying the reflected "echoes" on a monitor

4. _____ visual examination of the lungs, pleura, and pleural space with a scope inserted through a small incision between the ribs

5. _____ excision of a core sample of tissue for examination

6. _____ visual examination of a cavity or canal using a special lighted instrument

7. _____ use of a radioactive material and scanning device to determine, size, shape, location, and function of various organs and structures

8. _____ radiographic technique that directs x-rays to a fluorescent screen and displays "live" images on a monitor

9. _____ disease, or pertaining to disease

10. _____ substance that emits radiation spontaneously; also called *tracer*

11. _____ feverish; pertaining to a fever

12. _____ partial excision of a bone, organ, or other structure

13. _____ producing or associated with generation of pus

14. _____ destruction of tissue by electricity, freezing, heat, or corrosive chemicals

15. _____ removal of a part, pathway, or function by surgery, chemical destruction, electrocautery, freezing, or radiofrequency (RF)

✓ Check your answers in Appendix A. Review any material that you did not answer correctly.

**CORRECT ANSWERS** _____ × **6.67 =** _____ **% SCORE**

# MEDICAL RECORD ACTIVITIES

The two medical records included in the following activities use common clinical scenarios to show how medical terminology is used to document patient care. Complete the terminology and analysis sections for each activity to help you recognize and understand terms related to body structure.

## Medical Record Activity 4–1

### Radiologic consultation: Cervical and lumbar spine

#### Terminology

The terms listed in the chart come from the medical record *Radiologic Consultation: Cervical and Lumbar Spine* that follows. Use a medical dictionary such as *Taber's Cyclopedic Medical Dictionary*, the appendices of this book, or other resources to define each term. Then review the pronunciations for each term and practice by reading the medical record aloud.

| Term | Definition |
|------|------------|
| **AP** | |
| **atlantoaxial**<br>ăt-lăn-tō-ĂK-sē-ăl | |
| **cervical**<br>SĔR-vĭ-kăl | |
| **lateral**<br>LĂT-ĕr-ăl | |
| **lumbar**<br>LŬM-băr | |
| **lumbosacral junction**<br>lŭm-bō-SĀ-krăl | |
| **odontoid**<br>ō-DŎN-toyd | |
| **sacral**<br>SĀ-krăl | |
| **scoliosis**<br>skō-lē-Ō-sĭs | |
| **spasm**<br>SPĂZM | |
| **spina bifida occulta**<br>SPĪ-nă  BĬF-ĭ-dă  ŏ-KŬL-tă | |
| **vertebral bodies**<br>VĔR-tĕ-brăl | |

## RADIOLOGIC CONSULTATION: CERVICAL AND LUMBAR SPINE

Thank you for referring Chester Bowen to our office. Mr. Bowen presents with neck and lower back pain of more than 2 years' duration. Radiographic evaluation of June 14, 20xx, reveals the following.

AP, lateral, and odontoid views of the cervical spine demonstrate some reversal of normal cervical curvature, as seen on lateral projection. There is some right lateral scoliosis of the cervical spine. The vertebral bodies, however, appear to be well maintained in height; the intervertebral spaces are well maintained. The odontoid is visualized and appears to be intact. The atlantoaxial joint appears symmetrical.

**IMPRESSION:** Films of the cervical spine demonstrate some reversal of normal cervical curvature and a minimal scoliosis, possibly secondary to muscle spasm, without evidence of recent bony disease or injury. AP and lateral films of the lumbar spine, with spots of the lumbosacral junction, demonstrate an apparent minimal spina bifida occulta of the first sacral segment. The vertebral bodies, however, are well maintained in height; the intervertebral spaces appear well maintained.

**PATHOLOGICAL DIAGNOSIS:** Right lateral scoliosis with some reversal of normal cervical curvature.

### Analysis

**Review the medical record *Radiologic Consultation: Cervical and Lumbar Spine* to answer the following questions.**

1. Why was the x-ray film taken of the cervical spine?

   _____

2. Did the patient appear to have experienced any type of recent injury to the spine?

   _____

3. What cervical vertebrae form the atlantoaxial joint?

   _____

4. Was the odontoid process fractured?

   _____

5. What did the radiologist believe was the possible cause of the minimal scoliosis?

   _____

## Radiographic consultation: Injury of left wrist and hand

### Terminology

The terms listed in the chart come from the medical record *Radiographic Consultation: Injury of Left Wrist and Hand* that follows. Use a medical dictionary such as *Taber's Cyclopedic Medical Dictionary*, the appendices of this book, or other resources to define each term. Then review the pronunciations for each term and practice by reading the medical record aloud.

| Term | Definition |
|---|---|
| **anterior** <br> ăn-TĬR-ē-or | |
| **AP** | |
| **distal** <br> DĬS-tăl | |
| **dorsal** <br> DOR-săl | |
| **epicondyle** <br> ĕp-ĭ-KŎN-dīl | |
| **humerus** <br> HŪ-mĕr-ŭs | |
| **lucency** <br> LOO-sĕnt-sē | |
| **medial** <br> MĒ-dē-ăl | |
| **mm** | |
| **posterior** <br> pŏs-Tē-rē-or | |
| **radius** <br> RĀ-dē-ŭs | |
| **ulna** <br> ŬL-nă | |
| **ventral-lateral** <br> VĔN-trăl LĂT-ĕr-ăl | |

## RADIOGRAPHIC CONSULTATION: INJURY OF LEFT WRIST AND HAND

**LEFT WRIST IMAGES:** Obtained with the patient's arm taped to an arm board. There are fractures through the distal shafts of the radius and ulna. The radial fracture fragments show approximately 8 mm overlap with dorsal displacement of the distal radial fracture fragment. The distal ulnar shaft fracture shows ventral-lateral angulation at the fracture apex. There is no overriding at this fracture. No additional fracture is seen. Soft tissue deformity is present, correlating with the fracture sites.

**LEFT ELBOW AND LEFT HUMERUS:** Single view of the left elbow was obtained in the lateral projection. AP view of the humerus was obtained to include a portion of the elbow. A third radiograph was obtained but is not currently available for review. There is lucency through the distal humerus on the AP view along its medial aspect. It would be difficult to exclude fracture just above the medial epicondyle. On the lateral view, there is elevation of the anterior and posterior fat pad. These findings are of some concern. Repeat elbow study is recommended.

## Analysis

**Review the medical record *Radiographic Consultation: Injury of Left Wrist and Hand* to answer the following questions.**

1. What is the abbreviation for anteroposterior?

   _____

2. What caused the soft tissue deformity?

   _____

3. Why was an AP view of the humerus taken?

   _____

4. Where are the left wrist fractures located?

   _____

5. Did the radiologist take any side views of the left elbow?

   _____

# Chapter

# 5

# Integumentary System

## OBJECTIVES

*Upon completion of this chapter, you will be able to:*

- Locate and describe the structures of the integumentary system.
- Recognize, pronounce, spell, and build words related to the integumentary system.
- Describe pathological conditions, diagnostic and therapeutic procedures, and other terms related to the integumentary system.
- Explain pharmacology related to the treatment of skin disorders.
- Demonstrate your knowledge of this chapter by completing the learning and medical record activities.

## Key Terms

This section introduces important integumentary system terms and their definitions. Word analyses are also provided.

| Term | Definition |
|------|------------|
| **adipose**<br>ĂD-ĭ-pōs<br><br>*adip:* fat<br>*-ose:* pertaining to, relating to | Fatty; pertaining to fat |
| **androgen**<br>ĂN-drō-jĕn | Generic term for an agent, usually a hormone (testosterone) that stimulates activity of the accessory male sex organs or stimulates the development of male characteristics |
| **dorsal**<br>DOR-săl<br><br>*dors:* back (of body)<br>*-al:* pertaining to; relating to | Indicating a position; pertaining to the back or posterior (of a structure) |
| **ductule**<br>DŬK-tūl<br><br>*duct:* to lead; carry<br>*-ule:* small, minute | A very small duct |
| **homeostasis**<br>hō-mē-ō-STĀ-sĭs<br><br>*homeo-:* same, alike<br>*-stasis:* standing still | Relative constancy or equilibrium in the internal environment of the body, which is maintained by the ever-changing processes of feedback and regulation in response to external or internal changes |
| **hypodermis**<br>hi-pō-DĔR-mis<br><br>*hypo-:* under, below, deficient<br>*derm:* skin<br>*-is:* noun ending | Subcutaneous tissue layer below the dermis |
| **integument**<br>ĭn-TĔG-ū-mĕnt | A covering (the skin) consisting of the epidermis and dermis, or corium |
| **systemic**<br>sĭs-TĔM-ĭk | Pertaining to the entire body rather than to one of its individual parts |

## Anatomy and Physiology

The integumentary system consists of the skin and its epidermal structures (integumentary glands, hair, and nails). The skin, also called *integument,* covers and protects all outer surfaces of the body and performs many vital functions. Its elaborate system of distinct tissues includes glands that produce several types of secretions, nerves that transmit impulses, and blood vessels that help regulate body temperature. (See Figure 5–1.)

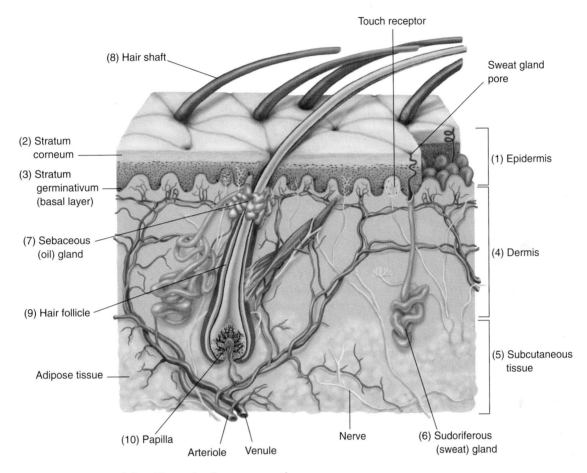

**Figure 5–1**   Structure of the skin and subcutaneous tissue.

## Skin

The skin protects underlying structures from injury and provides sensory information to the brain. Beneath the skin's surface is an intricate network of nerve fibers that register sensations of temperature, pain, and pressure. Other important functions of the skin are protecting the body against ultraviolet rays, regulating body temperature, and preventing dehydration. The skin also acts as a reservoir for food and water and is responsible for the synthesis of vitamin D when exposed to sunlight. The skin consists of two distinct layers: the epidermis and the dermis. A subcutaneous layer of tissue binds the skin to underlying structures.

### Epidermis

The outer layer, the (1) **epidermis,** is thick (comprised of five layers) on the palms of the hands and the soles of the feet but relatively thin over most other areas. Although the epidermis is composed of four or five sublayers called *strata*, the (2) **stratum corneum** and the (3) **stratum germinativum (basal layer)** are of greatest importance.

The stratum corneum is composed of dead flat cells that lack a blood supply and sensory receptors. Its thickness is correlated with normal wear of the area it covers. Only the stratum germinativum is composed of living cells and includes a basal layer where new cells are formed. As these cells move toward the stratum corneum to replace the cells that have been sloughed off, they die and become filled with a hard protein material called *keratin.* The relatively water-proof characteristic of keratin prevents body fluids from evaporating and moisture from entering the body. The entire process by which a cell forms in the basal layers, rises to the surface, becomes keratinized, and sloughs off takes about 1 month.

In the basal layer of the epidermis, specialized epithelial cells called *melanocytes* produce a dark pigment called *melanin.* Melanin filters ultraviolet radiation (light) and provides a protective barrier from the damaging effects of the sun. The number of melanocytes is about the same in all races. Differences in skin color are attributed to production of melanin. In people with dark skin, melanocytes continuously produce large amounts of melanin. In people with light skin, melanocytes produce less melanin. The activity of melanocytes is genetically regulated and, thus, inherited. Local accumulations of melanin are seen in pigmented moles and freckles. Environmental and physiological factors also play a role in skin color. An absence of pigment in the skin, eyes, and hair is most likely due to an inherited inability to produce melanin. This lack of melanin results in the condition known as *albinism.* A person with this condition is called an *albino.*

## Dermis

The second layer of the skin, the (4) **dermis** (corium), lies directly beneath the epidermis. It is composed of living tissue and contains numerous capillaries, lymphatic vessels, and nerve endings. Hair follicles, sebaceous (oil) glands, and sweat glands are also located in the dermis. The **hypodermis,** or (5) **subcutaneous tissue,** is composed primarily of loose connective tissue and adipose tissue interlaced with blood vessels. It binds the dermis to underlying structures. The hypodermis stores fats, insulates and cushions the body, and regulates temperature. The amount of fat in the hypodermis varies with the region of the body and a person's sex, age, and nutritional state.

## Accessory Organs of the Skin

The accessory organs of the skin consist of integumentary glands, hair, and nails. All of these structures are formed from the epidermis. The glands play an important role in body defense and maintaining homeostasis, whereas the hair and nails have more limited functional roles.

## Glands

Two important glands located in the dermis produce secretions: the (6) **sudoriferous glands** produce sweat, and the (7) **sebaceous glands** produce oil. These two glands are known as *exocrine glands* because they secrete substances through ducts to an outer surface of the body rather than directly into the bloodstream.

The sudoriferous glands secrete perspiration or sweat onto the surface of the skin through pores. Pores are most plentiful on the palms, soles, forehead, and armpits (axillae). The main functions of the sudoriferous glands are to cool the body by evaporation, excrete waste products, and moisten surface cells.

The sebaceous glands are filled with cells, the centers of which contain fatty droplets. As these cells disintegrate, they yield an oily secretion called **sebum.** The acidic nature of sebum helps to destroy harmful organisms on the skin thus preventing infection. When sebaceous **ductules** become blocked, acne may result. Congested sebum causes the formation of pimples or whiteheads, and if the sebum is dark, it forms blackheads. Sex hormones, particularly **andro-**

**gens,** regulate the production and secretion of sebum. During adolescence, the secretions increase; as the person ages, the secretions diminish. The loss of sebum, which lubricates the skin, may be one of the reasons for the formation of wrinkles that accompany old age. Sebaceous glands are present over the entire body, except on the soles of the feet and the palms of the hands. They are especially prevalent on the scalp and face; around openings such as the nose, mouth, external ear, and anus; and on the upper back and scrotum.

## Hair

Hair is found on nearly all parts of the body, except for the lips, nipples, palms of the hands, soles of the feet, and parts of the external genitalia. The visible part of the hair is the (8) **hair shaft;** the part that is embedded in the dermis is the **hair root.** The root, together with its coverings, forms the (9) **hair follicle.** At the bottom of the follicle is a loop of capillaries enclosed in a covering called the (10) **papilla.** The cluster of epithelial cells lying over the papilla reproduces and is responsible for the eventual formation of the hair shaft. As long as these cells remain alive, hair will regenerate even if it is cut, plucked, or otherwise removed. Baldness **(alopecia)** occurs when the hairs of the scalp are not replaced because of death of the papilla.

Like skin color, hair color is related to the amount of pigment produced by epidermal melanocytes. Melanocytes are found at the base of the hair follicle. Various amounts of melanin compounds of different colors (yellow, brown, and black) combine to produce hair color from blond to dark black. Both heredity and aging account for the loss of hair color due to the absence of melanin.

## Nails

The nails protect the tips of the fingers and toes from bruises and injuries. (See Figure 5–2.) Each nail is formed in the (1) **nail root** and is composed of keratinized stratified squamous epithelial cells producing a very tough covering. As the nail grows, it stays attached and slides forward over the layer of epithelium called the (2) **nail bed.** This epithelial layer is continuous with the epithelium of the skin. Most of the (3) **nail body** appears pink because of the underlying vascular tissue. The half-moon shaped area at the base of the nail, the (4) **lunula,** is the region where new growth occurs. The lunula has a whitish appearance because the vascular tissue underneath does not show through.

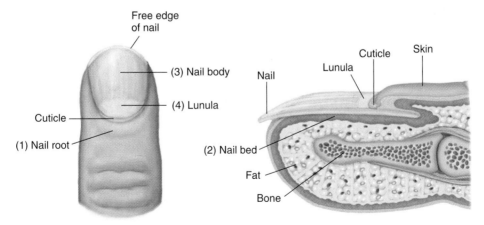

**Figure 5–2**   Structure of a fingernail.

 **It is time to review anatomy by completing Learning Activity 5–1.**

**Medical Word Elements**

This section introduces combining forms, suffixes, and prefixes related to the integumentary system. Word analyses are also provided.

| Element | Meaning | Word Analysis |
|---------|---------|---------------|
| **COMBINING FORMS** | | |
| **adip/o** | fat | adip/osis (ăd-ĭ-PŌ-sĭs): abnormal accumulation of fat in the body<br>*-osis:* abnormal condition; increase (used primarily with blood cells) |
| **lip/o** | | lip/o/cele (LĬP-ō-sēl): hernia containing fat or fatty tissue<br>*-cele:* hernia, swelling |
| **steat/o** | | steat/itis (stē-ă-TĪ-tĭs): inflammation of adipose (fatty) tissue<br>*-itis:* inflammation |
| **cutane/o** | skin | sub/cutane/ous (sŭb-kū-TĀ-nē-ŭs): beneath the skin<br>*sub-:* under, below<br>*-ous:* pertaining to, relating to |
| **dermat/o** | | dermat/o/plasty (DĔR-mă-tō-plăs-tē): plastic surgery of the skin, as in skin grafting<br>*-plasty:* surgical repair |
| **derm/o** | | hypo/derm/ic (hī-pō-DĔR-mĭk): under or inserted under the skin, as in a hypodermic injection<br>*hypo-:* under, below<br>*-ic:* pertaining to, relating to |
| **hidr/o** | sweat | hidr/aden/itis (hī-drăd-ĕ-NĪ-tĭs): inflammation of the sweat glands<br>*aden:* gland<br>*-itis:* inflammation<br>*Do not confuse hidr/o (sweat) with hydr/o (water).* |
| **sudor/o** | | sudor/esis (soo-dō-RĒ-sĭs): profuse sweating<br>*-esis:* condition |
| **ichthy/o** | dry, scaly | ichthy/osis (ĭk-thē-Ō-sĭs): any of several dermatologic conditions in which the skin is dry and hyperkeratotic (hardened), resembling fish scales<br>*-osis:* abnormal condition; increase (used primarily with blood cells)<br>*A mild form called* winter itch *is commonly seen on the legs of older patients, especially during the winter months.* |

| Element | Meaning | Word Analysis |
|---|---|---|
| **kerat/o** | horny tissue; hard; cornea | kerat/osis (kĕr-ă-TŌ-sĭs): thickened area of the epidermis; any horny growth on the skin (such as a callus or wart)<br><br>*-osis:* abnormal condition; increase (used primarily with blood cells) |
| **melan/o** | black | melan/oma (mĕl-ă-NŌ-mă): malignant tumor of melanocytes that commonly begins in a darkly pigmented mole and can metastasize widely<br><br>*-oma:* tumor |
| **myc/o** | fungus (plural, fungi) | dermat/o/myc/osis (dĕr-mă-tō-mĭ-KŌ-sĭs): fungal infection of the skin<br><br>*dermat/o:* skin<br>*-osis:* abnormal condition; increase (used primarily with blood cells) |
| **onych/o** | nail | onych/o/malacia (ŏn-ĭ-kō-mă-LĀ-shē-ă): abnormal softening of the nails<br><br>*-malacia:* softening |
| **ungu/o** | | ungu/al (ŬNG-gwăl): pertaining to the nails<br><br>*-al:* pertaining to, relating to |
| **pil/o** | hair | pil/o/nid/al (pī-lō-NĪ-dăl): a growth of hair in a cyst or other internal structure<br><br>*nid:* nest<br>*-al:* pertaining to, relating to<br><br>*A pilonidal cyst commonly develops in the skin of the sacral region.* |
| **trich/o** | | trich/o/pathy (trĭk-ŎP-ă-thē): any disease involving the hair<br><br>*-pathy:* disease |
| **scler/o** | hardening; sclera (white of eye) | scler/o/derma (sklĕr-ă-DĒR-mă): chronic hardening and thickening of the skin caused by new collagen formation<br><br>*-derma:* skin<br><br>*Scleroderma is most common in middle-aged women and may occur in a localized form or as a systemic disease.* |
| **seb/o** | sebum, sebaceous | seb/o/rrhea (sĕb-Ō-rē-ă): excessive secretion or discharge of sebum<br><br>*-rrhea:* discharge, flow<br><br>*Sebum is an oil secretion of the sebaceous glands.* |
| **squam/o** | scale | squam/ous (SKWĀ-mŭs): relating to or covered with scales<br><br>*-ous:* pertaining to, relating to |

*(Continued)*

| Element | Meaning | Word Analysis | (Continued) |
|---|---|---|---|
| **xer/o** | dry | xer/o/derma (zē-rō-DĔR-mă): chronic skin condition characterized by dryness and roughness<br>*-derma:* skin<br>*Xeroderma is a mild form of ichthyosis.* | |

**SUFFIXES**

| | | | |
|---|---|---|---|
| **-cyte** | cell | lip/o/cyte (LĬP-ō-sīt): fat cell<br>*lip/o:* fat | |
| **-derma** | skin | py/o/derma (pī-ō-DĔR-mă): any pyogenic infection of the skin<br>*py/o:* pus<br>*Pyoderma may be primary, such as impetigo, or secondary to a previous condition.* | |
| **-logist** | specialist in the study of | dermat/o/logist (dĕr-mă-TŎL-ō-jĭst): physician specializing in treatment of skin disorders<br>*dermat/o:* skin | |
| **-logy** | study of | dermat/o/logy (dĕr-mă-TŎL-ō-jē): study of the skin and its diseases<br>*dermat/o:* skin | |
| **-therapy** | treatment | cry/o/therapy (krī-ō-THĔR-ă-pē): destruction of tissue by freezing with liquid nitrogen<br>*cry/o:* cold<br>*Cutaneous warts and actinic keratosis are common skin disorders that are responsive to cryotherapy treatment.* | |

**PREFIXES**

| | | | |
|---|---|---|---|
| **an-** | without, not | an/hidr/osis (ăn-hī-DRŌ-sĭs): diminished or complete absence of sweat<br>*hidr:* sweat<br>*-osis:* abnormal condition; increase (used primarily with blood cells) | |
| **dia-** | through, across | dia/phoresis (dī-ă-fă-RĒ-sĭs): condition of profuse sweating; also called *sudoresis* or *hyperhidrosis*<br>*-phoresis:* carrying, transmission | |
| **epi-** | above, upon | epi/derm/is (ĕp-ĭ-DĔR-mĭs): outermost layer of the skin<br>*derm:* skin<br>*-is:* noun ending | |

| Element | Meaning | Word Analysis |
|---------|---------|---------------|
| **hyper-** | excessive, above normal | hyper/hidr/osis (hī-pĕr-hī-DRŌ-sĭs): excessive or profuse sweating; also called *diaphoresis* or *sudoresis* <br><br> *hidr:* sweat <br> *-osis:* abnormal condition; increase (used primarily with blood cells) |
| **sub-** | under, below | sub/ungu/al (sŭb-ŬNG-gwăl): pertaining to the area beneath the nail of a finger or toe <br><br> *ungu:* nail <br> *-al:* pertaining to, relating to |

 It is time to review medical word elements by completing Learning Activity 5–2.

 ## Pathology

The general appearance and condition of the skin are clinically important because they may provide clues to body conditions or dysfunctions. Pale skin may indicate shock; red, flushed, very warm skin may indicate fever and infection. A rash may indicate allergies or local infections. Even chewed fingernails may be a clue to emotional problems. For diagnosis, treatment, and management of skin disorders, the medical services of a specialist may be warranted. Dermatology is the branch of medicine concerned with skin disease, and the relationship of cutaneous lesions to **systemic** disease. The physician who specializes in the diagnosis and treatment of skin disease is known as a dermatologist.

### Skin Lesions

Lesions are areas of pathologically altered tissue caused by disease, injury, or a wound due to external factors or internal disease. Evaluation of skin lesions, injuries, or changes to tissue helps establish the diagnosis of skin disorders. Lesions are described as **primary** or **secondary.** *Primary* skin lesions are the initial reaction to pathologically altered tissue and may be flat or elevated. *Secondary* skin lesions are the changes that take place in the primary lesion due to infection, scratching, trauma, or various stages of a disease. Lesions are also described by their appearance, color, location, and size as measured in centimeters. Some of the major primary and secondary skin lesions are described and illustrated in Figure 5–3.

**PRIMARY LESIONS**

### FLAT LESIONS
*Flat, discolored, circumscribed lesions of any size*

**Macule**
Flat, pigmented, circumscribed area less than 1 cm in diameter.
**Examples:** freckle, flat mole, or rash that occurs in rubella.

---

### ELEVATED LESIONS

*Solid*

**Papule**
Solid, elevated lesion less than 1 cm in diameter that may be the same color as the skin or pigmented.
**Examples:** nevus, wart, pimple, ringworm, psoriasis, eczema.

**Nodule**
Palpable, circumscribed lesion; larger and deeper than a papule (0.6 to 2 cm in diameter); extends into the dermal area.
**Examples:** intradermal nevus, benign or malignant tumor.

**Tumor**
Solid, elevated lesion larger than 2 cm in diameter that extends into the dermal and subcutaneous layers.
**Examples:** lipoma, steatoma, dermatofibroma, hemangioma.

**Wheal**
Elevated, firm, rounded lesion with localized skin edema (swelling) that varies in size, shape, and color; paler in the center than its surrounding edges; accompanied by itching.
**Examples:** hives, insect bites, urticaria.

*Fluid-filled*

**Vesicle**
Elevated, circumscribed, fluid-filled lesion less than 0.5 cm in diameter.
**Examples:** poison ivy, shingles, chickenpox.

**Pustule**
Small, raised, circumscribed lesion that contains pus; usually less than 1 cm in diameter.
**Examples:** acne, furuncle, pustular psoriasis, scabies.

**Bulla**
A vesicle or blister larger than 1 cm in diameter.
**Examples:** second degree burns, severe poison oak, poison ivy.

---

**SECONDARY LESIONS**

### DEPRESSED LESIONS
*Depressed lesions caused by loss of skin surface*

**Excoriations**
Linear scratch marks or traumatized abrasions of the epidermis.
**Examples:** scratches, abrasions, chemical or thermal burns.

**Fissure**
Small slit or cracklike sore that extends into the dermal layer; could be caused by continuous inflammation and drying.

**Ulcer**
An open sore or lesion that extends to the dermis and usually heals with scarring.
**Examples:** pressure sore, basal cell carcinoma.

**Figure 5–3**  Primary and secondary lesions.

 **It is time to review skin lesions by completing Learning Activity 5–3.**

## Burns

Burns are tissue injuries caused by contact with thermal, chemical, electrical, or radioactive agents. Although burns generally occur on the skin, they can also involve the respiratory and digestive tract linings. Burns that have a *local* effect (local tissue destruction) are not as serious as those that have a *systemic* effect. Systemic effects are life threatening and may include dehydration, shock, and infection.

Burns are usually classified as first-, second-, or third-degree. The extent of injury and degree of severity determine a burn's classification. In *first-degree* burns, the epidermis is damaged. Symptoms are restricted to local effects, such as skin redness (erythema) and acute sensitivity to such sensory stimuli as touch, heat, or cold (hyperesthesia). A first-degree burn does not blister and heals without scar formation. Examples are damaged skin caused by sunburn or scalding with hot water. *Second-degree* burns are deep burns that damage both the epidermis and part of the dermis. They are characterized by the formation of fluid-filled blisters (vesicles or bullae), caused by the deeper penetration of heat. Second-degree burns are more painful, and recovery is usually slow but complete with no scar formation. In *third-degree* burns, both the epidermis and the dermis are destroyed and some of the underlying connective tissue is damaged, leaving the skin waxy and charred with insensitivity to touch. Because of such extensive destruction, ulcerating wounds develop and the body attempts to heal itself by forming scar tissue. Skin grafts (dermatoplasty) are frequently used to assist recovery.

An emergency method for estimating the extent of burn damage is to apply the *Rule of Nines.* This method calculates body surface involved in burns by assigning values of 9% or 18% of surface areas to specific regions. (See Figure 5–4.) Accurate estimation of damaged surface area is important for treatment with I.V. fluid, which replaces the fluids lost from tissue damage and destruction.

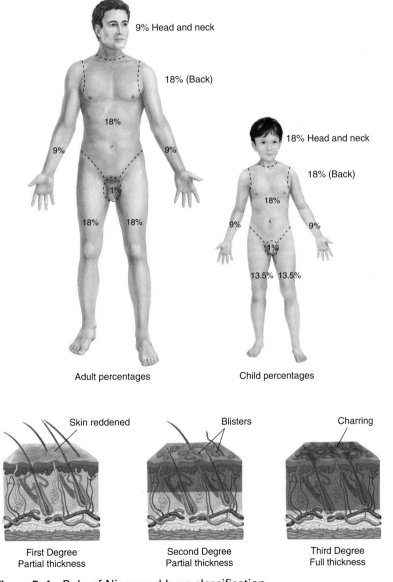

**Figure 5–4**  Rule of Nines and burn classification.

## Oncology

Neoplasms are abnormal growths of new tissue that can be benign or malignant. *Benign* neoplasms are noncancerous growths composed of the same type of cells as the tissue in which they are growing. They harm the individual only as much as they place pressure on surrounding structures. If the benign neoplasm remains small and places no pressure on adjacent structures, it commonly is not removed. When it becomes excessively large, causes pain, or places pressure on other organs or structures, excision is necessary. *Malignant* neoplasms are composed of cancerous cells that do not necessarily resemble the tissue in which they are growing. The cells show altered function, altered appearance, and uncontrolled growth, and the malignant tumor invades the surrounding tissue. Ultimately, malignant cells break loose from the primary tumor, enter blood and lymph vessels, and travel to remote regions of the body to form secondary tumor sites, a process called *metastasis*. The ability to invade surrounding tissues and spread to remote regions of body is a distinguishing feature of malignancy. If left untreated, malignant neoplasms are usually progressive and generally fatal.

Cancer treatment includes surgery, chemotherapy, immunotherapy, and radiation therapy. Immunotherapy, also called *biotherapy*, is a recent treatment approach that stimulates the body's own immune defenses to fight tumor cells. When combined with surgery, chemotherapy, or radiation, immunotherapy may be most effective in early cancer stages.

### Grading and Staging Systems

Pathologists grade and stage tumors for diagnostic and therapeutic purposes. A tumor grading system is used to evaluate the appearance and maturity of cancer cells in a tumor. Pathologists commonly describe tumors by four grades of severity based on microscopic appearance of cancer cells. (See Table 5–1.) A patient with a grade 1 tumor has the best prognosis; one with a grade 4 tumor has the worst prognosis.

The tumor, node, metastasis (TNM) system of staging is used to determine how much the cancer has spread (metastasis) within the body. The TNM system stages tumors according to three basic criteria. *T* refers to the size and extent of the primary *tumor*, *N* indicates number of area lymph *nodes* involved, *M* refers to any *metastases* of the primary tumor. A subscript number is used to indicate the size or spread of the tumor. For example, $T_2$ designates a small tumor; $M_0$ designates no metastasis. (See Table 5–2.)

| Table 5–1 | TUMOR GRADING |
|---|---|

The table below defines the four tumor grades and their characteristics.

| Grading | Tumor Characteristics |
|---|---|
| *Grade I* <br> Tumor cells well differentiated | Close resemblance to tissue of origin, thus, retaining some specialized functions |
| *Grade II* <br> Tumor cells moderately differentiated | Less resemblance to tissue of origin; more variation in size and shape of tumor cells; increased mitoses |
| *Grade III* <br> Tumor cells poorly to very poorly differentiated | Does not closely resemble tissue of origin; much variation in shape and size of tumor cells; greatly increased mitoses |
| *Grade IV* <br> Tumor cells very poorly differentiated | No resemblance to tissue of origin; great variation in size and shape of tumor cells |

## Table 5-2    TNM SYSTEM OF STAGING

The table below outlines the tumor, node, metastasis (TNM) system of staging, including designations, stages, and degrees of tissue involvement.

| Designation | Stage | Tissue involvement |
|---|---|---|
| **Tumor** | | |
| $T_0$ | | No evidence of primary tumor |
| $T_{is}$ | Stage I | Carcinoma *in situ*, which indicates no invasion of other tissues |
| $T_1, T_2, T_3, T_4,$ | Stage II | Primary tumor size and extent of local invasion, where $T_1$ is small with minimal invasion and $T_4$ is large with extensive local invasion into surrounding organs and tissues |
| **Node** | | |
| $N_0$ | | Regional lymph nodes with no abnormalities |
| $N_1, N_2, N_3, N_4$ | Stage III | Degree of lymph node involvement and spread to regional lymph nodes, where $N_1$ is less involved with minimal spreading and $N_4$ is more involved with extensive spreading |
| **Metastasis** | | |
| $M_0$ | | No evidence of metastasis |
| $M_1$ | Stage IV | Indicates metastasis |

## Basal Cell Carcinoma

Basal cell carcinoma, the most common type of skin cancer, is a malignancy of the stratum germinativum, basal cell layer of the epidermis (see Figure 5–1), or hair follicles that is commonly caused by overexposure to sunlight. (See Figure 5–5.) These tumors are locally invasive but rarely metastasize. Basal cell carcinoma is most prevalent in blond, fair-skinned men and is the most common malignant tumor affecting Caucasians. Although these tumors grow slowly, they commonly ulcerate as they increase in size and develop crusting that is firm to the touch. Metastases are uncommon with this type of cancer; however, the disease can invade the tissue sufficiently to destroy an ear, nose, or eyelid. Depending on the location, size, and depth of the lesion, treatment may include curettage and electrodesiccation, chemotherapy, surgical excision, irradiation, or chemosurgery.

**Figure 5–5**   Basal cell carcinoma.

## Squamous Cell Carcinoma

Squamous cell carcinoma of the skin arises from keratinizing epidermal cells. It is an invasive tumor with potential for metastasis and occurs most commonly in fair-skinned white men over age 60. Repeated overexposure to the sun's ultraviolet rays greatly increases the risk of squamous cell carcinoma. Other predisposing factors associated with this type of cancer include radiation therapy, chronic skin irritation and inflammation, exposure to local carcinogens (such as tar and oil), hereditary diseases (such as xeroderma pigmentosum and albinism), and the presence of premalignant lesions (such as actinic keratosis or Bowen disease).

There are two types of squamous cell carcinoma: *in situ* (confined to the original site) and *invasive.* Treatment may consist of surgical excision; curettage and electrodesiccation, which provide good cosmetic results for smaller lesions; radiation therapy, usually for older or debilitated patients; and chemotherapy, depending on the location, size, shape, degree of invasion, and condition of underlying tissue. A combination of these treatment methods may be required for a deeply invasive tumor.

## Malignant Melanoma

Malignant melanoma is a neoplasm composed of abnormal melanocytes that commonly begin in a darkly pigmented mole. Although malignant melanoma is relatively rare, the incidence is rising more rapidly than any other malignancy. It is the most lethal of the skin cancers and can metastasize extensively to the liver, lungs, or brain.

Several factors may influence the development of melanoma, but the persons at greatest risk have fair complexions, blue eyes, red or blonde hair, and freckles. Excessive exposure to sunlight and severe sunburn during childhood are believed to increase the risk of melanoma in later life. Avoiding the sun and using sunscreen have proved effective in preventing the disease.

Melanomas are diagnosed by biopsy along with histologic examination. Treatment requires surgery to remove the primary cancer, along with adjuvant therapies to reduce the risk of metastasis. The extent of surgery depends on the size and location of the primary tumor and is determined by staging the disease. (See Table 5–2.)

 **It is time to review burn and oncology terms by completing Learning Activity 5–4.**

## Diagnostic, Symptomatic, and Related Terms

This section introduces diagnostic, symptomatic, and related terms and their meanings. Word analyses for selected terms are also provided.

| Term | Definition |
|------|------------|
| **abscess**<br>ĂB-sĕs | Walled cavity containing pus and surrounded by inflamed or necrotic tissue<br>*If an abscess does not respond to treatment, it may require an incision to drain the purulent material.* |
| **acne**<br>ĂK-nē | Inflammatory disease of the sebaceous glands and hair follicles of the skin |
| **acne vulgaris** | Characterized by comedones (blackheads), papules, and pustules; usually associated with seborrhea<br>*In acne, cysts and nodules may develop and scarring is common. The face, neck, and shoulders are common sites for this condition.* |
| **Bowen disease**<br>BŌ-ĕn dĭ-ZĒZ | Form of intraepidermal carcinoma (squamous cells) characterized by red-brown scaly or crusted lesions that resemble a patch of psoriasis or dermatitis; also called *Bowen precancerous dermatosis*<br>*Treatment includes curettage and electrodesiccation.* |
| **carbuncle**<br>KĂR-bŭng-kĕl | Deep-seated pyogenic infection of the skin usually involving subcutaneous tissues<br>*A carbuncle consists of several furuncles developing in adjoining hair follicles with multiple drainage sinuses. The most common sites of these lesions are the nape of the neck, the upper back, and the buttocks. (See Figure 5–6.) See also furuncle.*<br><br>**Figure 5–6**  Carbuncle-furuncle. |
| **cellulitis**<br>sĕl-ū-LĪ-tĭs | Diffuse (widespread), acute infection of the skin and subcutaneous tissue<br>*Cellulitis is characterized by localized heat, redness, pain, swelling, and, occasionally, fever, malaise, chills, and headache.* |
| **chloasma**<br>klō-ĂZ-mă | Pigmentary skin discoloration usually occurring in yellowish-brown patches or spots |

*(Continued)*

| Term | Definition | (Continued) |
|------|-----------|-------------|
| **comedo**<br>KŎM-ē-dō | Typical small skin lesion of acne vulgaris caused by accumulation of keratin, bacteria, and dried sebum plugging an excretory duct of the skin<br><br>*The closed form of comedo, called a* whitehead, *consists of a papule from which the contents are not easily expressed.* | |
| **decubitus ulcer**<br>dē-KŪ-bĭ-tŭs  ŬL-sĕr | Skin ulceration caused by prolonged pressure, usually in a person who is bedridden; also known as a *bedsore*<br><br>*Decubitus ulcers are most commonly found in skin overlying a bony projection, such as the hip, ankle, heel, shoulder, and elbow.* | |
| **dermatomycosis**<br>dĕr-mă-tō-mĭ-KŌ-sĭs<br><br>  *dermat/o:* skin<br>  *myc:* fungus<br>  *-osis:* abnormal condition; increase (used primarily with blood cells) | Fungal infection of the skin | |
| **ecchymosis**<br>ĕk-ĭ-MŌ-sĭs | Skin discoloration consisting of a large, irregularly formed hemorrhagic area with colors changing from blue-black to greenish brown or yellow; commonly called a bruise (See Figure 5–7.)<br><br><br>**Figure 5–7**   Ecchymosis. | |
| **eczema**<br>ĔK-zĕ-mă | Acute or chronic skin inflammation characterized by erythema, papules, vesicles, pustules, scales, crusts, scabs and, possibly, itching<br>*Symptoms may occur alone or in combination.* | |
| **erythema**<br>ĕr-ĭ-THĒ-mă | Redness of the skin caused by swelling of the capillaries<br>*An example of erythema is a mild sunburn or nervous blushing.* | |
| **eschar**<br>ĔS-kăr | Damaged tissue following a severe burn | |
| **furuncle**<br>FŪ-rŭng-k'l | Bacterial infection of a hair follicle or sebaceous gland that produces a pus-filled lesion commonly called a *boil*<br>*Lesions drain a creamy pus when incised and may heal with scarring.* | |
| **hirsutism**<br>HĔR-soot-ĭzm | Condition characterized by the excessive growth of hair or presence of hair in unusual places, especially in women | |

| Term | Definition |
|------|------------|
| **impetigo**<br>ĭm-pĕ-TĪ-gō | Inflammatory skin disease characterized by isolated pustules that become crusted and rupture |
| **keratosis**<br>kĕr-ă-TŌ-sĭs<br><br>*kerat:* horny tissue; hard; cornea<br>*-osis:* abnormal condition; increase (used primarily with blood cells) | Thickened area of the epidermis; any horny growth on the skin (such as a callus or wart) |
| **lentigo**<br>lĕn-TĪ-gō | Small brown macules, especially on the face and arms with lesions distributed on sun-exposed areas of the skin |
| **pallor**<br>PĂL-or | Unnatural paleness or absence of color in the skin |
| **pediculosis**<br>pē-dĭk-ū-LŌ-sĭs | Infestation with lice, transmitted by personal contact or common use of brushes, combs, or headgear |
| **petechia**<br>pē-TĒ-kē-ă | Minute, pinpoint hemorrhage under the skin<br>*A petechia is a smaller version of an ecchymosis.* |
| **pruritus**<br>proo-RĪ-tŭs | Intense itching |
| **psoriasis**<br>sō-RĪ-ă-sĭs | Chronic skin disease characterized by circumscribed red patches covered by thick, dry, silvery, adherent scales that are the result of excessive development of the basal layer of the epidermis<br><br>*New lesions tend to appear at sites of trauma. They may be found in any location but commonly on the scalp, knees, elbows, umbilicus, and genitalia. Treatment includes topical application of various medications, keratolytics, phototherapy, and ultraviolet light therapy in an attempt to slow hyperkeratosis.* |
| **purpura**<br>PŬR-pū-ră | Any of several bleeding disorders characterized by hemorrhage into the tissues, particularly beneath the skin or mucous membranes, producing ecchymoses or petechiae<br><br>*Hemorrhage into the skin shows red darkening into purple and then brownish-yellow and finally disappearing in 2 to 3 weeks. Areas of discoloration do not disappear under pressure.* |
| **scabies**<br>SKĀ-bēz | Contagious skin disease transmitted by the itch mite, commonly through sexual contact<br><br>*Scabies manifests as papules, vesicles, pustules, and burrows and causes intense itching commonly resulting in secondary infections. The axillae, genitalia, inner aspect of the thighs, and areas between the fingers are most commonly affected.* |
| **tinea**<br>TĬN-ē-ăh | Any fungal skin disease whose name commonly indicates the body part affected; also called *ringworm*<br><br>*Examples include tinea barbae (beard), tinea corporis (body), tinea pedis (athlete's foot), tinea versicolor (skin), tinea cruris (jock itch).* |

*(Continued)*

| Term | Definition | (Continued) |
|------|-----------|---------|
| **urticaria** ŭr-tĭ-KĀ-rē-ă | Allergic reaction of the skin characterized by the eruption of pale red elevated patches called wheals (hives) | |
| **vitiligo** vĭt-ĭl-Ī-gō | Localized loss of skin pigmentation characterized by milk-white patches | |
| **verruca** vĕr-ROO-kă | Epidermal growth caused by a virus, such as plantar warts, juvenile warts, and venereal warts *Warts may be removed by cryosurgery, electrocautery, or acids; however, they may regrow if virus remains in the skin.* | |

# Diagnostic and Therapeutic Procedures

This section introduces procedures used to diagnose and treat skin disorders. Descriptions are provided as well as pronunciations and word analyses for selected terms.

| Procedure | Description |
|-----------|-------------|
| **DIAGNOSTIC PROCEDURES** | |
| Clinical | |
| **skin test (ST)** | Any test in which a suspected allergen or sensitizer is applied to or injected into the skin to determine the patient's reaction to it *The most commonly used tests are the intradermal, patch, and scratch tests. The intensity of the response is determined by the wheal-and-flare reaction 10 minutes after the suspected allergen is applied. Positive and negative controls are used to verify normal skin reactivity.* |
| **intradermal test** | Identifies suspected allergens by subcutaneously injecting small amounts of extracts of the suspected allergens and observing the skin for a subsequent reaction; used to determine immunity to diphtheria (Schick test) or tuberculosis (Mantoux test) |
| **patch test** | Identifies suspected allergens by topical application of substance to be tested (e.g., food, pollen, animal fur), usually on the forearm and observing for subsequent reaction *After the patch is removed, a lack of noticeable reaction indicates a negative result; skin reddening or swelling indicates a positive result.* |

| Procedure | Description |
|---|---|
| **scratch test** | Identifies suspected allergens by placing a small quantity of suspected allergen on a lightly scratched area of the skin |
| | *Redness or swelling at the scratch sites within 10 minutes indicates allergy to the substance indicating the test result is positive. If no reaction occurs, the test result is negative.* |

### Surgical

| | |
|---|---|
| **biopsy**<br>BĪ-ŏp-sē | Representative tissue sample removed from a body site for microscopic examination, usually to establish a diagnosis |
| | *Skin biopsies are used to establish or confirm a diagnosis, estimate prognosis, or follow the course of disease. Any lesion suspected of malignancy is removed and sent to the pathology laboratory.* |
|    **needle** | Removal of small tissue sample for examination using a hollow needle, usually attached to a syringe |
|    **punch** | Removal of a small core of tissue using a hollow punch |
|    **shave** | Removal of tissue using a surgical blade to shave elevated lesions |
|    **frozen section (FS)** | Ultra-thin slice of tissue cut from a frozen specimen for immediate pathological examination |
| | *Frozen section is commonly used for rapid diagnosis of malignancy after the patient has been anesthetized to determine conservative or radical approach.* |

## THERAPEUTIC PROCEDURES

| Procedure | Description |
|---|---|
| **debridement**<br>dā-brēd-MŎN | Removal of foreign material and dead or damaged tissue, especially in a wound; used to promote healing and prevent infection |
| **dermabrasion**<br>DĔRM-ă-brā-zhŭn | Removal of acne scars, nevi, tattoos, or fine wrinkles on the skin through the use of sandpaper, wire brushes, or other abrasive materials on the anesthetized epidermis |
| **fulguration**<br>fŭl-gū-RĀ-shŭn | Tissue destruction by means of high-frequency electric sparks; also called *electrodesiccation* |

### Surgical

| | |
|---|---|
| **chemical peel** | Chemical removal of the outer layers of skin to treat acne scarring and general keratoses; also used for cosmetic purposes to remove fine wrinkles on the face; also called *chemabrasion* |
| **cryosurgery**<br>krī-ō-SĔR-jĕr-ē | Use of subfreezing temperature (commonly with liquid nitrogen) to destroy or eliminate abnormal tissue cells, such as tumors, warts, and unwanted, cancerous, or infected tissue |
| **incision and drainage (I&D)** | Incision in a lesion such as an abscess and drainage of its contents |

## Pharmacology

Various medications are available to treat skin disorders. (See Table 5–3.) Because of their superficial nature and location, many skin disorders respond well to topical drug therapy. Mild skin diseases such as contact dermatitis, acne, poison ivy, and diaper rash can be effectively treated with topical agents available as over-the-counter products. These products provide relief in mild, localized skin disorders.

Widespread or particularly severe dermatologic disorders may require systemic treatment. For example, poison ivy with large areas of open, weeping lesions may be difficult to treat with topical medication and may require a prescription-strength drug. In this case, an oral steroid or antihistamine might be prescribed to relieve inflammation and severe itching.

### Table 5–3    DRUGS USED TO TREAT SKIN DISORDERS

This table lists common drug classifications used to treat skin disorders, their therapeutic actions, and selected generic and trade names.

| Classification | Therapeutic Action | Generic and Trade Names |
|---|---|---|
| anesthetics | Block the sensation of pain by numbing the skin layers and mucous membranes<br><br>*These topical drugs can be administered directly by means of sprays, creams, gargles, suppositories, and other preparations. They provide temporary symptomatic relief for minor burns, sunburns, rashes, and insect bites.* | **bupivacaine**<br>bū-PĬV-ă-kān<br>*Marcaine*<br>**lidocaine**<br>LĬ-dō-kān<br>*Xylocaine*<br>**procaine**<br>PRŌ-kān<br>*Novocain* |
| antifungals | Alter the cell wall of fungi or disrupt enzyme activity, resulting in cell death<br><br>*Antifungals provide effective treatment for ringworm (tinea corporis), athlete's foot (tinea pedis), and fungal infection of the nail (onychomycosis). When topical antifungals are not effective, oral or intravenous antifungal drugs may be necessary.* | **clotrimazole**<br>clō-TRĬ-mă-zōl<br>*Lotrimin, Mycelex*<br>**miconazole**<br>mĭ-KŎN-ă-zōl<br>*Micatin, Monistat-Derm*<br>**nystatin**<br>NĬS-tă-tĭn<br>*Mycostatin, Nystex, Pedi-Dri*<br>**itraconazole**<br>ĭt-ră-KŎN-ă-zōl<br>*Sporanox* |
| antihistamines | Inhibit inflammation, redness, and itching caused by allergic skin reaction and the release of histamine<br><br>*In case of severe itching, antihistamines may be given orally. As a group, these drugs are also known as antipruritics.* | **diphenhydramine**<br>di-fēn-HĬ-dră-mēn<br>*Benadryl*<br>**hydroxyzine**<br>hi-DRŎK-si-zēn<br>*Atarax, Vistaril* |
| antiseptics | Topically applied agents that inhibit the growth of bacteria, thus preventing infections in cuts, scratches, and surgical incisions | **chlorhexidine**<br>klor-HĔKS-ĭ-dēn<br>*Hibiclens*<br>**ethyl or isopropyl alcohol**<br>ĔTH-ĭl, ī-sō-PRŌ-pĭl<br>**hydrogen peroxide**<br>HĬ-drō-jĕn pĕ-RŎK-sĭd |

## Table 5–3    DRUGS USED TO TREAT SKIN DISORDERS

| Classification | Therapeutic Action | Generic and Trade Names |
|---|---|---|
| **corticosteroid anti-inflam- matories** | Decrease inflammation and itching by suppressing the immune system's response to tissue damage<br><br>*Topical corticosteroids are used to treat contact dermatitis, poison ivy, insect bites, psoriasis, seborrhea, and eczema. Oral corticosteroids may be given for systemic treatment of severe or widespread inflammation or itching.* | **hydrocortisone***<br>hī-drō-KOR-tĭ-sōn<br>  *Cortaid, Dermolate, Locoid*<br>**triamcinolone**<br>trī-ăm-SĬN-ō-lōn<br>  *Aristocort, Kenalog* |
| **keratolytics** | Destroy and soften the outer layer of skin so that it is sloughed off or shed<br><br>*Strong keratolytics effectively remove warts and corns and aid in penetration of antifungal drugs. Milder keratolytics promote shedding of scales and crusts in eczema, psoriasis, seborrheic dermatitis, and other dry, scaly conditions. Very weak keratolytics irritate inflamed skin, acting as a tonic to accelerate healing.* | **tretinoin**<br>TRĔT-ĭ-noyn<br>  *Retin-A, Vesanoid*<br>**erythromycin**<br>ĕ-rith-rō-MĪ-sĭn<br>  *EryDerm, Staticin*<br>**tetracycline**<br>tĕt-ră-SĪ-klēn<br>  *Topicycline* |
| **parasiticides** | Kill insect parasites, such as mites and lice<br><br>*Parasiticides are used to treat scabies (mites) and pediculosis (lice). The drug is applied as a cream or lotion to the body and as a shampoo to treat the scalp (rare in scabies).* | **lindane**<br>LĬN-dān<br>  *Kwell*<br>**permethrin**<br>pĕr-MĔTH-rĭn<br>  *Nix* |
| **protectives** | Cover, cool, dry, or soothe inflamed skin<br><br>*Protectives do not penetrate the skin or soften it; rather, they allow the natural healing process to occur by forming a long-lasting film that protects the skin from air, water, and clothing.* | **lotions**<br>  *Cetaphil moisturizing lotion*<br>**creams**<br>  *Neutrogena hand cream*<br>**ointments**<br>  *Vaseline* |

*The suffixes *-sone*, *-olone*, and *-onide* are common to generic corticosteroids.

 It is time to review diagnostic, symptomatic, procedure, and pharmacology terms by completing Learning Activity 5–5.

## Abbreviations

This section introduces integumentary-related abbreviations and their meanings.

| Abbreviation | Meaning |
| --- | --- |
| Bx, bx | biopsy |
| BCC | basal cell carcinoma |
| cm | centimeter |
| decub | decubitus (ulcer); bedsore |
| derm | dermatology |
| FS | frozen section |
| ID | intradermal |
| I&D | incision and drainage |
| IMP | impression (synonymous with *diagnosis*) |
| Sub Q, sub Q* | subcutaneous (injection) |
| ung | ointment |
| XP, XDP | xeroderma pigmentosum |

*Although these abbreviations are currently found in medical records and clinical notes, the Joint Commission on Accreditation of Healthcare Organizations (JCAHO) requires their discontinuance. Instead, write out their meanings.

# LEARNING ACTIVITIES

The following activities provide review of the integumentary system terms introduced in this chapter. Complete each activity and review your answers to evaluate your understanding of the chapter.

## Learning Activity 5–1

### Identifying integumentary structures

*Label the following illustration using the terms listed below.*

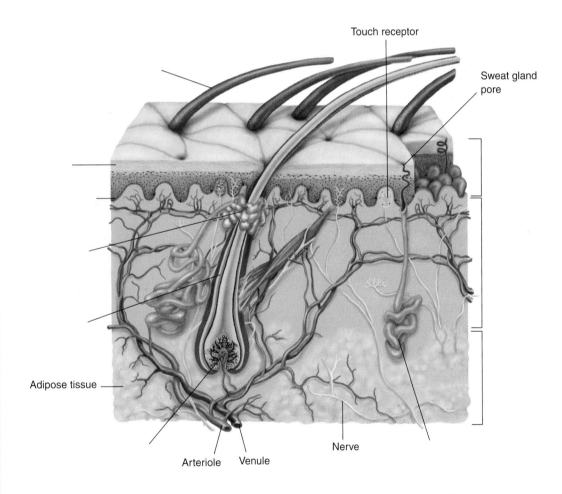

| dermis | papilla | subcutaneous tissue |
|--------|---------|---------------------|
| epidermis | sebaceous (oil) gland | sudoriferous (sweat) gland |
| hair follicle | stratum corneum | |
| hair shaft | stratum germinativum | |

 Check your answers by referring to Figure 5–1 on page 77. Review material that you did not answer correctly.

Learning Activity 5–2

## Building medical words

*Use* **adip/o** *or* **lip/o** *(fat) to build words that mean:*

1. tumor consisting of fat _____

2. hernia containing fat _____

3. resembling fat _____

4. fat cell _____

*Use* **dermat/o** *(skin) to build words that mean:*

5. inflammation of the skin _____

6. instrument to incise the skin _____

*Use* **onych/o** *(nail) to build words that mean:*

7. tumor of the nails _____

8. softening of the nails _____

9. abnormal condition of the nails _____

10. abnormal condition of the nails caused by a fungus _____

11. abnormal condition of a hidden (ingrown) nail _____

12. disease of the nails _____

*Use* **trich/o** *(hair) to build words that mean:*

13. disease of the hair _____

14. abnormal condition of hair caused by a fungus _____

*Use* **-logy** *or* **-logist** *to build words that mean:*

15. study of the skin _____

16. specialist in skin (diseases) _____

*Build surgical words that mean:*

17. excision of fat (adipose tissue) _____

18. removal of a nail _____

19. incision of a nail _____

20. surgical repair (plastic surgery) of the skin _____

✓ Check your answers in Appendix A. Review material that you did not answer correctly.

**CORRECT ANSWERS** _____ × 5 = _____ **% SCORE**

Learning Activity 5–3

## Identifying skin lesions

*Label the following skin lesions on the lines provided, using the terms listed below.*

| | | | |
|---|---|---|---|
| *bulla* | *macule* | *pustule* | *vesicle* |
| *excoriations* | *nodule* | *tumor* | *wheal* |
| *fissure* | *papule* | *ulcer* | |

**PRIMARY LESIONS**

**FLAT LESIONS**
*Flat, discolored, circumscribed lesions of any size*

Flat, pigmented, circumscribed area less than 1 cm in diameter.
**Examples:** freckle, flat mole, or rash that occurs in rubella.

**ELEVATED LESIONS**

*Solid*                                                                 *Fluid-filled*

Solid, elevated lesion less than 1 cm in diameter that may be the same color as the skin or pigmented.
**Examples:** nevus, wart, pimple, ringworm, psoriasis, eczema.

Elevated, circumscribed, fluid-filled lesion less than 0.5 cm in diameter.
**Examples:** poison ivy, shingles, chickenpox.

Palpable, circumscribed lesion; larger and deeper than a papule (0.6 to 2 cm in diameter); extends into the dermal area.
**Examples:** intradermal nevus, benign or malignant tumor.

Small, raised, circumscribed lesion that contains pus; usually less than 1 cm in diameter.
**Examples:** acne, furuncle, pustular psoriasis, scabies.

Solid, elevated lesion larger than 2 cm in diameter that extends into the dermal and subcutaneous layers.
**Examples:** lipoma, steatoma, dermatofibroma, hemangioma.

A vesicle or blister larger than 1 cm in diameter.
**Examples:** second degree burns, severe poison oak, poison ivy.

Elevated, firm, rounded lesion with localized skin edema (swelling) that varies in size, shape, and color; paler in the center than its surrounding edges; accompanied by itching.
**Examples:** hives, insect bites, urticaria.

**SECONDARY LESIONS**

**DEPRESSED LESIONS**
*Depressed lesions caused by loss of skin surface*

Linear scratch marks or traumatized abrasions of the epidermis.
**Examples:** scratches, abrasions, chemical or thermal burns.

Small slit or cracklike sore that extends into the dermal layer; could be caused by continuous inflammation and drying.

An open sore or lesion that extends to the dermis and usually heals with scarring.
**Examples:** pressure sore, basal cell carcinoma.

 Check your answers by referring to Figure 5–3 on page 84. Review material that you did not answer correctly.

## Learning Activity 5–4

### Matching burn and oncology terms

*Match each term on the left with its meaning on the right.*

1. _____ erythema
2. _____ $T_0$
3. _____ malignant
4. _____ first-degree burn
5. _____ grading
6. _____ squamous cell carcinoma
7. _____ benign
8. _____ $T_1$
9. _____ $M_0$
10. _____ third-degree burns

a. develops from keratinizing epidermal cells
b. noncancerous
c. no evidence of metastasis
d. extensive damage to underlying connective tissue
e. no evidence of primary tumor
f. determines degree of abnormal cancer cells compared with normal cells
g. heals without scar formation
h. cancerous; may be life-threatening
i. redness of skin
j. primary tumor size, small with minimal invasion

Check your answers in Appendix A. Review any material that you did not answer correctly.

**CORRECT ANSWERS** _____ × 10 = _____ **% SCORE**

## Learning Activity 5–5

### Matching diagnostic, symptomatic, procedure, and pharmacology terms

*Match the following terms with the definitions in the numbered list.*

| | | |
|---|---|---|
| *alopecia* | *fulguration* | *petechiae* |
| *antifungals* | *impetigo* | *scabies* |
| *autograft* | *intradermal test* | *tinea* |
| *chloasma* | *keratolytics* | *urticaria* |
| *corticosteroids* | *parasiticides* | *vitiligo* |
| *dermabrasion* | *patch test* | *xenograft* |
| *ecchymosis* | *pediculosis* | |

1. _____ infestation with lice
2. _____ depigmentation in areas of the skin characterized by milk-white patches
3. _____ any fungal skin disease, also called *ringworm*

4. _____ contagious skin disease transmitted by the itch mite

5. _____ skin infection characterized by vesicles that become pustular and crusted and then rupture

6. _____ severe itching of the skin, also known as hives

7. _____ hyperpigmentation of the skin, characterized by yellowish-brown patches or spots

8. _____ hemorrhagic spot or bruise on the skin

9. _____ minute or small hemorrhagic spots on the skin

10. _____ loss or absence of hair

11. _____ topical agents to treat athlete's foot and onychomycosis

12. _____ tissue destruction by means of high-frequency electric sparks

13. _____ agents that decrease inflammation or itching

14. _____ use of wire brushes, or other abrasive materials, to remove scars, tattoos, or fine wrinkles

15. _____ agents that kill parasitic skin infestations

16. _____ agents that soften the outer layer of skin so that it sloughs off

17. _____ extracts of suspected allergens are subcutaneously injected

18. _____ allergens are applied topically, usually on forearm

19. _____ graft transferred from one part of a person's body to another part

20. _____ graft transferred from one species to a different species

Check your answers in Appendix A. Review material that you did not answer correctly.

**CORRECT ANSWERS** _____ × 5 = _____ **% SCORE**

# MEDICAL RECORD ACTIVITIES

The two medical records included in the following activities use common clinical scenarios to show how medical terminology is used to document patient care. Complete the terminology and analysis sections for each activity to help you recognize and understand terms related to the integumentary system.

## Medical Record Activity 5-1

### Pathology report of skin lesion

#### Terminology

The terms listed in the chart come from the medical record *Pathology Report of Skin Lesion* that follows. Use a medical dictionary such as *Taber's Cyclopedic Medical Dictionary,* the appendices of this book, or other resources to define each term. Then review the pronunciations for each term and practice by reading the medical record aloud.

| Term | Definition |
| --- | --- |
| **atypia**<br>ā-TĬP-ē-ă | |
| **atypical**<br>ā-TĬP-ĭ-kăl | |
| **basal cell layer**<br>BĀ-săl | |
| **Bowen disease**<br>BŌ-ĕn dĭ-ZĒZ | |
| **carcinoma**<br>kăr-sĭ-NŌ-mă | |
| **dermatitis**<br>dĕr-mă-TĪ-tĭs | |
| **dermis**<br>DĔR-mĭs | |
| **dorsum**<br>DOR-sŭm | |
| **epidermal hyperplasia**<br>ĕp-ĭ-DĔR-măl hī-pĕr-PLĀ-zē-ă | |
| **fibroplasia**<br>fī-brō-PLĀ-sē-ă | |

| Term | Definition |
|---|---|
| hyperkeratosis<br>hi-pĕr-kĕr-ă-TŌ-sĭs | |
| infiltrate<br>ĭn-FĬL-trāt | |
| keratinocytes<br>kĕ-RĂT-ĭ-nō-sīts | |
| lymphocytic<br>lĭm-fō-SĬT-ĭk | |
| neoplastic<br>nē-ō-PLĂS-tĭk | |
| papillary<br>PĂP-ĭ-lăr-ē | |
| pathological<br>păth-ō-LŎJ-ĭk-ăl | |
| solar elastosis<br>SŌ-lăr ĕ-lăs-TŌ-sĭs | |
| squamous<br>SKWĀ-mŭs | |

## PATHOLOGY REPORT OF SKIN LESION

**SPECIMEN:** Skin on (a) dorsum left wrist and (b) left forearm, ulnar, near elbow.

**CLINICAL DIAGNOSIS:** Bowen disease versus basal cell carcinoma versus dermatitis.

**MICROSCOPIC DESCRIPTION:** (a) There is mild hyperkeratosis and moderate epidermal hyperplasia with full-thickness atypia of squamous-keratinocytes. Squamatization of the basal cell layer exists. A lymphocytic inflammatory infiltrate is present in the papillary dermis. Solar elastosis is present. (b) Nests, strands, and columns of atypical neoplastic basaloid keratinocytes grow down from the epidermis into the underlying dermis. Fibroplasia is present. Solar elastosis is noted.

**PATHOLOGICAL DIAGNOSIS:** (a) Bowen disease of left wrist; (b) nodular and infiltrating basal cell carcinoma of left forearm, near elbow.

### Analysis

**Review the medical record *Pathology Report of Skin Lesion* to answer the following questions.**

1. In the specimen section, what does "skin on dorsum left wrist" mean?

2. What was the inflammatory infiltrate?

3. What was the pathologist's diagnosis for the left forearm?

4. Provide a brief description of Bowen disease, the pathologist's diagnosis for the left wrist.

Medical Record Activity 5-2

## Patient referral letter: Onychomycosis

### Terminology

The terms listed in the chart come from the medical record *Patient Referral Letter: Onychomycosis* that follows. Use a medical dictionary such as *Taber's Cyclopedic Medical Dictionary*, the appendices of this book, or other resources to define each term. Then review the pronunciations for each term and practice by reading the medical record aloud.

| Term | Definition |
| --- | --- |
| alkaline phosphatase<br>ĂL-kă-lĭn  FŎS-fă-tās | |
| bilaterally<br>bī-LĂT-ĕr-ăl-ē | |
| CA | |
| debridement<br>dā-brēd-MŎN | |
| hypertension<br>hī-pĕr-TĔN-shŭn | |
| mastectomy<br>măs-TĔK-tŏ-mē | |
| neurological<br>noor-ō-LŎJ-ĭk-ăl | |
| onychomycosis<br>ŏn-ĭ-kō-mi-KO-sĭs | |
| Sporanox*<br>SPOR-ă-nŏks | |
| vascular<br>VĂS-kū-lăr | |

*Refer to Table 5–3 to determine the drug classification and the generic name for Sporanox.

### PATIENT REFERRAL LETTER: ONYCHOMYCOSIS

Dear Doctor Meyers:

Thank you for referring Alicia Gonzoles to my office. Mrs. Gonzoles presents to the office for evaluation and treatment of onychomycosis with no previous treatment. Past pertinent medical history does reveal hypertension and breast CA. Pertinent surgical history does reveal mastectomy.

Examination of patient's feet does reveal onychomycosis 1–5 bilaterally. Vascular and neurological examinations are intact. Previous laboratory work was within normal limits except for an elevated alkaline phosphatase of 100.

Tentative diagnosis: Onychomycosis 1–5 bilaterally

Treatment consisted of debridement of mycotic nails bilateral feet as well as dispensing a prescription for Sporanox, Pulse Pack, to be taken times three months to treat the onychomycotic infection. I have also asked her to repeat her liver enzymes in approximately 4 weeks. Mrs. Gonzoles will reappoint in 2 months for follow-up, and I will keep you informed of any changes in her progress. If you have any questions, please let me know.

## Analysis

**Review the medical record *Patient Referral Letter: Onychomycosis* to answer the following questions.**

1. What pertinent disorders were identified in the past medical history?

   _____

2. What pertinent surgery was identified in the past surgical history?

   _____

3. Did the doctor identify any problems in the vascular system or nervous system?

   _____

4. What was the significant finding in the laboratory results?

   _____

5. What treatment did the doctor employ for the onychomycosis?

   _____

6. What did the doctor recommend regarding the abnormal laboratory finding?

   _____

# Chapter

**6**

# Digestive System

## OBJECTIVES

*Upon completion of this chapter, you will be able to:*

■ Locate and describe the structures of the digestive system.

■ Recognize, pronounce, spell, and build words related to the digestive system.

- Describe pathological conditions, diagnostic and therapeutic procedures, and other terms related to the digestive system.
- Explain pharmacology related to the treatment of digestive disorders.
- Demonstrate your knowledge of this chapter by completing the learning and medical record activities.

 **Key Terms**

This section introduces important digestive system terms and their definitions. Word analyses are also provided.

| Term | Definition |
|------|------------|
| **asymptomatic**<br>ā-sĭmp-tō-MĂT-ĭk | Without symptoms |
| **defecation**<br>dĕf-ĕ-KĀ-shŭn | Elimination of feces from the gastrointestinal tract through the rectum |
| **duodenal bulb**<br>dū-ō-DĒ-năl BŬLB | Upper duodenal area just beyond the pylorus |
| **endoscope**<br>ĔN-dō-skōp<br><br>*endo-:* in, within<br>*-scope:* instrument for examining | Instrument consisting of a rigid or flexible fiberoptic tube and optical system for observing the inside of a hollow organ or cavity |
| **exocrine**<br>ĔKS-ō-krĭn<br><br>*exo-:* outside, outward<br>*-crine:* secrete | Pertaining to a gland that secretes outwardly through excretory ducts to the surface of an organ or tissue or into a vessel |
| **friable**<br>FRĪ-ă-bŭl | Easily broken or pulverized |
| **pepsin**<br>PĔP-sĭn | Enzyme secreted in the stomach that begins the digestion of proteins |
| **punctate**<br>PŬNK-tāt | Having pinpoint punctures or depressions on the surface; marked with dots |
| **varices**<br>VĂR-ĭ-sēz | Tortuous dilations of a vein |
| **sphincter**<br>SFĬNGK-tĕr | Circular muscle constricting an orifice, such as the pyloric sphincter around the opening of the stomach into the duodenum |

## Anatomy and Physiology

The digestive system, also called the *gastrointestinal* (GI) system, consists of a digestive tube called the *GI tract,* or *alimentary canal,* and several accessory organs whose primary function is to break down food, prepare it for absorption, and eliminate waste. The GI tract, extending from the mouth to the anus, varies in size and structure in several distinct regions:

- mouth
- pharynx (throat)
- esophagus
- stomach
- small intestine
- large intestine
- rectum
- anus

Food passing along the GI tract is mixed with digestive enzymes and broken down into nutrient molecules, which are absorbed in the bloodstream. Undigested waste materials that cannot be absorbed in the blood are then eliminated from the body through defecation. Included in the digestive system are the accessory organs of digestion: the liver, gallbladder, and pancreas.

## Mouth

The process of digestion begins in the mouth. (See Figure 6–1.) The mouth, also known as the (1) **oral cavity** or *buccal cavity,* is a receptacle for food. It is formed by the cheeks (bucca), lips, teeth, tongue, and hard and soft palates. Located around the oral cavity are three pairs of salivary glands, which secrete saliva. Saliva contains important digestive enzymes that help begin the chemical breakdown of food. In the mouth, food is broken down mechanically (by the teeth) and chemically (by saliva), and then formed into a *bolus.*

**Figure 6–1**  Sagittal view of the head showing oral, nasal, and pharyngeal components of the digestive system.

## Teeth

The (2) **teeth** play an important role in initial stages of digestion by mechanically breaking down food (mastication) into smaller pieces as it mixes it with saliva. Teeth are covered by a hard enamel, giving them a smooth, white appearance. Beneath the enamel is the *dentin,* the main structure of the tooth. The innermost part of the tooth is the pulp, which contains nerves and blood vessels. The teeth are embedded in pink, fleshy tissue known as gums (gingiva).

## Tongue

The (3) **tongue** assists in this mechanical digestion process by manipulating the bolus of food during chewing and moving it to the back of the mouth for swallowing (deglutition). The tongue also aids in speech production and taste. Rough projections on the surface of the tongue called *papillae* contain taste buds. The four basic taste sensations registered by chemical stimulation of the taste buds are sweet, sour, salty, and bitter. All other taste perceptions are combinations of these four basic flavors. In addition, sense of taste is intricately linked with sense of smell, making taste perception very complex.

## Hard and Soft Palates

The two structures forming the roof of the mouth are the (4) **hard palate** (anterior portion) and the (5) **soft palate** (posterior portion). The soft palate, which forms a partition between the mouth and the nasopharynx, is continuous with the hard palate. The entire oral cavity, like the rest of the GI tract, is lined with mucous membranes.

## Pharynx, Esophagus, and Stomach

As the bolus is pushed by the tongue into the (6) **pharynx** (throat), it is guided by the soft, fleshy, V-shaped structure called the (7) **uvula.** The funnel-shaped pharynx serves as a passageway to the respiratory and GI tracts and provides a resonating chamber for speech sounds. The lowest portion of the pharynx divides into two tubes: one that leads to the lungs, called the (8) **trachea,** and one that leads to the stomach, called the (9) **esophagus.** A small flap of cartilage, the (10) **epiglottis,** folds back to cover the trachea during swallowing, forcing food to enter the esophagus. At all other times, the epiglottis remains upright, allowing air to freely pass through the respiratory structures.

The **stomach,** a saclike structure located in the left upper quadrant (LUQ) of the abdominal cavity, serves as a food reservoir that continues mechanical and chemical digestion. (See Figure 6–2.) The stomach extends from the (1) **esophagus** to the first part of the small intestine, the (2) **duodenum.** The terminal portion of the esophagus, the (3) **lower esophageal (cardiac) sphincter,** is composed of muscle fibers that constrict once food has passed into the stomach. It prevents the stomach contents from regurgitating back into the esophagus. The (4) **body** of the stomach, the large central portion, together with the (5) **fundus,** the upper portion, are mainly storage areas. Most digestion takes place in the funnel-shaped terminal portion, the (6) **pylorus.** The interior lining of the stomach is composed of mucous membranes (mucosa) and contains numerous macroscopic longitudinal folds called (7) **rugae** that gradually unfold as the stomach fills. Located within the rugae, digestive glands produce hydrochloric acid (HCl) and enzymes. Secretions from these glands coupled with the mechanical churning of the stomach turn the bolus into a semiliquid form called *chyme* that slowly leaves the stomach through the (8) **pyloric sphincter** to enter the duodenum. This sphincter regulates the speed and movement of chyme into the small intestine and prohibits backflow. Food is propelled through the entire GI tract by coordinated, rhythmic muscle contractions called **peristalsis.**

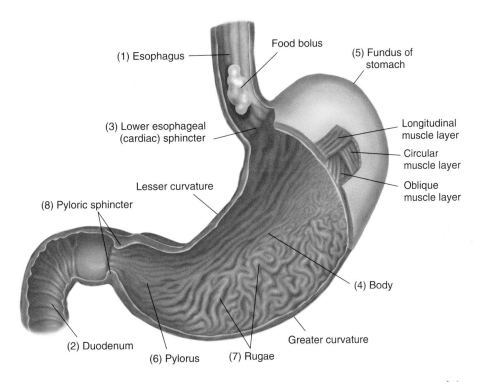

**Figure 6–2**    Anterior view of the stomach showing muscle layers and rugae of the mucosa.

## Small Intestine

The small intestine is a coiled, 20′-long tube that begins at the pyloric sphincter and extends to the large intestine. (See Figure 6–3.) It consists of three parts:

- the (1) **duodenum,** the uppermost segment, which is about 10″ long
- the (2) **jejunum,** which is approximately 8′ long
- the (3) **ileum,** which is about 12′ long

Digestion is completed in the small intestine with the help of additional enzymes and secretions from the (4) **pancreas** and (5) **liver.** Nutrients in chyme are absorbed through microscopic, fingerlike projections called villi to enter the bloodstream and lymphatic system for distribution to the rest of the body. At the terminal end of the small intestine, a sphincter muscle called the *ileocecal valve* joins the ileum to the large intestine's cecum. When the sphincter muscle is relaxed, undigested or unabsorbed material from the small intestine is passed to the large intestine to be excreted from the body.

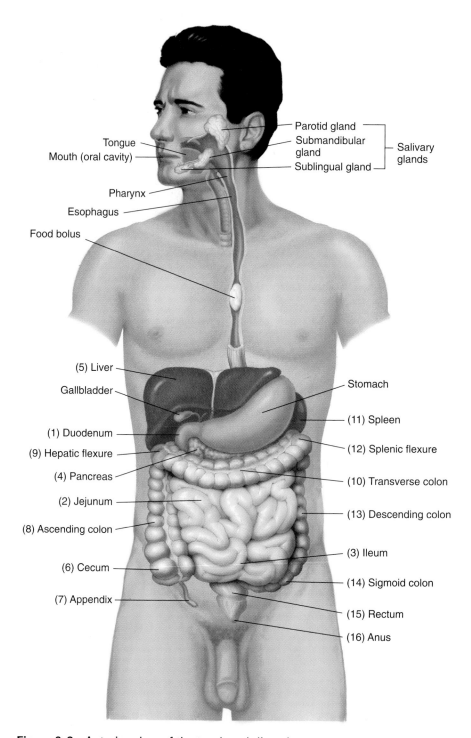

**Figure 6–3**   Anterior view of the trunk and digestive organs.

## Large Intestine

The large intestine is about 5′ long. It begins at the ileum and extends to the anus. No digestion takes place in the large intestine. The only secretion is mucus in the colon, which lubricates fecal material so it can pass from the body. The large intestine is divided into four major

regions: cecum, colon, rectum, and anus. The first 2″ or 3″ of the large intestine is called the (6) **cecum,** a pouchlike structure located below the ileocecal opening. Projecting downward from the cecum is a wormlike projection, called the (7) **appendix.** The function of the appendix is unknown; however, problems arise if it becomes infected or inflamed. The cecum merges with the colon. The main functions of the colon are to absorb water and minerals and eliminate undigested material. The colon is divided into ascending, transverse, descending, and sigmoid portions:

- The (8) **ascending colon** extends from the cecum to the lower border of the liver and turns abruptly to form the (9) **hepatic flexure.**
- The colon continues across the abdomen to the left side as the (10) **transverse colon** curving beneath the lower end of the (11) **spleen** to form the (12) **splenic flexure.**
- As the transverse colon turns downward, it becomes the (13) **descending colon.**
- The descending colon continues until it forms the (14) **sigmoid colon** and the (15) **rectum.** The rectum, the last part of the GI tract, terminates at the (16) **anus.**

 **It is time to review digestive structures by completing Learning Activity 6–1.**

## Accessory Organs of Digestion

Although the liver, gallbladder, and pancreas lie outside the GI tract, they play a vital role in the proper digestion and absorption of nutrients. (See Figure 6–4.)

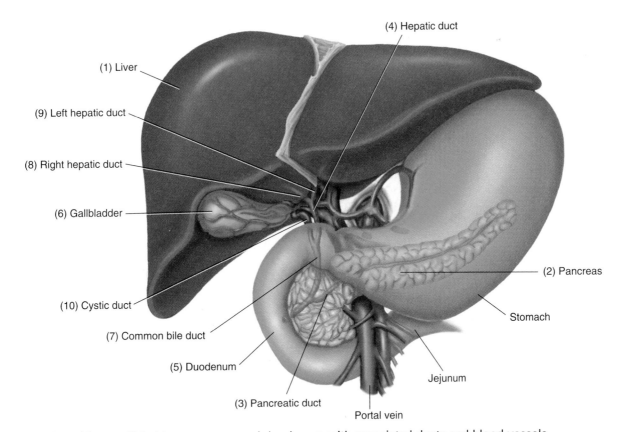

**Figure 6–4** Liver, gallbladder, pancreas, and duodenum with associated ducts and blood vessels.

## Liver

The (1) **liver,** the largest glandular organ in the body, weighs approximately 3 to 4 lb. It is located beneath the diaphragm in the right upper quadrant (RUQ) of the abdominal cavity. The liver performs many vital activities and death occurs if it ceases to function. Some of its important activities include:

- producing bile, used in the small intestine to emulsify and absorb fats
- removing **glucose** (sugar) from blood to synthesize glycogen (starch) and retain it for later use
- storing vitamins, such as $B_{12}$, A, D, E, and K
- destroying or transforming toxic products into less harmful compounds
- maintaining normal glucose levels in the blood
- destroying old erythrocytes and releasing bilirubin
- producing various blood proteins, such as prothrombin and fibrinogen, that aid in blood clotting

## Pancreas

The (2) **pancreas** is an elongated, somewhat flattened organ that lies posterior and slightly inferior to the stomach. It performs both endocrine and exocrine functions. As an endocrine gland, the pancreas secretes insulin directly into the bloodstream to maintain normal blood glucose levels. For a comprehensive discussion of the endocrine function of the pancreas, review Chapter 13. As an exocrine gland, the pancreas produces digestive enzymes that pass into the duodenum through the (3) **pancreatic duct.** The pancreatic duct extends along the pancreas and, together with the (4) **hepatic duct** from the liver, enters the (5) **duodenum.** The digestive enzymes produced by the pancreas contain trypsin, which breaks down proteins; amylase, which breaks down carbohydrates; and lipase, which breaks down fat.

## Gallbladder

The (6) **gallbladder,** a saclike structure on the inferior surface of the liver, serves as a storage area for bile. When bile is needed for digestion, the gallbladder releases it into the duodenum through the (7) **common bile duct.** Bile is also drained from the liver through the (8) **right hepatic duct** and the (9) **left hepatic duct.** These two structures eventually form the hepatic duct. The (10) **cystic duct** of the gallbladder merges with the hepatic duct to form the common bile duct, which leads into the duodenum. Bile production is stimulated by hormone secretions, which are produced in the duodenum, as soon as food enters the small intestine. Without bile, fat digestion is not possible.

 **It is time to review anatomy of the accessory organs of digestion by completing Learning Activity 6–2.**

**Medical Word Elements**

This section introduces combining forms, suffixes, and prefixes related to the digestive system. Word analyses are also provided.

| Element | Meaning | Word Analysis |
|---------|---------|---------------|
| **COMBINING FORMS** | | |
| **Mouth** | | |
| **or/o** | mouth | or/al (OR-ăl): pertaining to the mouth<br>*-al:* pertaining to, relating to |
| **stomat/o** | | stomat/itis (stŏ-mă-TĪ-tĭs): inflammation of the mouth<br>*-itis:* inflammation |
| **gloss/o** | tongue | gloss/ectomy (glŏs-ĔK-tō-mē): removal of all or part of the tongue<br>*-ectomy:* excision, removal |
| **lingu/o** | | lingu/al (LĬNG-gwăl): pertaining to the tongue<br>*-al:* pertaining to, relating to |
| **bucc/o** | cheek | bucc/al (BŬK-ăl): pertaining to the cheek<br>*-al:* pertaining to, relating to |
| **cheil/o** | lip | cheil/o/plasty (KĪ-lō-plăs-tē): surgical repair of a defect of the lip<br>*-plasty:* surgical repair |
| **labi/o** | | labi/al (LĀ-bē-ăl): pertaining to the lips, particularly the lips of the mouth<br>*-al:* pertaining to, relating to |
| **dent/o** | teeth | dent/ist (DĔN-tĭst): specialist who diagnoses and treats diseases and disorders of teeth and tissues of the oral cavity<br>*-ist:* specialist |
| **odont/o** | | orth/odont/ist (or-thō-DŎN-tĭst): dentist who specializes in correcting and preventing irregularities of abnormally positioned or aligned teeth<br>*orth:* straight<br>*-ist:* specialist |

*(Continued)*

| Element | Meaning | Word Analysis | _(Continued)_ |
|---------|---------|---------------|---------------|
| **gingiv/o** | gum(s) | gingiv/ectomy (jĭn-jĭ-VĔK-tō-mē): excision of diseased gingival tissue in surgical treatment of periodontal disease<br>_-ectomy:_ excision, removal | |
| **sial/o** | saliva, salivary gland | sial/o/lith (sī-ĂL-ō-lĭth): calculus formed in a salivary gland or duct<br>_-lith:_ stone, calculus | |

### Esophagus, Pharynx, and Stomach

| Element | Meaning | Word Analysis | |
|---------|---------|---------------|---|
| **esophag/o** | esophagus | esophag/o/scope (ē-SŎF-ă-gō-skōp): endoscope used to examine the esophagus<br>_-scope:_ instrument for examining | |
| **pharyng/o** | pharynx (throat) | pharyng/o/tonsill/itis (fă-rĭng-gō-tŏn-sĭ-LĪ-tĭs): inflammation of the pharynx and tonsils<br>_tonsill:_ tonsils<br>_-itis:_ inflammation | |
| **gastr/o** | stomach | gastr/algia (găs-TRĂL-jē-ă): pain in the stomach from any cause; also called _stomachache_<br>_-algia:_ pain | |
| **pylor/o** | pylorus | pylor/o/spasm (pī-LOR-ō-spăzm): involuntary contraction of the pyloric sphincter of the stomach, as in pyloric stenosis<br>_-spasm:_ involuntary contraction, twitching | |

### Small Intestine

| Element | Meaning | Word Analysis | |
|---------|---------|---------------|---|
| **duoden/o** | duodenum (first part of small intestine) | duoden/o/scopy (dū-ŏd-ē-NŎS-kō-pē): visual examination of the duodenum<br>_-scopy:_ visual examination | |
| **enter/o** | intestine (usually small intestine) | enter/o/pathy (ĕn-tĕr-ŎP-ă-thē): any intestinal disease<br>_-pathy:_ disease | |
| **jejun/o** | jejunum (second part of small intestine) | jejun/o/rrhaphy (jĕ-joo-NOR-ă-fē): suture of the jejunum<br>_-rrhaphy:_ suture | |

| Element | Meaning | Word Analysis |
|---------|---------|---------------|
| **ile/o** | ileum (third part of small intestine) | ile/o/stomy (ĭl-ē-ŎS-tō-mē): creation of an opening between the ileum and the abdominal wall<br><br>*-stomy\**: forming an opening (mouth)<br><br>*An ileostomy creates an opening on the surface of the abdomen to allow feces to be discharged into a bag worn on the abdomen.* |
| **Large Intestine** | | |
| **append/o** | appendix | append/ectomy (ăp-ĕn-DĔK-tō-mē): excision of the appendix<br><br>*-ectomy:* excision, removal<br><br>*Appendectomy is performed to remove a diseased appendix in danger of rupturing.* |
| **appendic/o** | | appendic/itis (ă-pĕn-dĭ-SĪ-tĭs): inflammation of the appendix<br><br>*-itis:* inflammation |
| **col/o** | colon | col/o/stomy (kō-LŎS-tō-mē): creation of an opening between the colon and the abdominal wall<br><br>*-stomy\**: forming an opening (mouth)<br><br>*A colostomy creates a place for fecal matter to exit the body other than through the anus.* |
| **colon/o** | | colon/o/scopy (kō-lŏn-ŎS-kō-pē): visual examination of the colon using a colonoscope, an elongated endoscope<br><br>*-scopy:* visual examination |
| **sigmoid/o** | sigmoid colon | sigmoid/o/tomy (sĭg-moyd-ŎT-ō-mē): incision of the sigmoid colon<br><br>*-tomy:* incision |
| **Terminal End of Large Intestine** | | |
| **rect/o** | rectum | rect/o/cele (RĔK-tō-sēl): herniation or protrusion of the rectum; also called *proctocele*<br><br>*-cele:* hernia, swelling |
| **proct/o** | anus, rectum | proct/o/logist (prŏk-TŎL-ō-jĭst): physician who specializes in treating disorders of the colon, rectum, and anus.<br><br>*-logist:* specialist in the study of |
| **an/o** | anus | peri/an/al (pĕr-ē-Ā-năl): pertaining to the area around the anus<br><br>*peri-:* around<br>*-al:* pertaining to, relating to |

*(Continued)*

| Element | Meaning | Word Analysis | (Continued) |
|---|---|---|---|

### Accessory Organs of Digestion

| Element | Meaning | Word Analysis |
|---|---|---|
| **hepat/o** | liver | hepat/o/megaly (hĕp-ă-tō-MĔG-ă-lē): enlargement of the liver, usually a sign of disease<br>  *-megaly:* enlargement |
| **pancreat/o** | pancreas | pancreat/o/lysis (păn-krē-ă-TŎL-ĭ-sĭs): destruction of the pancreas by pancreatic enzymes<br>  *-lysis:* separation; destruction; loosening |
| **cholangi/o** | bile vessel | cholangi/ole (kō-LĂN-jē-ōl): small terminal portion of the bile duct<br>  *-ole:* small, minute |
| **chol/e**** | bile, gall | chol/e/lith (KŌ-lē-lĭth): gallstone<br>  *-lith:* calculus, stone<br>*Gallstones are solid accumulations of bile and cholesterol that form in the gallbladder and common bile duct.* |
| **cholecyst/o** | gallbladder | cholecyst/ectomy (kō-lē-sĭs-TĔK-tō-mē): removal of the gallbladder by laparoscopic or open surgery<br>  *-ectomy:* excision, removal |
| **choledoch/o** | bile duct | choledoch/o/plasty (kō-LĔD-ō-kō-plăs-tē): surgical repair of the common bile duct<br>  *-plasty:* surgical repair |

### SUFFIXES

| Element | Meaning | Word Analysis |
|---|---|---|
| **-emesis** | vomit | hyper/emesis (hī-pĕr-ĔM-ĕ-sĭs): excessive vomiting<br>  *hyper-:* excessive, above normal |
| **-iasis** | abnormal condition (produced by something specified) | chol/e/lith/iasis (kō-lē-lĭ-THĪ-ă-sĭs): presence or formation of gallstones in the gallbladder or common bile duct<br>  *chol/e:* bile, gall<br>  *lith:* stone, calculus<br>*When gallstones form in the common bile duct, the condition is called* choledocholithiasis. |
| **-megaly** | enlargement | hepat/o/megaly (hĕp-ă-tō-MĔG-ă-lē): enlargement of the liver, usually a sign of disease<br>  *hepat/o:* liver<br>*Hepatomegaly may be caused by hepatitis or infection, fatty infiltration (as in alcoholism), biliary obstruction, or malignancy.* |

| Element | Meaning | Word Analysis |
|---------|---------|---------------|
| **-orexia** | appetite | an/orexia (ăn-ō-RĔK-sē-ă): loss of appetite<br>*an-:* without, not<br>*Anorexia can result from various conditions, such as adverse effects of drugs or various physical or psychological causes.* |
| **-pepsia** | digestion | dys/pepsia (dĭs-PĔP-sē-ă): epigastric discomfort felt after eating; also called *indigestion*<br>*dys-:* bad; painful; difficult |
| **-phagia** | swallowing, eating | aer/o/phagia (ĕr-ō-FĀ-jē-ă): swallowing of air<br>*aer/o:* air |
| **-prandial** | meal | post/prandial (pōst-PRĂN-dē-ăl): following a meal<br>*post-:* after, behind |
| **-rrhea** | discharge, flow | steat/o/rrhea (stē-ă-tō-RĒ-ă): excessive amount of fat discharged in fecal matter<br>*-rrhea:* discharge, flow |
| **PREFIXES** | | |
| **dia-** | through, across | dia/rrhea (dī-ă-RĒ-ă): abnormally frequent discharge or flow of fluid fecal matter from the bowel<br>*-rrhea:* discharge, flow |
| **peri-** | around | peri/sigmoid/itis (pĕr-ĭ-sĭg-moy-DĪ-tĭs): inflammation of peritoneal tissue around the sigmoid colon<br>*peri-:* around |
| **sub-** | under, below | sub/lingu/al (sŭb-LĬNG-gwăl): pertaining to the area under the tongue<br>*lingu:* tongue<br>*-al:* pertaining to, relating to |

*When the suffix *-stomy* is used with a combining form that denotes an organ, it refers to a surgical opening to the outside of the body.

**The *e* in *chol/e* is an exception to the rule of using the connecting vowel *o*.

 **It is time to review medical word elements by completing Learning Activities 6–3 and 6–4.**

## Pathology

Although some digestive disorders may be asymptomatic, many are associated with such symptoms as nausea, vomiting, bleeding, pain, and weight loss. Clinical signs, such as jaundice and edema, may indicate a hepatic disorder. Severe infection, drug toxicity, hepatic disease, and changes in fluid and electrolyte balance can cause behavioral abnormalities. Disorders of the GI tract or any of the accessory organs (liver, gallbladder, pancreas) may result in far-reaching metabolic or systemic problems that can eventually threaten life itself. Assessment of a suspected digestive disorder must include a thorough history and physical examination. A range of diagnostic tests assist in identifying abnormalities of the GI tract, liver, gallbladder, and pancreas.

For diagnosis, treatment, and management of digestive disorders, the medical services of a specialist may be warranted. Gastroenterology is the branch of medicine concerned with digestive diseases. The physician who specializes in the diagnoses and treatment of digestive disorders is known as a *gastroenterologist*. Gastroenterologists do not perform surgeries; however, under the broad classification of surgery, they do perform such procedures as liver biopsy and endoscopic examination.

## Ulcer

An ulcer is a circumscribed lesion (open sore) of the skin or mucous membrane. Peptic ulcers are the most common type of ulcer that occurs in the digestive system. There are two main types of peptic ulcers: gastric ulcers, which develop in the stomach, and duodenal ulcers, which develop in the duodenum, usually in the area nearest the stomach. A third type of ulceration that affects the digestive system is associated with a disorder called colitis. As the name implies, it occurs in the colon.

### Peptic Ulcer Disease

Peptic ulcer disease (PUD) develops in the parts of the GI tract that are exposed to hydrochloric acid and pepsin. Both of these products are found in gastric juice and normally act on food to begin the digestive process. The strong action of these digestive products can destroy the protective defenses of the mucous membranes of the stomach and duodenum, causing the lining to erode. Eventually, an ulcer forms. If left untreated, mucosal destruction forms a hole (perforation) in the wall lining.

Current scientific studies have identified bacterial infection with *Helicobacter pylori* as a leading cause of PUD. Its spiral shape helps the bacterium burrow into the mucosa, weakening it and making it more susceptible to the action of pepsin and stomach acid. These studies have also found that *H. pylori* releases a toxin that promotes mucosal inflammation and ulceration. Antibiotics and antacids are used to treat peptic ulcers. Patients are advised to avoid nonsteroidal anti-inflammatory drugs (NSAIDs), caffeine, smoking, and alcohol, which exacerbate the symptoms of gastric ulcers.

### Ulcerative Colitis

Ulcerative colitis, a chronic inflammatory disease of the large intestine and rectum, commonly begins in the rectum or sigmoid colon and extends upward into the entire colon. It is characterized by profuse, watery diarrhea containing varying amounts of blood, mucus, and pus. Ulcerative colitis is distinguished from other closely related bowel disorders by its characteristic inflammatory pattern. The inflammation involves only the mucosal lining of the colon, and the affected portion of the colon is uniformly involved, with no patches of healthy mucosal tissue evident. Ulcerative colitis is associated with a higher risk of colon cancer. Severe cases may require surgical creation of an opening (stoma) for bowel evacuation to a bag worn on the abdomen.

## Hernia

A hernia is a protrusion of any organ, tissue, or structure through the wall of the cavity in which it is naturally contained. (See Figure 6–5.) In general, though, the term is applied to the protrusion of an abdominal organ (viscus) through the abdominal wall.

An (1) **inguinal hernia** develops in the groin where the abdominal folds of flesh meet the thighs. In initial stages, it may be hardly noticeable and appears as a soft lump under the skin, no larger than a marble. In early stages, an inguinal hernia is usually reducible; that is, it can be pushed gently back into its normal place. With this type of hernia, pain may be minimal. As time passes, pressure of the abdomen against the weak abdominal wall may increase the size of the opening as well as the size of the hernia lump. If the blood supply to the hernia is cut off because of pressure, a (2) **strangulated hernia** with gangrene (necrosis) may develop. An (3) **umbilical hernia** is a protrusion of part of the intestine at the navel. It occurs more commonly in obese women and among those who have had several pregnancies. Hernias also occur in newborn infants (congenital) or during early childhood. If the defect has not corrected itself by age 2, the deformity can be surgically corrected. Treatment consists of surgical repair of the hernia (hernioplasty) with suture of the abdominal wall (herniorrhaphy).

Although hernias most commonly occur in the abdominal region, they may develop in the diaphragm. Two forms of hernia of the diaphragm include (4) **diaphragmatic hernia,** a congenital disorder, and (5) **hiatal hernia,** in which the lower part of the esophagus and the top of the stomach slides through an opening (hiatus) in the diaphragm into the thorax. With hiatal hernia, stomach acid backs up into the esophagus causing heartburn, chest pain, and swallowing difficulty. Although many hiatal hernias are asymptomatic, if the disease continues for a prolonged period, it may cause gastroesophageal reflux disease (GERD).

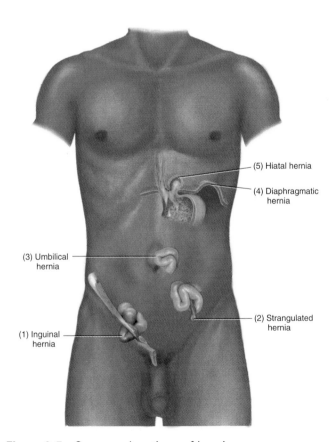

**Figure 6–5**  Common locations of hernia.

## Bowel Obstruction

A life-threatening obstruction in which the bowel twists on itself (volvulus) with occlusion of the blood supply occurs most frequently in middle-aged and elderly men. The accumulation of gas and fluid coupled with loss of blood supply (ischemia) in the trapped bowel eventually leads to tissue death (necrosis), perforation, and an inflammation of the peritoneum (peritonitis). Surgery is required to untwist the bowel.

Telescoping of the intestine within itself (intussusception) occurs when one part of the intestine slips into another part located below it, much as a telescope is shortened by pushing one section into the next. This is a rare type of intestinal obstruction more common in infants 10 to 15 months of age than in adults. Surgery is usually necessary to correct this obstruction.

## Hemorrhoids

Enlarged veins in the mucous membrane of the anal canal are called *hemorrhoids*—especially when they bleed, hurt, or itch. They may occur inside (internal) or outside (external) the rectal area. Hemorrhoids are usually caused by abdominal pressure, such as from straining during bowel movement, pregnancy, and standing or sitting for long periods. They may also be associated with some disorders of the liver or the heart.

A high-fiber diet as well as drinking plenty of water and juices plays a pivotal role in hemorrhoid prevention. Temporary relief from hemorrhoids can usually be obtained by cold compresses, sitz baths, stool softeners, or analgesic ointments. Treatment of an advanced hemorrhoidal condition involves surgical removal (hemorrhoidectomy).

## Liver Disorders

A growing public health concern is the increasing incidence of viral **hepatitis.** Even though its mortality rate is low, the disease is easily transmitted and can cause significant morbidity and prolonged loss of time from school or employment. The two most common forms of hepatitis are hepatitis A, also called *infectious hepatitis,* and hepatitis B, also called *serum hepatitis.* The most common causes of hepatitis A are ingestion of contaminated food, water, or milk. Hepatitis B is usually transmitted by routes other than the mouth (parenteral), such as from blood transfusions and sexual contact. Because of patient exposure, health-care personnel are at increased risk for contracting hepatitis B, but a vaccine that provides immunity to hepatitis B is available.

One of the major symptoms of many liver disorders, including hepatitis and cirrhosis, is a yellowing of the skin (jaundice). Because the liver is no longer able to remove bilirubin, a yellow product formed when erythrocytes are destroyed, bilirubin appears in the skin and mucous membranes. This condition is also known as *icterus.* Jaundice may also result when the bile duct is blocked, causing bile to enter the bloodstream.

## Diverticulosis

Diverticulosis is a condition in which small, blisterlike pockets (diverticula) develop in the inner lining of the large intestine and may balloon through the intestinal wall. These pockets occur most commonly in the sigmoid colon. They commonly do not cause any problem unless they become inflamed (diverticulitis). (See Figure 6–6.) Signs and symptoms of diverticulitis include pain, usually in the left lower quadrant (LLQ) of the abdomen; extreme constipation (**obstipation**) or diarrhea; fever; abdominal swelling; and occasional blood in bowel movements. The usual treatment for diverticulitis consists of bed rest, antibiotics, and a soft diet. In severe cases, however, excision of the diverticulum (diverticulectomy) may be advised.

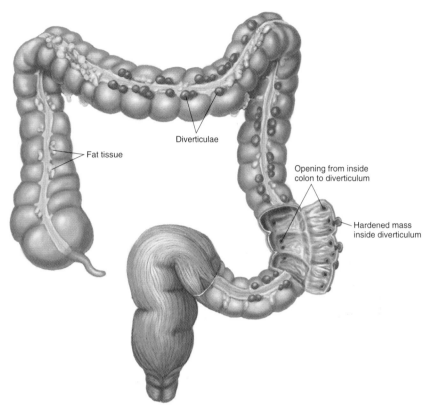

Diverticulae

Fat tissue

Opening from inside
colon to diverticulum

Hardened mass
inside diverticulum

**Figure 6–6**   Diverticula of the colon.

## Oncology

Although stomach cancer is rare in the United States, it is common in many parts of the world where food preservation is problematic. It is an important medical problem because of its high mortality rate. Men are more susceptible to stomach cancer than women. The neoplasm nearly always develops from the epithelial or mucosal lining of the stomach in the form of a cancerous glandular tumor (gastric adenocarcinoma). Persistent indigestion is one of the important warning signs of stomach cancer. Other types of GI carcinomas include esophageal carcinomas, hepatocellular carcinomas, and pancreatic carcinomas.

Colorectal cancer arises from the epithelial lining of the large intestine. Signs and symptoms, which depend largely on the location of the malignancy, include changes in bowel habits, passage of blood and mucus in stools, rectal or abdominal pain, anemia, weight loss, obstruction, and perforation. A suddenly developing obstruction may be the first symptom of cancer involving the colon between the cecum and the sigmoid because in this region, where bowel contents are liquid, a slowly developing obstruction will not become evident until the lumen is almost closed. Cancer of the sigmoid and rectum causes earlier symptoms of partial obstruction with constipation alternating with diarrhea, lower abdominal cramping pain, and distention.

## Diagnostic, Symptomatic, and Related Terms

This section introduces diagnostic, symptomatic, and related terms and their meanings. Word analyses for selected terms are also provided.

| Term | Definition |
|------|-----------|
| **anorexia**<br>ăn-ō-RĔK-sē-ă<br><br>  *an-:* without, not<br>  *-orexia:* appetite | Lack or loss of appetite, resulting in the inability to eat<br><br>*Anorexia should not be confused with anorexia nervosa, which is a complex psychogenic eating disorder characterized by an all-consuming desire to remain thin. Anorexia nervosa and a similar eating disorder called bulimia nervosa are discussed in Chapter 14.* |
| **appendicitis**<br>ă-pĕn-dĭ-SĪ-tĭs<br><br>  *appendic:* appendix<br>  *-itis:* inflammation | Inflammation of the appendix, usually due to obstruction or infection<br><br>*If left undiagnosed, appendicitis rapidly leads to perforation and peritonitis. Treatment is appendectomy within 24 to 48 hours of the first symptoms because delay usually results in rupture and peritonitis as fecal matter is released into the peritoneal cavity. (See Figure 6–7.)* |
| **ascites**<br>ă-SĪ-tēz | Accumulation of serous fluid in the abdomen<br><br>*Ascites is associated primarily with cirrhosis of the liver, venous hypertension (high blood pressure), cancer, and heart failure.* |
| **borborygmus**<br>bor-bō-RĬG-mŭs | Rumbling or gurgling noises that are audible at a distance and caused by passage of gas through the liquid contents of the intestine |
| **cachexia**<br>kă-KĔKS-ē-ă | General lack of nutrition and wasting occurring in the course of a chronic disease or emotional disturbance |

A. Diseased appendix

B. Incision site

C. Excision of diseased appendix

**Figure 6–7**   Appendectomy.

| Term | Definition |
|---|---|
| **cholelithiasis**<br>kō-lē-li̇-THĪ-ă-sĭs<br><br>*chol/e:* bile, gall<br>*lith:* stone, calculus<br>*-iasis:* abnormal condition<br>(produced by something<br>specified) | Presence or formation of gallstones in the gallbladder or common bile duct<br><br>*Cholelithiasis may or may not produce symptoms. (See Figure 6–8.)* |
| **Crohn disease, regional enteritis**<br>KRŌN dĭ-ZĒZ, RĒ-jŭn-ăl<br>ĕn-tĕr-Ī-tĭs | Chronic inflammation, usually of the ileum, but possibly affecting any portion of the intestinal tract<br><br>*Crohn disease is a chronic disease distinguished from closely related bowel disorders by its inflammatory pattern that causes fever, cramping, diarrhea, and weight loss.* |
| **cirrhosis**<br>sĭr-RŌ-sĭs | Chronic, irreversible, degenerative disease of the liver<br><br>*Cirrhosis is most commonly caused by chronic alcoholism but may also be caused by toxins, infectious agents, metabolic diseases, and circulatory disorders. In this disorder, hepatic cells are replaced by fibrous tissue that impairs the flow of blood and lymph within the liver, resulting in hepatic insufficiency.* |
| **colic**<br>KŎL-ĭk | Spasm in any hollow or tubular soft organ accompanied by pain, especially in the colon |
| **deglutition**<br>dē-gloo-TĬSH-ŭn | Act of swallowing |

*(Continued)*

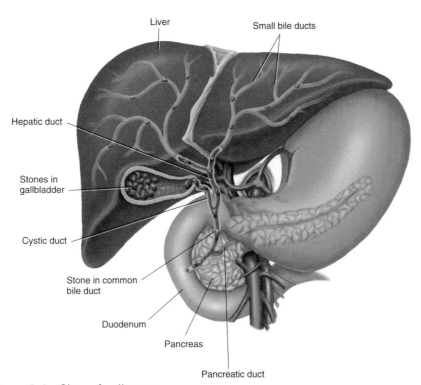

**Figure 6–8**  Sites of gallstones.

| Term | Definition | (Continued) |
|---|---|---|

| Term | Definition |
|---|---|
| **dysentery**<br>DĬS-ĕn-tĕr-ē | Inflammation of the intestine, especially the colon, possibly caused by ingesting water or food containing chemical irritants, bacteria, protozoa, or parasites, that results in bloody diarrhea<br>*Dysentery is common in underdeveloped countries and in times of disaster when sanitary living conditions, clean food, and safe water are not available.* |
| **dyspepsia**<br>dis-PĔP-sē-ă<br><br>*dys-:* bad; painful; difficult<br>*-pepsia:* digestion | Epigastric discomfort felt after eating; also called *indigestion* |
| **dysphagia**<br>dĭs-FĀ-jē-ă<br><br>*dys-:* bad; painful; difficult<br>*-phagia:* swallowing, eating | Inability or difficulty in swallowing; also called *aphagia* |
| **eructation**<br>ĕ-rūk-TĀ-shŭn | Producing gas from the stomach, usually with a characteristic sound; also called *belching* |
| **fecalith**<br>FĒ-kă-lĭth | Fecal concretion |
| **flatus**<br>FLĀ-tŭs | Gas in the GI tract; expelling of air from a body orifice, especially the anus |
| **gastroesophageal reflux disease (GERD)**<br>găs-trō-ĕ-sŏf-ă-JĒ-ăl RĒ-flŭks dĭ-ZĔZ<br><br>*gastr/o:* stomach<br>*esophag:* esophagus<br>*-eal:* pertaining to, relating to | Backflow of gastric contents into the esophagus due to a malfunction of the sphincter muscle at the inferior portion of the esophagus<br>*GERD may occur whenever pressure in the stomach is greater than that in the esophagus and may be associated with heartburn, esophagitis, or chest pain.* |
| **halitosis**<br>hăl-ĭ-TŌ-sĭs | Offensive or "bad" breath |
| **hematemesis**<br>hĕm-ăt-ĔM-ĕ-sĭs<br><br>*hemat:* blood<br>*-emesis:* vomiting | Vomiting of blood<br>*The vomiting of bright red blood, indicating upper GI bleeding, is commonly associated with esophageal varices or peptic ulcer.* |
| **irritable bowel syndrome (IBS)** | Symptom complex marked by abdominal pain and altered bowel function (typically constipation, diarrhea, or alternating constipation and diarrhea) for which no organic cause can be determined; also called *spastic colon*<br>*Contributing or aggravating factors of IBS include anxiety and stress.* |
| **obstipation**<br>ŏb-stĭ-PĀ-shŭn | Intestinal obstruction; also called *severe constipation* |

| Term | Definition |
|------|------------|
| **malabsorption syndrome**<br>măl-ăb-SORP-shŭn  SĬN-drōm | Symptom complex of the small intestine characterized by the impaired passage of nutrients, minerals, or fluids through intestinal villi into the blood or lymph<br><br>*Malabsorption syndrome may be associated with or due to a number of diseases, including those affecting the intestinal mucosa. It may also be due to surgery, such as gastric resection and ileal bypass, or antibiotic therapy.* |
| **oral leukoplakia**<br>OR-ăl  loo-kō-PLĀ-kē-ă<br><br>*leuk/o:* white<br>*-plakia:* plaque | Formation of white spots or patches on the mucous membrane of the tongue, lips, or cheek caused primarily by irritation<br><br>*This precancerous condition is usually associated with pipe or cigarette smoking or ill-fitting dentures.* |
| **melena**<br>MĔL-ĕ-nă | Passage of dark-colored, tarry stools, due to the presence of blood altered by intestinal juices |
| **peristalsis**<br>pĕr-ĭ-STĂL-sĭs | Progressive, wavelike movement that occurs involuntarily in hollow tubes of the body, especially the GI tract |
| **pyloric stenosis**<br>pi-LOR-ĭk  stĕ-NŌ-sĭs<br><br>*pylor:* pylorus<br>*-ic:* pertaining to, relating to<br>*sten:* narrowing, stricture<br>*-osis:* abnormal condition; increase (used primarily with blood cells) | Stricture or narrowing of the pyloric orifice, possibly due to excessive thickening of the pyloric sphincter (circular muscle of the pylorus)<br><br>*Treatment for pyloric stenosis involves surgical section of the thickened muscle around the pyloric orifice.* |
| **regurgitation**<br>rē-gŭr-jĭ-TĀ-shŭn | Backward flowing, as in the return of solids or fluids to the mouth from the stomach or the backward flow of blood through a defective heart valve |
| **steatorrhea**<br>stē-ă-tō-RĒ-ă<br><br>*steat/o:* fat<br>*-rrhea:* discharge, flow | Passage of fat in large amounts in the feces due to failure to digest and absorb it<br><br>*Steatorrhea may occur in pancreatic disease when pancreatic enzymes are not sufficient. It also occurs in malabsorption syndrome.* |

 **It is time to review pathological, diagnostic, symptomatic, and related terms by completing Learning Activity 6–5.**

## Diagnostic and Therapeutic Procedures

This section introduces procedures used to diagnose and treat digestive system disorders. Descriptions are provided as well as pronunciations and word analyses for selected terms.

| Procedure | Description |
|---|---|
| **DIAGNOSTIC PROCEDURES** | |
| Endoscopic | |
| **endoscopy**<br>ĕn-DŎS-kō-pē<br><br>*endo-:* in, within<br>*-scopy:* visual examinination | Visual examination of a cavity or canal using a specialized lighted instrument called an *endoscope*<br><br>*The organ, cavity, or canal being examined dictates the name of the endoscopic procedure. (See Figure 4–5.) A camera and video recorder are commonly used during the procedure to provide a permanent record.* |
| **upper GI** | Endoscopy of the esophagus (esophagoscopy), stomach (gastroscopy), and duodenum (duodenoscopy)<br><br>*Endoscopy of the upper GI tract is performed to identify tumors, esophagitis, gastroesophageal varices, peptic ulcers, and the source of upper GI bleeding. It is also used to confirm the presence and extent of varices in the lower esophagus and stomach in patients with liver disease.* |
| **lower GI** | Endoscopy of the colon (colonoscopy), sigmoid colon (sigmoidoscopy), and rectum and anal canal (proctoscopy) (See Figure 6–9.)<br><br>*Endoscopy of the lower GI tract is used to identify pathological conditions in the colon. It may also be used to remove polyps. When polyps are discovered in the colon, they are retrieved and tested for cancer.* |

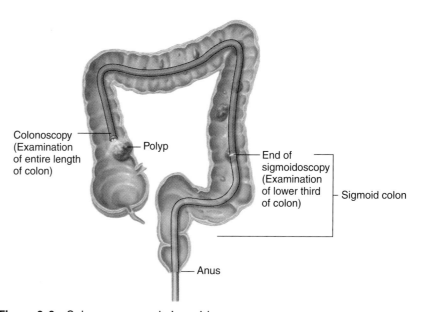

**Figure 6–9**   Colonoscopy and sigmoidoscopy.

| Procedure | Description |
|---|---|
| **Laboratory** | |
| **hepatitis panel**<br>hĕp-ă-TĪ-tĭs<br><br>  *hepat:* liver<br>  *-itis:* inflammation | Panel of blood tests that identify the specific virus—hepatitis A (HAV), hepatitis B (HBV), or hepatitis C (HCV)—causing hepatitis by testing serum using antibodies to each of these antigens |
| **liver function tests (LFTs)**<br>LĬV-ĕr FŬNGK-shŭn tĕsts | Tests involving measurement of the levels of certain enzymes, bilirubin, and various proteins<br><br>*LFTs are used to evaluate metabolism, storage, filtration, and excretory functions.* |
| **serum bilirubin**<br>SĒ-rŭm bĭl-ĭ-ROO-bĭn | Measurement of the level of bilirubin in the blood<br><br>*Elevated serum bilirubin indicates excessive destruction of erythrocytes, liver disease, or biliary tract obstruction. Bilirubin is a breakdown product of hemoglobin and is normally excreted from the body as bile. Excessive bilirubin causes yellowing of the skin and mucous membranes, a condition called* jaundice. |
| **stool culture** | Microbiological procedure in which microorganisms in feces are grown on media or nutrient material to identify specific pathogens |
| **stool guaiac**<br>GWĪ-ăk | Applying a substance called guaiac to a stool sample to detect the presence of blood in the feces; also called *Hemoccult* (trade name of a modified guaiac test)<br><br>*This stool test is performed to detect the presence of blood in the feces that is not apparent on visual inspection (obscure, hidden, or occult blood). It also helps detect colon cancer and determine bleeding in digestive disorders.* |

*(Continued)*

| Procedure | Description | *(Continued)* |
|---|---|---|

### Radiographic

**barium enema**
BĂ-rē-ŭm  ĔN-ĕ-mă

Radiographic examination of the rectum and colon following enema administration of barium sulfate (contrast medium) into the rectum; also called *lower GI series*

*Barium sulfate is used as the contrast medium in a barium enema. It is retained in the lower GI tract during fluoroscopic and radiographic studies. Barium enema is used for diagnosing obstructions, tumors, or other abnormalities of the colon. (See Figure 6–10.)*

**Figure 6–10**    Barium enema done poorly (A) and correctly (B).

**barium swallow**
BĂ-rē-ŭm  SWĂL-ō

Radiographic examination of the esophagus, stomach, and small intestine following oral administration of barium sulfate (contrast medium); also called *esophagram* and *upper GI series*

*Barium swallow is used to diagnose structural defects of the esophagus and vessels, such as esophageal varices. It may also be used to locate swallowed objects.*

**cholecystography**
kō-lē-sĭs-TŎG-ră-fē

chol/e: bile, gall
cyst/o: bladder
-graphy: process of recording

Radiographic images taken of the gallbladder after administration of a contrast material containing iodine, usually in the form of a tablet

*Cholecystography is used to evaluate gallbladder function and determine the presence of disease or gallstones.*

| Procedure | Description |
|---|---|
| **computed tomography (CT) scan** kŏm-PŪ-tĕd tō-MŎG-ră-fē  *tom/o:* to cut  *-graphy:* process of recording | Imaging technique achieved by rotating an x-ray emitter around the area to be scanned and measuring the intensity of transmitted rays from different angles; formerly called *computerized axial tomography*  *In CT scanning, a computer is used to generate a detailed cross-sectional image that appears as a slice. (See Figure 4–4D.) In the digestive system, CT scans are used to view the gallbladder, liver, bile ducts, and pancreas. It is used to diagnose tumors, cysts, inflammation, abscesses, perforation, bleeding, and obstructions.* |
| **endoscopic retrograde cholangiopancreatography (ERCP)** ĕn-dō-SKŎ-pĭk RĔT-rō-grād kŏ-lăn-jē-ō-păn-krē-ă-TŎG-ră-fē  *cholangi/o:* bile vessel  *pancreat/o:* pancreas  *-graphy:* process of recording | Endoscopic procedure that provides radiographic visualization of the bile and pancreatic ducts  *A flexible fiberoptic duodenoscope is placed into the common bile duct. A radiopaque substance is instilled directly into the duct and serial x-ray films are taken. ERCP is useful in identifying partial or total obstruction of these ducts as well as stones, cysts, and tumors.* |
| **percutaneous transhepatic cholangiography** pĕr-kū-TA-nē-ŭs trăns-hĕ-PĂT-ĭk kō-lăn-jē-ŎG-ră-fē  *per-:* through  *cutane:* skin  *-ous:* pertaining to, relating to  *trans-:* through, across  *hepat:* liver  *-ic:* pertaining to, relating to  *cholangi/o:* bile vessel  *-graphy:* process of recording | Radiographic examination of the structure of the bile ducts  *A contrast medium is injected through a needle passed directly into the hepatic duct. The bile duct structure can be viewed for obstructions, anatomic variations, and cysts.* |
| **sialography** sī-ă-LŎG-ră-fē  *sial/o:* saliva, salivary glands  *-graphy:* process of recording | Radiologic examination of the salivary glands and ducts  *Sialography may be performed with or without a contrast medium.* |

*(Continued)*

| Procedure | Description | (Continued) |
|---|---|---|

**ultrasonography (US)**
ŭl-tră-sŏn-ŎG-ră-fē

   *ultra-:* excess, beyond
   *son/o:* sound
   *-graphy:* process of recording

Image produced by using high-frequency sound waves (ultrasound) and displaying the reflected "echoes" on a monitor (A computer analyzes the reflected echos and converts them into an image on a video monitor.); also called *ultrasound, sonography, echo,* and *echogram*

*US is used to detect diseases and deformities in digestive organs, such as the gallbladder, liver, and pancreas. It is also used to locate abdominal masses outside the digestive organs.*

**abdominal**
ăb-DŎM-ĭ-năl

   *abdomin:* abdomen
   *-al:* pertaining to, relating to

Ultrasound visualization of the abdominal aorta, liver, gallbladder, bile ducts, pancreas, kidneys, ureters, and bladder

*Abdominal ultrasound is used to diagnose and locate cysts, tumors, and malformations. It is also used to document the progression of various diseases and guide the insertion of instruments during surgical procedures.*

## Surgical

**biopsy**
BĪ-ŏp-sē

Representative tissue sample removed from a body site for microscopic examination, usually to establish a diagnosis

   **liver**

Use of a large-bore needle to remove a core of liver tissue for histological examination

## THERAPEUTIC PROCEDURES

**nasogastric intubation**
nā-zō-GĂS-trĭk
ĭn-tū-BĀ-shŭn

   *nas/o:* nose
   *gastr:* stomach
   *-ic:* pertaining to, relating to

Insertion of a nasogastric tube through the nose into the stomach to relieve gastric distention by removing gas, gastric secretions, or food; to instill medication, food, or fluids; or to obtain a specimen for laboratory analysis

## Surgical

**anastomosis**
ă-năs-tō-MŌ-sĭs

Surgical joining of two ducts, vessels, or bowel segments to allow flow from one to another

   **ileorectal**
   ĭl-ē-ō-RĔK-tăl

      *ile/o:* ileum
      *rect:* rectum
      *-al:* pertaining to, relating to

Surgical connection of the ileum and rectum after total colectomy, as is sometimes performed in the treatment of ulcerative colitis

   **intestinal**
   ĭn-TĔS-tĭ-năl

Surgical connection of two portions of the intestines; also called *enteroenterostomy*

| Procedure | Description |
|---|---|
| **colostomy**<br>kō-LŎS-tō-mē<br><br>*col/o:* colon<br>*-stomy:* forming an opening (mouth) | Creation of an opening of some portion of the colon through the abdominal wall to its outside surface in order to divert fecal flow to a colostomy bag (See Figure 6–11.) |
| **lithotripsy**<br>LĬTH-ō-trĭp-sē<br><br>*lith/o:* stone, calculus<br>*-tripsy:* crushing | Procedure for eliminating a stone within the urinary system or gallbladder by crushing the stone surgically or using a noninvasive method, such as ultrasonic shock waves, to shatter it |
| **extracorporeal shockwave**<br>ĕks-tră-kor-POR-ē-ăl  SHŎK-wāv | Use of shock waves as a noninvasive method to break up stones in the gallbladder or biliary ducts<br><br>*In extracorporeal shockwave lithotripsy (ESWL), ultrasound is used to locate the stone or stones and to monitor the destruction of the stones. The patient is usually placed on a course of oral dissolution drugs to ensure complete removal of all stones and stone fragments.* |

*(Continued)*

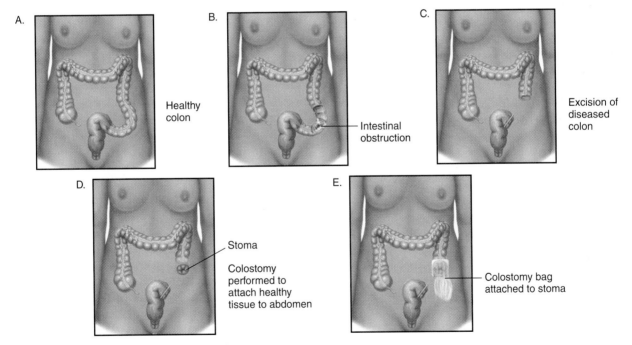

A. Healthy colon

B. Intestinal obstruction

C. Excision of diseased colon

D. Stoma
Colostomy performed to attach healthy tissue to abdomen

E. Colostomy bag attached to stoma

**Figure 6–11**   Colostomy.

| Procedure | Description | (Continued) |
|---|---|---|
| **polypectomy**<br>pŏl-i-PĔK-tō-mē<br><br>*polyp:* small growth<br>*-ectomy:* excision, removal | Excision of a polyp<br><br>*When polyps are discovered during sigmoidoscopy or colonoscopy, polypectomy is used to retrieve them to test for cancer. (See Figure 6–12.)* | |
| **pyloromyotomy**<br>pi-lō-rō-mī-ŎT-ō-mē<br><br>*pylor/o:* pylorus<br>*my/o:* muscle<br>*-tomy:* incision | Incision of the longitudinal and circular muscles of the pylorus; used to treat hypertrophic pyloric stenosis | |

Polyps are removed from
colon for examination

**Figure 6–12**   Polypectomy.

## Pharmacology

Various pharmaceutical agents are available to counteract abnormal conditions that occur in the GI tract. Antacids counteract or decrease excessive stomach acid, which is responsible for heartburn, gastric discomfort, and gastric reflux. Antidiarrheals and antiemetics are used to preserve water and electrolytes, which are essential for body hydration because they control the rapid elimination of digestive materials from the body. Medications that increase or decrease peristalsis are used to regulate the speed at which food passes through the GI tract. These drugs include agents that relieve "cramping" (antispasmodics) and those that help in the movement of material through a sluggish bowel (laxatives). (See Table 6–1.)

## Table 6-1    DRUGS USED TO TREAT DIGESTIVE DISORDERS

This table lists common drug classifications use to treat digestive disorders, their therapeutic actions, and selected generic and trade names.

| Classification | Therapeutic Action | Generic and Trade Names |
|---|---|---|
| **antacids** | Neutralize stomach acid<br><br>*Antacids are used for the treatment and prevention of heartburn and acid reflux and for short-term treatment of active duodenal ulcers and benign gastric ulcers.* | **cimetidine**<br>sĭ-MĔT-ĭ-dēn<br>  *Tagamet, Tagamet HB*<br>**famotidine**<br>fă-MŌ-tĭ-dēn<br>  *Mylanta AR, Pepcid, Pepcid AC* |
| **antidiarrheals** | Control loose stools; relieve diarrhea<br><br>*Antidiarrheals produce a therapeutic effect by absorbing excess water in the stool or slowing peristalsis in the intestinal tract.* | **loperamide**<br>lō-PĔR-ă-mĭd<br>  *Imodium, Imodium A-D, Kaopectate II Caplets, Maalox Antidiarrheal Caplets, Pepto Diarrhea Control*<br>**kaolin/pectin**<br>KĀ-ō-lĭn/PĔK-tĭn<br>  *Donnagel-MB, Kao-Spen, Kapectolin, K-P* |
| **antiemetics** | Control nausea and vomiting<br><br>*The majority of antiemetics block nerve impulses to the vomiting center in the brain.* | **prochlorperazine**<br>prō-klor-PĔR-ă-zēn<br>  *Compazine, Ultrazine*<br>**trimethobenzamide**<br>trī-mĕth-ō-BĔN-ză-mĭd<br>  *T-Gen, Ticon, Tigan, Trimazide* |
| **antispasmodics** | Decrease gastrointestinal spasms<br><br>*Antispasmodics are anticholinergics that decrease spasms by slowing peristalsis and motility throughout the GI tract. They are used in the treatment of irritable bowel syndrome (IBS), spastic colon, and diverticulitis.* | **glycopyrrolate**<br>glĭ-kō-PĬR-rō-lāt<br>  *Robinul, Robinul-Forte*<br>**propantheline**<br>prō-PĂN-thĕ-lēn<br>  *Pro-Banthine* |
| **laxatives** | Treat constipation<br><br>*Laxatives produce a therapeutic effect by increasing peristaltic activity in the large intestine or increasing water and electrolyte secretion into the bowel to induce defecation.* | **senna, sennosides**<br>SĔN-ă, SĔN-ō-sĭdz<br>  *Dosaflex, Senna-Gen, Senokot, Senolax*<br>**psyllium**<br>SĬL-ē-ŭm<br>  *Fiberall, Hydrocil, Metamucil, Mylanta Natural Fiber Supplement* |

## Abbreviations

This section introduces digestive-related abbreviations and their meanings.

| Abbreviation | Meaning |
|---|---|
| **COMMON** | |
| **ABC** | aspiration biopsy cytology |
| **alk phos** | alkaline phosphatase |
| **ALT** | alanine aminotransferase (elevated in liver and heart disease); formerly *SGPT* |
| **AST** | angiotensin sensitivity test; aspartate aminotransferase (cardiac enzyme, formerly called *SGOT*) |
| **Ba** | barium |
| **BaE** | barium enema |
| **BM** | bowel movement |
| **CT** | computed tomography |
| **CT scan, CAT scan** | computed tomography scan |
| **EGD** | esophagogastroduodenoscopy |
| **ERCP** | endoscopic retrograde cholangiopancreatography |
| **GB** | gallbladder |
| **GBS** | gallbladder series |
| **GER** | gastroesophageal reflux |
| **GERD** | gastroesophageal reflux disease |
| **GI** | gastrointestinal |
| **HAV** | hepatitis A virus |
| **HBV** | hepatitis B virus |
| **HCV** | hepatitis C virus |
| **HDV** | hepatitis D virus |
| **HEV** | hepatitis E virus |
| **IBS** | irritable bowel syndrome |
| **NG** | nasogastric |
| **PUD** | peptic ulcer disease |
| **R/O** | rule out |

| Abbreviation | Meaning |
|---|---|
| **DOSAGE SCHEDULES*** | |
| **ac** | before meals |
| **bid** | twice a day |
| **npo** | nothing by mouth |
| **pc, pp** | after meals (postprandial) |
| **po** | by mouth (per os) |
| **prn** | as required |
| **qam, qm** | every morning |
| **qh** | every hour<br><br>*This abbreviation may also contain a number to indicate the number of hours between administration of medication or therapy, as in q8h.* |
| **q2h** | every 2 hours |
| **qid** | four times a day |
| **qod**** | every other day |
| **qpm, qn** | every night |
| **stat** | immediately |
| **tid** | three times a day |

*Because many of these abbreviations deal with pharmacology and the administration of medication, they are not unique to the digestive system.

**Although this abbreviation is currently found in medical records and clinical notes, the Joint Commission on Accreditation of Healthcare Organizations (JCAHO) requires its discontinuance. Instead, write out its meaning.

**It is time to review procedures, pharmacology, and abbreviations by completing Learning Activity 6–6.**

# LEARNING ACTIVITIES

The following activities provide review of the digestive system terms introduced in this chapter. Complete each activity and review your answers to evaluate your understanding of the chapter.

## Learning Activity 6–1

### Identifying digestive structures

*Label the illustration on page 139 using the terms listed below.*

| | | |
|---|---|---|
| anus | hepatic flexure | rectum |
| appendix | ileum | sigmoid colon |
| ascending colon | jejunum | spleen |
| cecum | liver | splenic flexure |
| descending colon | pancreas | transverse colon |
| duodenum | | |

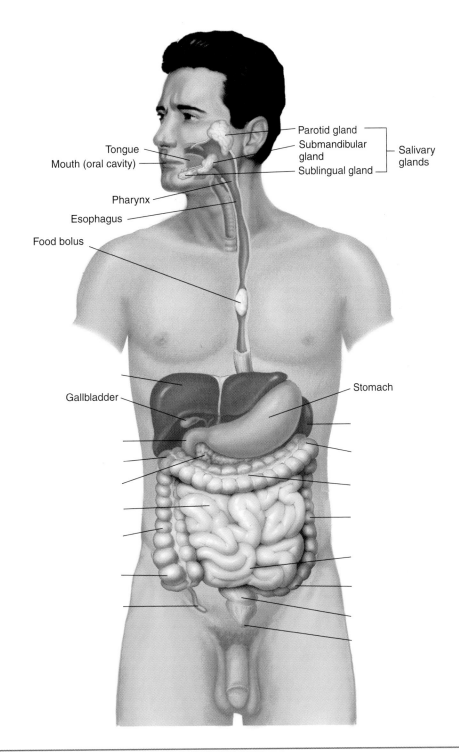

Parotid gland
Submandibular gland
Sublingual gland
Salivary glands
Tongue
Mouth (oral cavity)
Pharynx
Esophagus
Food bolus
Gallbladder
Stomach

 Check your answers by referring to Figure 6–3 on page 112. Review material that you did not answer correctly.

Learning Activity 6–2

## Identifying accessory organs of digestion

*Label the following illustration using the terms listed below.*

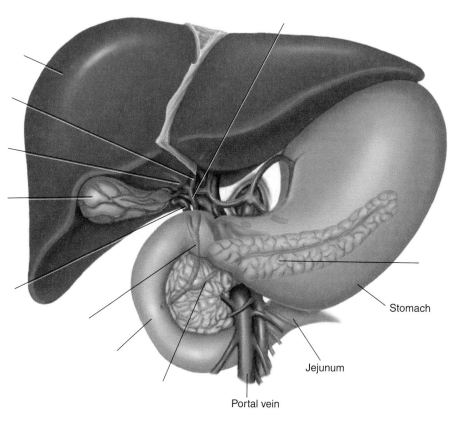

Stomach

Jejunum

Portal vein

| | | |
|---|---|---|
| *common bile duct* | *hepatic duct* | *pancreas* |
| *cystic duct* | *left hepatic duct* | *pancreatic duct* |
| *duodenum* | *liver* | *right hepatic duct* |
| *gallbladder* | | |

Check your answers by referring to Figure 6–4 on page 113. Review material that you did not answer correctly.

# Learning Activity 6-3

## Building medical words

*Use* **esophag/o** *(esophagus) to build words that mean:*

1. pain in the esophagus _____
2. spasm of the esophagus _____
3. stricture or narrowing of the esophagus _____

*Use* **gastr/o** *(stomach) to build words that mean:*

4. inflammation of the stomach _____
5. pain in the stomach _____
6. disease of the stomach _____

*Use* **duoden/o** *(duodenum),* **jejun/o** *(jejunum), or* **ile/o** *(ileum) to build words that mean:*

7. excision of all or part of the jejunum _____
8. relating to the duodenum _____
9. inflammation of the ileum _____
10. concerning the jejunum and ileum _____

*Use* **enter/o** *(usually small intestine) to build words that mean:*

11. inflammation of the small intestine _____
12. disease of the small intestine _____

*Use* **col/o** *(colon) to build words that mean:*

13. inflammation of the colon _____
14. pertaining to the colon and rectum _____
15. inflammation of the small intestine and colon _____
16. prolapse or downward displacement of the colon _____
17. disease of the colon _____

*Use* **proct/o** *(anus, rectum) or* **rect/o** *(rectum) to build words that mean:*

18. narrowing or constriction of the rectum _____
19. herniation of the rectum _____
20. paralysis of the anus (anal muscles) _____

*Use* **chol/e** *(bile, gall) to build words that mean:*

21. inflammation of the gallbladder _____
22. abnormal condition of a gallstone _____

*Use* **hepat/o** *(liver) or* **pancreat/o** *(pancreas) to build words that mean:*

23. tumor of the liver _____
24. enlargement of the liver _____
25. inflammation of the pancreas _____

✓ Check your answers in Appendix A. Review material that you did not answer correctly.

**CORRECT ANSWERS** _____ × 4 = _____ **% SCORE**

Learning Activity 6–4

## Building surgical words

*Build a surgical word that means:*

1. excision of gums (tissue) _____

2. partial or complete excision of the tongue _____

3. repair of the esophagus _____

4. removal of part or all of the stomach _____

5. forming an opening between the stomach and jejunum _____

6. excision of (part of) the esophagus _____

7. forming an opening between the stomach, small intestine, and colon _____

8. surgical repair of the small intestine _____

9. fixation of the small intestine (to the abdominal wall) _____

10. suture of the bile duct _____

11. forming an opening into the colon _____

12. fixation of a movable liver (to the abdominal wall) _____

13. surgical repair of the anus or rectum _____

14. removal of the gallbladder _____

15. surgical repair of a bile duct _____

Check your answers in Appendix A. Review material that you did not answer correctly.

**CORRECT ANSWERS** _____ × **6.67** = _____ **% SCORE**

## Learning Activity 6–5

### Matching pathological, diagnostic, symptomatic, and related terms

*Match the following terms with the definitions in the numbered list.*

| | | |
|---|---|---|
| anorexia | dysphagia | hematemesis |
| cachexia | dyspnea | lesion |
| cirrhosis | fecalith | melena |
| dyspepsia | halitosis | obstipation |

1. _____ vomiting blood
2. _____ difficulty swallowing or inability to swallow
3. _____ fecal concretion
4. _____ "bad" breath
5. _____ loss of appetite
6. _____ poor digestion
7. _____ degenerative liver disease
8. _____ state of ill health, malnutrition, and wasting
9. _____ intractable constipation
10. _____ open sore

✓ Check your answers in Appendix A. Review any material that you did not answer correctly.

**CORRECT ANSWERS** _____ × 10 = _____ **% SCORE**

# Learning Activity 6–6

## Matching procedures, pharmacology, and abbreviations

*Match the following terms with the definitions in the numbered list.*

| | | | |
|---|---|---|---|
| *anastomosis* | *emetics* | *liver function tests* | *qid* |
| *antacids* | *endoscopy* | *lower GI series* | *stat* |
| *bid* | *gastroscopy* | *pc, pp* | *stool guaiac* |
| *bilirubin* | *intubation* | *ultrasonography* | *stomatoplasty* |
| *choledochoplasty* | *laxatives* | *proctosigmoidoscopy* | *upper GI series* |

1. _____ after meals

2. _____ breakdown of hemoglobin, normally excreted from the body as bile

3. _____ agents that produce vomiting

4. _____ twice a day

5. _____ surgical reconstruction of a bile duct

6. _____ an enema with a barium solution is administered while a series of radiographs are taken of the large intestine

7. _____ visual examination of the stomach

8. _____ surgical reconstruction of the mouth

9. _____ insertion of a tube into any hollow organ

10. _____ surgical formation of a passage or opening between two hollow viscera or vessels

11. _____ detects presence of blood in the feces; also called Hemoccult

12. _____ visual examination of a cavity or canal using a specialized lighted instrument

13. _____ used to treat constipation

14. _____ neutralize excess acid in the stomach and help to relieve gastritis and ulcer pain

15. _____ procedure in which high-frequency sound waves produce images of internal body structures that are displayed on a monitor

16. _____ measures the levels of certain enzymes, bilirubin, and various proteins

17. _____ four times a day

18. _____ immediately

19. _____ endoscopic procedure for visualization of the rectosigmoid colon

20. _____ barium solution swallowed for a radiographic examination of the esophagus, stomach, and duodenum

✓ Check your answers in Appendix A. Review material that you did not answer correctly.

**CORRECT ANSWERS** _____ × 5 = _____ **% SCORE**

# MEDICAL RECORD ACTIVITIES

The two medical records included in the following activities use common clinical scenarios to show how medical terminology is used to document patient care. Complete the terminology and analysis sections for each activity to help you recognize and understand terms related to the digestive system.

## Medical Record Activity 6–1

### GI evaluation

#### Terminology

The terms listed in the chart come from the medical record *GI Evaluation* that follows. Use a medical dictionary such as *Taber's Cyclopedic Medical Dictionary*, the appendices of this book, or other resources to define each term. Then review the pronunciations for each term and practice by reading the medical record aloud.

| Term | Definition |
|---|---|
| **appendectomy***<br>ăp-ĕn-DĔK-tō-mē | |
| **cholecystectomy**<br>kō-lē-sis-TĔK-tō-mē | |
| **cholecystitis**<br>kō-lē-sĭs-TĪ-tĭs | |
| **cholelithiasis***<br>kō-lē-lĭ-THĪ-ă-sĭs | |
| **crescendo**<br>kră-SHĔN-dō | |
| **decrescendo**<br>dā-kră-SHĔN-dō | |
| **defecate**<br>DĔF-ĕ-kāt | |
| **flatus**<br>FLĀ-tŭs | |
| **heme-negative stool**<br>hēm-NĔG-ă-tĭv | |
| **hepatomegaly**<br>hĕp-ă-tō-MĔG-ă-lē | |
| **intermittent**<br>ĭn-tĕr-MĬT-ĕnt | |

*(Continued)*

| Term | Definition | (Continued) |
|---|---|---|
| **nausea**<br>NAW-sē-ă | | |
| **PMH** | | |
| **postoperative**<br>pōst-ŎP-ĕr-ă-tǐv | | |
| **R/O** | | |
| **splenomegaly**<br>splē-nō-MĔG-ă-lē | | |
| **tonsillectomy**<br>tōn-sǐl-ĔK-tō-mē | | |

*Refer to Figure 6–5 and Figure 6–8 for a visual illustration of these terms.

## GI EVALUATION

**HISTORY OF PRESENT ILLNESS:**  The patient's abdominal pain began 2 years ago when she first had intermittent, sharp epigastric pain. Each episode lasted 2 to 4 hours. Eventually, she was diagnosed as having cholecystitis with cholelithiasis and underwent cholecystectomy. Three to five large calcified stones were found.

Her postoperative course was uneventful until 4 months ago, when she began having continuous deep right-sided pain.

This pain followed a crescendo pattern and peaked several weeks ago, at a time when family stress was also at its climax. Since then, the pain has been following a decrescendo pattern. It does not cause any nausea or vomiting, does not trigger any urge to defecate, and was not alleviated by passage of flatus. Her PMH is significant only for tonsillectomy, appendectomy, and the cholecystectomy. Her PE findings indicate that there was no hepatomegaly or splenomegaly. The rectal examination confirmed normal sphincter tone and heme-negative stool.

**IMPRESSION:**  Abdominal pain. R/O hepatomegaly and splenomegaly.

**PLAN:**  Schedule a complete barium workup for possible obstruction.

### Analysis

**Review the medical record *GI Evaluation* to answer the following questions.**

1. While referring to Figure 6–3, describe the location of the gallbladder in relation to the liver.

   _____

2. Why did the patient undergo the cholecystectomy?

   _____

3. List the patient's prior surgeries.

   _____

4. How does the patient's most recent postoperative episode of discomfort (pain) differ from the initial pain she described?

   _____

Medical Record Activity 6-2

## Esophagogastroduodenoscopy with biopsy

### Terminology

The terms listed in the chart come from the medical record *Esophagogastroduodenoscopy with Biopsy* that follows. Use a medical dictionary such as *Taber's Cyclopedic Medical Dictionary*, the appendices of this book, or other resources to define each term. Then review the pronunciations for each term and practice by reading the medical record aloud.

| Term | Definition |
|------|------------|
| **Demerol**<br>DĔM-ĕr-ŏl | |
| **duodenal bulb**<br>dū-ō-DĒ-năl BŬLB | |
| **duodenitis**<br>dū-ŏd-ĕ-NĪ-tĭs | |
| **erythema**<br>ĕr-ĭ-THĒ-mă | |
| **esophageal varices**<br>ē-sŏf-ă-JĒ-ăl VĂR-ĭ-sēz | |
| **esophagogastroduodenoscopy**<br>ĕ-SŎF-ă-gō-GĂS-trō-doo-ō-dĕn-ŎS-kō-pē | |
| **etiology**<br>ē-tē-ŎL-ō-jē | |
| **friability**<br>frī-ă-BĬL-ĭ-tē | |
| **gastric antrum**<br>GĂS-trĭk ĂN-trŭm | |
| **gastritis**<br>găs-TRĪ-tĭs | |
| **hematemesis**<br>hĕm-ăt-ĔM-ĕ-sĭs | |
| **lateral recumbent**<br>LĂT-ĕr-ăl rē-KŬM-bĕnt | |
| **oximeter**<br>ŏk-SĬM-ĕ-tĕr | |
| **punctate erythema**<br>PŬNK-tāt ĕr-ĭ-THĒ-mă | |

*(Continued)*

| Term | Definition | (Continued) |
|------|-----------|-------------|
| tomography<br>tŏ-MŎG-ră-fē | | |
| Versed<br>VĔR-sĕd | | |
| videoendoscope<br>vĭd-ē-ō-ĔND-ō-skōp | | |

## ESOPHAGOGASTRODUODENOSCOPY WITH BIOPSY

**POSTOPERATIVE DIAGNOSIS:** Diffuse gastritis and duodenitis.

**PROCEDURE:** Esophagogastroduodenoscopy with biopsy.

**TISSUE TO LABORATORY:** Biopsies from gastric antrum and duodenal bulb.

**ESTIMATED BLOOD LOSS:** Nil.

**COMPLICATIONS:** None.

**TIME UNDER SEDATION:** 20 minutes.

**INDICATIONS FOR PROCEDURE:** This is a patient with hematemesis of unknown etiology.

**FINDINGS AND PROCEDURE:** After obtaining informed consent regarding the procedure, its risks, and its alternatives, the patient was taken to the GI Laboratory, where she was placed on the examining table in the left lateral recumbent position. She was given nasal oxygen at 3 liters per minute throughout the procedure and monitored with a pulse oximeter throughout the procedure. Through a previously inserted intravenous line, the patient was sedated with a total of 50 mg of Demerol intravenously plus 4 mg of Versed intravenously throughout the procedure.

The Fujinon computed tomography scan videoendoscope was then readily introduced.

*Esophagus:* The esophageal mucosa appeared normal throughout. No other abnormalities were seen. Specifically, there was prior evidence of esophageal varices.

*Stomach:* There was diffuse erythema with old blood seen within the stomach. No ulcerations, erosions, or fresh bleeding was seen. A representative biopsy was obtained from the gastric antrum and submitted to the pathology laboratory.

*Duodenum:* Punctate erythema was noted in the duodenal bulb. There was some friability. No ulcerations, erosions, or active bleeding was seen. A bulbar biopsy was obtained. The second portion of the duodenum appeared normal.

## Analysis

Review the medical record *Esophagogastroduodenoscopy with Biopsy* to answer the following questions.

1. What caused the hematemesis?

_____

2. What procedures were carried out to determine the cause of bleeding?

_____

3. How much blood did the patient lose during the procedure?

   _____

4. Were there any ulcerations or erosions found during the exploratory procedure that might account for the bleeding?

   _____

5. What type of sedation was used during the procedure?

   _____

6. What did the doctors find when they examined the stomach and duodenum?

   _____

# Chapter

# 7

# Respiratory System

## CHAPTER OUTLINE

## OBJECTIVES

*Upon completion of this chapter, you will be able to:*

- Locate and describe the structures of the respiratory system.
- Recognize, pronounce, spell, and build words related to the respiratory system.
- Describe pathological conditions, diagnostic and therapeutic procedures, and other terms related to the respiratory system.
- Explain pharmacology related to the treatment of respiratory disorders.
- Demonstrate your knowledge of this chapter by completing the learning and medical record activities.

**Key Terms**

This section introduces important respiratory system terms and their definitions. Word analyses are also provided.

| Term | Definition |
|---|---|
| **cytoplasm**<br>SĪ-tō-plăzm<br><br>*cyt/o:* cell<br>*-plasm:* formation, growth | All the material within the cell membrane other than the nucleus |
| **carbon dioxide (CO₂)**<br>KĂR-bŏn dī-ŎK-sīd | Tasteless, colorless, odorless gas produced by body cells during the metabolic process<br><br>*A product of cell respiration, carbon dioxide is carried by the blood to the lungs and exhaled.* |
| **granuloma**<br>grăn-ū-LŌ-mă<br><br>*granul:* granule<br>*-oma:* tumor | Any type of nodular, inflammatory lesion; usually small; may be granular, firm, and persistent and may contain compactly grouped mononuclear phagocytes |
| **mucosa**<br>mū-KŌ-să | Moist tissue layer lining hollow organs and cavities of the body that open to the environment; also called *mucous membrane* |
| **mucus**<br>MŪ-kŭs | Viscous, slippery secretion of mucous membranes that acts as a lubricant and coats and protects many epithelial surfaces, especially the respiratory and genital tracts |
| **naris**<br>NĀ-rĭs | Nostril; opening to the nasal cavity |
| **oxygen (O₂)**<br>ŎK-sĭ-jĕn | Tasteless, odorless, colorless gas essential for human respiration |
| **pH** | Symbol that indicates the degree of acidity or alkalinity of a substance<br><br>*Increasing acidity is expressed as a number less than 7; increasing alkalinity as a number greater than 7, with 7 being neutral. Normal blood is slightly alkaline with a pH range from 7.37 to 7.43. When blood pH is less than 7.37 it is called acidosis; greater than 7.43, alkalosis.* |
| **respiratory failure**<br>RĔS-pĭ-ră-tō-rē | Inability of the cardiac and pulmonary systems to maintain an adequate exchange of oxygen and carbon dioxide in the lungs |
| **septum**<br>SĔP-tŭm | Wall dividing two cavities; for example, the nasal septum that separates the nostrils |
| **sputum**<br>SPŪ-tŭm | Secretions produced in the lungs and bronchi that are expelled by coughing and may contain such pathological elements as cellular debris, mucus, blood, pus, caseous material, and microorganisms |

| Term | Definition |
|------|------------|
| **status asthmaticus**<br>STĀ-tŭs  ăz-MĂ-tĭk-ŭs | Severe, prolonged asthma attack that does not respond to repeated doses of bronchodilators and may lead to respiratory failure and death |
| **surfactant**<br>sŭr-FĂK-tănt | Lipoprotein that decreases the surface tension of alveoli and contributes to their elasticity, thereby reducing the work of breathing |

## Anatomy and Physiology

The organs and structures of the respiratory system are responsible for the exchange of the respiratory gases oxygen and carbon dioxide. Oxygen, essential for life, is delivered to all cells of the body in exchange for carbon dioxide, a waste product. The cardiovascular system assists in this vital function by providing blood vessels, the pathways for transporting these gases. Failure of or deficiency in either system has the same effect on the body: disruption of homeostasis and oxygen starvation in tissues that may result in death.

The lungs and airways bring in fresh, oxygen-enriched air and expel waste carbon dioxide by a process called breathing, or ventilation. Breathing is an important method of regulating the pH of the blood, thereby maintaining homeostasis.

### Upper Respiratory Tract

The breathing process begins with inhalation. (See Figure 7–1.) Air is drawn into the (1) **nasal cavity,** a chamber lined with mucous membranes and tiny hairs called *cilia*. Here, air is filtered, heated, and moistened to prepare it for its journey to the lungs. The nasal cavity is divided into a right and left side by a vertical partition of cartilage called the *nasal septum.*

The receptors for the sense of smell are located in the nasal cavity. These receptors, called the *olfactory neurons,* are found among the epithelial cells lining the nasal tract and are covered with a layer of mucus. Because these receptors are located higher in the nasal passage than air normally inhaled during breathing, a person must sniff or inhale deeply to identify weak odors.

Air passes from the nasal cavity to a muscular tube called the *pharynx,* or *throat,* that serves as a passageway for food and air. It consists of three sections: the (2) **nasopharynx,** posterior to the nose; the (3) **oropharynx,** posterior to the mouth; and the (4) **laryngopharynx,** superior to the larynx.

Within the nasopharynx is a collection of lymphatic tissue known as (5) **adenoids,** or *pharyngeal tonsils.* The (6) **palatine tonsils,** more commonly known as *tonsils,* are located in the oropharynx. They protect the opening to the respiratory tract from microscopic organisms that may attempt entry by this route. The (7) **larynx** (voice box) contains the structures that make vocal sounds possible. A leaf-shaped structure on top of the larynx, the (8) **epiglottis,** seals off the air passage to the lungs during swallowing. This function ensures that food or liquids do not obstruct the flow of air to the lungs. The larynx is a short passage that joins the pharynx with the (9) **trachea** (windpipe). The trachea is composed of smooth muscle embedded with C-shaped rings of cartilage, which provide rigidity to keep the air passage open.

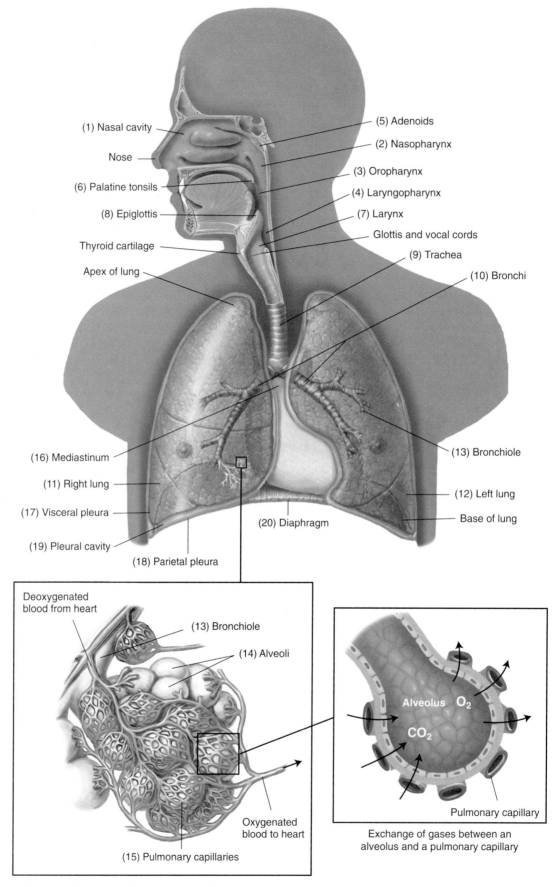

(1) Nasal cavity

Nose

(6) Palatine tonsils

(8) Epiglottis

Thyroid cartilage

Apex of lung

(5) Adenoids

(2) Nasopharynx

(3) Oropharynx

(4) Laryngopharynx

(7) Larynx

Glottis and vocal cords

(9) Trachea

(10) Bronchi

(16) Mediastinum

(11) Right lung

(17) Visceral pleura

(19) Pleural cavity

(18) Parietal pleura

(20) Diaphragm

(13) Bronchiole

(12) Left lung

Base of lung

Deoxygenated
blood from heart

(13) Bronchiole

(14) Alveoli

Oxygenated
blood to heart

(15) Pulmonary capillaries

Alveolus  $O_2$

$CO_2$

Pulmonary capillary

Exchange of gases between an
alveolus and a pulmonary capillary

**Figure 7–1** • Anterior view of the upper and lower respiratory tracts.

## Lower Respiratory Tract

The trachea divides into two branches called (10) **bronchi** (singular, **bronchus**). One branch leads to the (11) **right lung** and the other to the (12) **left lung.** The inner walls of the trachea and bronchi are composed of a mucous membrane embedded with cilia. This membrane traps incoming particles, and the cilia move the entrapped material upward into the pharynx, where it is coughed out, sneezed out, or swallowed. Like the trachea, bronchi contain C-shaped rings of cartilage.

Each bronchus divides into smaller and smaller branches, eventually forming (13) **bronchioles.** Where bronchioles terminate, tiny air sacs called (14) **alveoli** (singular, **alveolus**) are formed. An alveolus resembles a small balloon because it expands and contracts with inflow and outflow of air. The (15) **pulmonary capillaries** lie adjacent to the thin tissue membranes of the alveoli. Carbon dioxide diffuses from the blood within the pulmonary capillaries and enters the alveolar spaces. Simultaneously, oxygen from the alveoli diffuses into the blood. After the exchange of gases, freshly oxygenated blood returns to the heart. It is now ready for delivery to all body tissues.

The lungs are divided into lobes: three lobes in the right lung and two lobes in the left lung. The space between the right and left lungs, called the (16) **mediastinum,** contains the heart, aorta, esophagus, and bronchi. A serous membrane, the **pleura,** envelops the lobes of the lungs and folds over to line the walls of the thoracic cavity. The innermost membrane lying next to the lung is the (17) **visceral pleura;** the outermost membrane, which lines the thoracic cavity, is the (18) **parietal pleura.** Between these two membranes is the (19) **pleural cavity.** It contains a small amount of lubricating fluid, which permits the visceral pleura to glide smoothly over the parietal pleura during breathing.

Ventilation depends on a pressure differential between the atmosphere and chest cavity. A large muscular partition, the (20) **diaphragm,** lies between the chest and abdominal cavities. The diaphragm assists in changing the volume of the thoracic cavity to produce the needed pressure differential for ventilation. When the diaphragm contracts, it partially descends into the abdominal cavity, thus decreasing the pressure within the chest and drawing air into the lungs. When the diaphragm relaxes, it slowly re-enters the thoracic cavity, thus increasing the pressure within the chest **(inspiration).** As the pressure increases, air leaves the lungs **(expiration).** The **intercostal** muscles assist the diaphragm in changing the volume of the thoracic cavity by elevating and lowering the rib cage. (See Figure 7–2.)

## Respiration

Respiration is the overall process by which oxygen is taken from air and transported to body cells for the metabolic process, while carbon dioxide and water, the waste products generated by these cells, are returned to the environment.

Respiration includes four separate processes:

1. ventilation (breathing), the largely involuntary movement of air into (inspiration) and out of (expiration) the lungs in response to changes in oxygen and carbon dioxide levels in the blood and nervous stimulation of the diaphragm and intercostal muscles
2. external respiration, the exchange of oxygen and carbon dioxide between the alveoli and the blood in the pulmonary capillaries
3. transport of respiratory gases through the body by blood in the cardiovascular system
4. internal respiration, the exchange of oxygen and carbon dioxide between tissue cells and the blood in systemic capillaries

 **It is time to review respiratory structures by completing Learning Activity 7–1.**

**Figure 7–2**   Breathing muscles.

## Medical Word Elements

This section introduces combining forms, suffixes, and prefixes related to the integumentary system. Word analyses are also provided.

| Element | Meaning | Word Analysis |
|---|---|---|
| **COMBINING FORMS** | | |
| **Upper Respiratory Tract** | | |
| **nas/o** | nose | nas/al (NĀ-zl): pertaining to the nose <br> *-al:* pertaining to, relating to |
| **rhin/o** | | rhin/o/plasty (RĪ-nō-plăs-tē): plastic surgery of the nose to correct a birth defect or breathing problem or for cosmetic purposes <br> *-plasty:* surgical repair |
| **sept/o** | septum | sept/o/plasty (sĕp-tō-PLĂS-tē): plastic surgery to correct a deviated septum <br> *-plasty:* surgical repair |
| **sinus/o** | sinus, cavity | sinus/o/tomy (sī-nŭs-ŎT-ō-mē): incision of any of the sinuses to improve ventilation or drainage in unresponsive sinusitis <br> *-tomy:* incision |

| Element | Meaning | Word Analysis |
|---------|---------|---------------|
| **adenoid/o** | adenoids | adenoid/ectomy (ăd-ĕ-noyd-ĔK-tō-mē): excision of the adenoids<br>*-ectomy:* excision, removal |
| **tonsill/o** | tonsils | peri/tonsill/ar (pĕr-ĭ-TŎN-sĭ-lăr): pertaining to the area surrounding the tonsils<br>*peri-:* around<br>*-ar:* pertaining to, relating to |
| **pharyng/o** | pharynx (throat) | pharyng/o/scope (făr-ĬN-gō-skōp): instrument used to examine the pharynx<br>*-scope:* instrument for examining |
| **epiglott/o** | epiglottis | epiglott/itis (ĕp-ĭ-glŏt-Ī-tĭs): inflammation of the epiglottis that can lead to severe airway obstruction<br>*-itis:* inflammation |
| **laryng/o** | larynx (voice box) | laryng/o/plegia (lă-rĭn-gō-PLĒ-jē-ă): paralysis of the vocal cords and larynx<br>*-plegia:* paralysis |
| **trache/o** | trachea (windpipe) | trache/o/stomy (trā-kē-ŎS-tō-mē): opening created through the neck and into the trachea into which a breathing tube may be inserted<br>*-stomy:* forming an opening (mouth)<br>*A tracheostomy is usually performed to bypass an obstructed upper airway; clean and remove secretions from the airway; and deliver oxygen to the lungs.* |

## Lower Respiratory Tract

| Element | Meaning | Word Analysis |
|---------|---------|---------------|
| **bronchi/o** | bronchus | bronchi/ectasis (brŏng-kē-ĔK-tă-sĭs): abnormal dilation of one or more bronchi<br>*-ectasis:* dilation, expansion<br>*Bronchiectasis is associated with various lung conditions and is commonly accompanied by chronic infection.* |
| **bronch/o** | | bronch/o/scope (BRŎNG-kō-skōp): flexible tube that is passed into the lungs through the nose or mouth<br>*-scope:* instrument for examining<br>*A bronchoscope allows inspection of the lungs and collection of tissue biopsies and secretions for analysis.* |
| **bronchiol/o** | bronchiole | bronchiol/itis (brŏng-kē-ō-LĪ-tĭs): inflammation of the bronchioles (small passages of the bronchial tree); usually caused by a viral infection<br>*-itis:* inflammation |

*(Continued)*

| Element | Meaning | Word Analysis | (Continued) |
|---|---|---|---|
| **alveol/o** | alveolus | alveol/ar (ăl-VĒ-ō-lăr): pertaining to the alveoli<br><br>*-ar:* pertaining to, relating to | |
| **pneum/o**<br><br><br>**pneumon/o** | air; lung | pneum/ectomy (nūm-ĔK-tō-mē): excision of all or part of a lung<br><br>*-ectomy:* excision<br><br>pneumon/ia (nū-MŌ-nē-ă): inflammation of the lungs usually due to bacteria, viruses, or other pathogenic organisms<br><br>*-ia:* condition | |
| **pulmon/o** | lung | pulmon/o/logist (pŭl-mă-NŎL-ă-jĭst): physician specializing in the treatment of lung and respiratory diseases<br><br>*-logist:* specialist in the study of | |
| **pleur/o** | pleura | pleur/o/clysis (ploo-RŎK-lă-sĭs): injection and removal of a fluid into the pleural cavity to wash it out<br><br>*-clysis:* irrigation, washing | |
| Other | | | |
| **anthrac/o** | coal, coal dust | anthrac/osis (ăn-thră-KŌ-sĭs): chronic lung disease characterized by the deposit of coal dust in the lungs and the formation of black nodules on the bronchioles<br><br>*-osis:* abnormal condition; increase (used primarily with blood cells) | |
| **atel/o** | incomplete; imperfect | atel/ectasis (ăt-ĕ-LĔK-tă-sĭs): partial or complete collapse of the lung; airless lung<br><br>*-ectasis:* dilation, expansion | |
| **coni/o** | dust | pneum/o/coni/osis (nū-mō-kō-nē-Ō-sĭs): any disease of the lungs caused by chronic inhalation of dust, usually mineral dust of occupational or environmental origin<br><br>*pneum/o:* air; lung<br>*-osis:* abnormal condition; increase (used primarily with blood cells)<br><br>*Forms of pneumoconiosis include silicosis, asbestosis, and anthracosis.* | |
| **cyan/o** | blue | cyan/osis (sī-ă-NŌ-sĭs): abnormal blueness of the skin and mucous membranes associated with a decrease of oxygen in the blood<br><br>*-osis:* abnormal condition; increase (used primarily with blood cells)<br><br>*Cyanosis is associated with cold temperatures, heart failure, lung diseases, and smothering.* | |

| Element | Meaning | Word Analysis |
|---------|---------|---------------|
| **lob/o** | lobe | lob/ectomy (lō-BĚK-tō-mē): surgical removal of a lobe of an organ or gland (such as the lungs, liver, and thyroid gland)<br><br>*-ectomy:* excision<br><br>*A lobectomy is performed when a malignancy is confined to a single lobe of the lung.* |
| **orth/o** | straight | orth/o/pnea (or-THŎP-nē-ă): condition in which the patient experiences difficulty breathing in any position other than sitting or standing erect<br><br>*-pnea:* breathing |
| **ox/o** | oxygen | hyp/ox/emia (hī-pŏks-Ē-mē-ă): abnormal decrease of oxygen in arterial blood resulting in hypoxia<br><br>*hyp-:* under, below, deficient<br>*-emia:* blood condition |
| **ox/i** | | ox/i/meter (ŏk-SĬM-ĕ-tĕr): device used to measure the oxygen saturation of arterial blood<br><br>*-meter:* instrument for measuring<br><br>*The oximeter is usually attached to the tip of a finger but may also be placed on a toe or earlobe.* |
| **pector/o** | chest | pector/algia (pĕk-tō-RĂL-jē-ă): pain in the chest<br><br>*-algia:* pain |
| **steth/o** | | steth/o/scope (STĔTH-ō-skōp): instrument used to evaluate the sounds of the chest and abdomen<br><br>*-scope:* instrument for examining |
| **thorac/o** | | thorac/algia (thō-răk-ĂL-jē-ă): pain in the chest wall; also called *thoracodynia*<br><br>*-algia:* pain |
| **phren/o** | diaphragm; mind | phren/o/ptosis (frĕn-ŏp-TŌ-sĭs): abnormal downward displacement of the diaphragm<br><br>*-ptosis:* prolapse, downward displacement |
| **spir/o** | breathe | spir/o/meter (spī-RŎM-ĕt-ĕr): instrument that measures how much air the lungs can hold (vital capacity) as well as how much and how quickly air can be exhaled<br><br>*-meter:* instrument for measuring |

## SUFFIXES

| Element | Meaning | Word Analysis |
|---------|---------|---------------|
| **-capnia** | carbon dioxide ($CO_2$) | hyper/capnia (hī-pĕr-KĂP-nē-ă): excess of $CO_2$ in the blood<br><br>*hyper-:* excessive, above normal |
| **-osmia** | smell | an/osmia (ăn-ŎZ-mē-ă): loss or impairment of the sense of smell<br><br>*an-:* without, not |

*(Continued)*

| Element | Meaning | Word Analysis | (Continued) |
|---------|---------|---------------|-------------|
| **-phonia** | voice | dys/phonia (dĭs-FŌ-nē-ă): altered or impaired voice quality<br>  *dys-:* bad; painful; difficult<br>*Dysphonia includes hoarseness, voice fatigue, or decreased projection.* | |
| **-pnea** | breathing | a/pnea (ăp-NĒ-ă): temporary loss of breathing<br>  *a-:* without, not<br>*Types of apnea include sleep apnea, cardiac apnea, and apnea of the newborn.* | |
| **-ptysis** | spitting | hem/o/ptysis (hē-MŎP-tĭ-sĭs): coughing up of blood or bloody sputum from the lungs or airway<br>  *hem/o:* blood | |
| **-thorax** | chest | py/o/thorax (pī-ō-THŌ-răks): accumulation of pus in the chest cavity; also called *empyema*<br>  *py/o:* pus<br>*Pyothorax is usually caused by a penetrating chest wound or spread of infection from another part of the body.* | |
| **PREFIXES** | | | |
| **brady-** | slow | brady/pnea (brăd-ĭp-NĒ-ă): abnormally slow respiratory rate<br>  *-pnea:* breathing | |
| **dys-** | bad; painful; difficult | dys/pnea (dĭsp-NĒ-ă): breathing discomfort or significant breathlessness<br>  *-pnea:* breathing | |
| **eu-** | good, normal | eu/pnea (ūp-NĒ-ă): normal, unlabored breathing<br>  *-pnea:* breathing<br>*The normal range for a resting adult respiratory rate is 12 to 20 breaths/minute.* | |
| **tachy-** | rapid | tachy/pnea (tăk-ĭp-NĒ-ă): abnormally rapid respiratory rate<br>  *-pnea:* breathing | |

 It is time to review word elements by completing Learning Activity 7–2.

 **Pathology**

Common signs and symptoms for many respiratory disorders include cough (dry or productive), chest pain, altered breathing patterns, breathlessness, cyanosis, and fever. Many disorders of the respiratory system, including bronchitis and emphysema, begin as an acute problem but become chronic over time. Chronic respiratory diseases are commonly difficult to treat, and their damaging effects become irreversible.

For diagnosis, treatment, and management of respiratory disorders, the medical services of a specialist may be warranted. **Pulmonology** is the medical specialty concerned with disorders of the respiratory system. The physician who treats these disorders is called a **pulmonologist.**

## Chronic Obstructive Pulmonary Disease

Chronic obstructive pulmonary disease (COPD), also called *chronic obstructive lung disease (COLD)*, includes respiratory disorders characterized by a chronic partial obstruction of the air passages. The patient experiences difficulty breathing **(dyspnea)** on exertion and often exhibits a chronic cough. The three major disorders included in COPD are asthma, chronic bronchitis, and emphysema. (See Figure 7–3.)

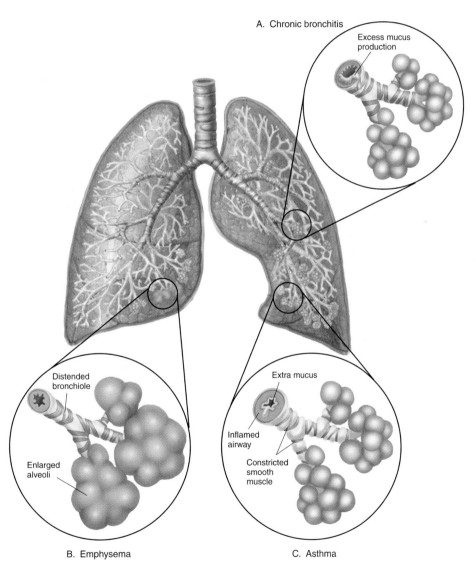

**Figure 7–3**    COPD. (A) Chronic bronchitis with inflamed airways and excessive mucus. (B) Emphysema with distended bronchioles and alveoli. (C) Asthma with narrowed bronchial tubes and swollen mucous membranes.

## Asthma

Asthma produces spasms in the bronchial passages **(bronchospasms)** that are typically sudden and violent **(paroxysmal)**, causing dyspnea. Asthma is commonly caused by exposure to allergens or irritants. Other causes include stress, cold, and exercise. During recovery, coughing episodes produce large amounts of mucus **(productive cough)**. Over time, the epithelium of the bronchial passages thickens, making breathing difficult. Treatment includes agents that loosen and break down mucus **(mucolytics)** and medications that open up the bronchi **(bronchodilators)** by relaxing their smooth muscles. If bronchospasms are not reversed by usual measures, the patient is said to have **status asthmaticus.**

## Chronic Bronchitis

Chronic bronchitis is an inflammation of the bronchi caused primarily by smoking and air pollution. However, other agents, such as viruses and bacteria, may also be responsible for the disorder. Bronchitis is characterized by swelling of the mucosa and a heavy, productive cough commonly accompanied by chest pain. Patients usually seek medical attention when they suffer exercise intolerance, wheezing, and shortness of breath. Bronchodilators and medications that facilitate the removal of mucus **(expectorants)** help to widen air passages. Steroids are commonly needed as the disease progresses.

## Emphysema

Emphysema is characterized by decreased elasticity of the alveoli. They expand **(dilate)** but are unable to contract to their original size. Residual air becomes trapped, resulting in a characteristic "barrel-chested" appearance. This disease is often found in combination with another respiratory disorder, such as asthma, tuberculosis, or chronic bronchitis. It is also associated with long-term heavy smoking. Emphysema sufferers often find it easier to breathe when sitting or standing erect **(orthopnea)**. As the disease progresses, however, the patient no longer finds relief even in the orthopneic position. Treatment for emphysema is similar to that for chronic bronchitis.

## Influenza

Influenza (flu) is an acute infectious respiratory disease caused by viruses. Three major viral types are responsible: type A, type B, and type C. Type A is of primary concern because it is commonly associated with worldwide epidemics **(pandemics)** and is extremely pathogenic **(virulent)**. The type A swine flu epidemic of 1918 was responsible for 20 to 40 million deaths worldwide. Influenza type A epidemics occur about every 2 to 3 years. Type B flu is usually limited geographically and tends to be less severe than type A. Both viruses undergo antigenic variations; consequently, new vaccines must continually be developed in anticipation of outbreaks. Type C flu is a mild flu and is not associated with epidemics.

The onset of the flu is usually very rapid. The patient experiences fever, chills, headache, generalized muscle pain **(myalgia)**, and loss of appetite. The patient is ill during the acute phase but recovery occurs in about 7 to 10 days. The flu virus rarely causes death. Should death occur, it is usually the result of a secondary pneumonia caused by a lower respiratory invasion by bacteria or viruses. Children should avoid using aspirin for relief of symptoms caused by viruses. An apparent relationship exists between Reye syndrome and the use of aspirin by children 2 to 15 years of age.

# Pleural Effusions

Any abnormal fluid in the pleural cavity, the space between the visceral and parietal pleura, is called a *pleural effusion*. The pleural cavity normally contains only a small amount of lubricating fluid but, in many disorders, an abnormal increase in fluid occurs. These disorders include failure of the heart to pump adequate amounts of blood to body tissues **(heart failure),** liver diseases associated with an accumulation of fluid in the abdominal and pleural cavities **(ascites),** infectious lung diseases, and trauma. Different types of pleural effusions include pus in the pleural space **(empyema),** serum in the pleural space **(hydrothorax),** blood in the pleural space **(hemothorax),** air in the pleural space **(pneumothorax),** and a mixture of pus and air in the pleural space **(pyopneumothorax).** (See Figure 7–4.)

A.

Normal lung

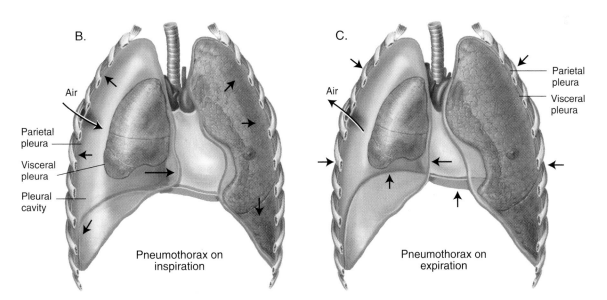

B.

Air

Parietal pleura

Visceral pleura

Pleural cavity

Pneumothorax on inspiration

C.

Air

Parietal pleura

Visceral pleura

Pneumothorax on expiration

**Figure 7–4**   Pneumothorax. (A)  Normal. (B)  Open pneumothorax during inspiration. (C)  Open pneumothorax during expiration.

Depending on the amount and type of fluid, treatment may include surgical puncture of the chest **(thoracocentesis, thoracentesis)** to remove excess fluid from the pleural cavity using a hollow bore needle. (See Figure 7–5.) Sometimes chest tubes are inserted to facilitate removal of the fluid. Two noninvasive techniques used in the diagnosis of pleural effusion are listening to the sounds of the chest cavity with a stethoscope **(auscultation)** and gently tapping the chest with the fingers to determine the position, size, or consistency of the underlying structures **(percussion).**

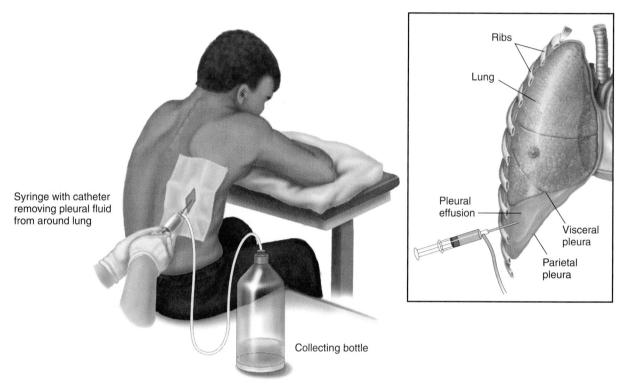

**Figure 7–5** • Thoracentesis.

## Tuberculosis

An alarming increase in tuberculosis occurred in the United States between 1985 and 1992. This increase corresponded with the escalation of drug-resistant TB strains, the number of people with acquired immunodeficiency syndrome (AIDS), and those who were homeless or living in poverty. Since 1992, incidence of the disease has declined primarily because of active surveillance and new treatment methods.

TB is highly communicable and spreads by droplets of respiratory secretions **(aerosol transmission)** or particles of dry sputum containing the TB organism. The waxy coat of the TB organism allows it to remain alive **(viable)** and infectious for 6 to 8 months outside the body.

The first time the TB organism enters the body **(primary tuberculosis),** the disease develops slowly. It eventually produces unique focal **granulomas** called *tubercles*. These granulomas usually remain dormant for years, during which time the patient is asymptomatic. When the immune system becomes impaired **(immunocompromised)** or when the patient is reintroduced to the bacterium, the full-blown disease may develop.

Although primarily a lung disease, TB can infect the bones, genital tract, meninges, and peritoneum. Many of the TB strains that infect AIDS patients are not responsive to standard medications **(drug resistant),** and treatment commonly includes simultaneous use of several antibiotics **(combination therapy).**

## Pneumonia

The term *pneumonia* refers to any inflammatory disease of the lungs. Pneumonia may be caused by bacteria, viruses, fungi, chemicals, and other agents. Infectious pneumonias are primarily attributed to bacteria or viruses. A type of pneumonia associated with influenza is sometimes fatal. Other potentially fatal pneumonias may result from food or liquid inhalation **(aspiration pneumonias).** Some pneumonias affect only a lobe of the lung **(lobar pneumonia),** but some are more diffuse **(bronchopneumonia).** Chest pain, mucopurulent sputum, and spitting of blood **(hemoptysis)** are frequent symptoms of the disease. The lungs may undergo solidification **(consolidation)** because of a pathological engorgement.

*Pneumocystis carinii* pneumonia (PCP) is a type of pneumonia closely associated with AIDS. Recent evidence suggests that it is caused by a fungus that resides in or on most people **(normal flora)** but causes no harm as long as the individual remains healthy. When the immune system becomes compromised, however, this organism becomes infectious **(opportunistic).** Diagnosis relies on examination of biopsied lung tissue or bronchial washings **(lavage).**

## Cystic Fibrosis

**Cystic fibrosis** is a hereditary disorder of the exocrine glands that causes the body to secrete extremely thick **(viscous)** mucus that clogs ducts or tubes of the pancreas, digestive tract, and sweat glands. In the lungs, this mucus blocks airways and impedes natural infection-fighting mechanisms, eventually turning the body's immune system against its own lung tissue. Medication in the form of mists **(aerosols)** along with postural drainage provides relief.

An important diagnostic finding in cystic fibrosis is an increase in the amount of salt excreted in sweat. A laboratory test called a *sweat test* analyzes the amount of chloride in sweat and, when elevated, is indicative of cystic fibrosis. Although the disease is fatal, improved methods of treatment have extended life expectancy, and patient survival is approximately 30 years.

## Respiratory Distress Syndrome

**Respiratory distress syndrome (RDS)** is most commonly caused by absence or impairment in the production of a phospholipid substance of the lungs called **surfactant** that allows the lungs to expand with ease **(compliance).** Without surfactant, the alveoli collapse and inhalation becomes extremely difficult.

When RDS is found in newborn infants, it is called **infant respiratory distress syndrome (IRDS)** or **hyaline membrane disease (HMD).** IRDS is most commonly seen in premature infants or infants born to diabetic mothers. If the amount of surfactant is inadequate at birth, clinical symptoms include blueness **(cyanosis)** of the extremities, rapid breathing **(tachypnea),** flaring of the nostrils **(nares),** intercostal retraction, and a characteristic grunt audible during exhalation. Radiography shows a membrane that has a ground-glass appearance **(hyaline membrane).** Although severe cases of IRDS result in death, some forms of therapy are effective.

**Acute respiratory distress syndrome (ARDS)** is caused by an impairment of surfactant production or by exposure to substances that remove surfactant from the lungs. Accidental inhalation of foreign substances, water, smoke, chemical fumes, or vomit is commonly the cause.

## Oncology

The most common form of lung cancer is bronchogenic carcinoma, also called *primary pulmonary cancer.* This cancer is most commonly associated with tobacco use. In this type of cancer, the cells at the base of the epithelium **(basal cells)** divide repeatedly until, eventually, the entire epithelium is involved. Within a short time, the epithelium begins to invade the underlying tissues. As masses form, they block air passages and alveoli. Bronchogenic carcinoma spreads (**metastasizes**) rapidly to other areas of the body, commonly to lymph nodes, liver, bones, brain, or kidney. Only about 10% of lung cancers are found in the early stages when the cure rate is high. Treatment of lung cancer includes surgery, radiation, and chemotherapy or a combination of these methods. Nevertheless, lung cancer is difficult to control and survival rates are extremely low.

## Diagnostic, Symptomatic, and Related Terms

This section introduces diagnostic, symptomatic, and related terms and their meanings. Word analyses for selected terms are also provided.

| Term | Definition |
|---|---|
| **acidosis**<br>ăs-ĭ-DO-sĭs | Excessive acidity of body fluids, commonly associated with pulmonary insufficiency and the subsequent retention of carbon dioxide |
| **anosmia**<br>ăn-ŎZ-mē-ă<br><br>*an-:* without, not<br>*-osmia:* smell | Absence of or decrease in the sense of smell<br><br>*Anosmia usually occurs as a temporary condition resulting from an upper respiratory infection or a condition that causes intranasal swelling.* |
| **apnea**<br>ăp-NĒ-ă<br><br>*a-:* without, not<br>*-pnea:* breathing | Temporary loss of breathing<br><br>*There are three types of apnea: obstructive (enlarged tonsils and adenoids), central (failure of the brain to transmit impulses for breathing), and mixed (combination of obstructive and central apnea).* |
| **sleep** | One of several disorders in which breathing during sleep stops for more than 10 seconds and usually more than 20 times/hour, causing measurable blood deoxygenation |
| **asphyxia**<br>ăs-FĬK-sē-ă<br><br>*a-:* without, not<br>*-sphyxia:* pulse | Condition caused by insufficient intake of oxygen<br><br>*Some common causes of asphyxia are drowning, electrical shock, lodging of a foreign body in the respiratory tract, inhalation of toxic smoke, and poisoning.* |
| **atelectasis**<br>ăt-ĕ-LĔK-tă-sĭs<br><br>*atel-:* incomplete; imperfect<br>*-ectasis:* dilation, expansion | Collapsed or airless state of the lung, which may be acute or chronic and affect all or part of a lung<br><br>*Atelectasis is a potential complication of some surgical procedures, especially those of the chest because breathing is commonly shallow after surgery to avoid pain from the surgical incision. In fetal atelectasis, the lungs fail to expand normally at birth.* |
| **Cheyne-Stokes respiration**<br>CHĀN-STŌKS | Repeated breathing pattern characterized by fluctuation in the depth of respiration, first deeply, then shallow, then not at all<br><br>*Cheyne-Stokes respiration is usually caused by diseases that affect the respiratory centers of the brain (such as heart failure and brain damage).* |

| Term | Definition |
|---|---|
| **compliance**<br>kŏm-PLĪ-ăns | Ease with which lung tissue can be stretched<br>*Low compliance means lungs are less elastic; therefore, more effort is required to inflate the lungs.* |
| **coryza**<br>kŏ-RĪ-ză | Head cold; upper respiratory infection (URI) |
| **croup**<br>CROOP | Common childhood condition involving inflammation of the larynx, trachea, bronchial passages and, sometimes, lungs characterized by resonant, barking cough; suffocative and difficult breathing; laryngeal spasm; and, sometimes, the formation of a membrane |
| **deviated nasal septum**<br>DĒ-vē-āt-ĕd<br>NĀ-zl SĔP-tŭm | Displacement of cartilage dividing the nostrils |
| **epiglottitis**<br>ĕp-i-glŏt-Ī-tĭs<br><br>*epiglott:* epiglottis<br>*-itis:* inflammation | Severe, life-threatening infection of the epiglottis and supraglottic structures that occurs most commonly in children between 2 and 12 years of age<br>*Symptoms of epiglottitis include fever, dysphagia, inspiratory stridor, and severe respiratory distress. Intubation or tracheostomy may be required to open the obstructed airway.* |
| **epistaxis**<br>ĕp-ĭ-STĂK-sĭs | Nosebleed; nasal hemorrhage |
| **finger clubbing**<br>KLŬB-ĭng | Enlargement of the terminal phalanges of the fingers and toes, commonly associated with pulmonary disease |
| **hypoxemia**<br>hī-pŏks-Ē-mē-ă<br><br>*hyp-:* under, below, deficient<br>*ox:* oxygen<br>*-emia:* blood condition | Deficiency of oxygen in the blood; also called *anoxemia*<br>*Hypoxemia is usually a sign of respiratory impairment.* |
| **hypoxia**<br>hī-PŎKS-ē-ă<br><br>*hyp-:* under, below, deficient<br>*-oxia:* oxygen | Absence or deficiency of oxygen in the tissues; also called *anoxia*<br>*Hypoxia is usually a sign of respiratory impairment.* |
| **pertussis**<br>pĕr-TŬS-ĭs | Acute infectious disease characterized by a cough that has a "whoop" sound; also called *whooping cough*<br>*Immunization of infants as part of the diphtheria-pertussis-tetanus (DPT) vaccination is very effective in the prevention of this disease.* |
| **pleurisy**<br>PLOO-rĭs-ē<br><br>*pleur:* pleura<br>*-isy:* state of; condition | Inflammation of the pleural membrane characterized by a stabbing pain that is intensified by coughing or deep breathing; also called *pleuritis* |

*(Continued)*

| Term | Definition | (Continued) |
|---|---|---|
| **pneumoconiosis**<br>nū-mō-kō-nē-Ō-sĭs<br><br>*pneum/o:* air; lung<br>*coni:* dust<br>*-osis:* abnormal condition; increase (used primarily with blood cells) | Generally occupational disease caused by inhaling dust particles, including coal dust (anthracosis), stone dust (chalicosis), iron (siderosis), and asbestos (asbestosis) | |
| **pulmonary edema**<br>PŬL-mō-nĕ-rē<br>ĕ-DĒ-mă<br><br>*pulmon:* lung<br>*-ary:* pertaining to, relating to | Accumulation of extravascular fluid in lung tissues and alveoli, caused most commonly by heart failure<br>*The excessive fluid in the lungs induces coughing and dyspnea.* | |
| **pulmonary embolus**<br>PŬL-mō-nĕ-rē<br>ĔM-bō-lŭs<br><br>*pulmon:* lung<br>*-ary:* pertaining to, relating to<br>*embol:* plug<br>*-us:* condition, structure | Mass of undissolved matter (such as a blood clot, tissue, air bubbles, and bacteria) in the pulmonary arteries or its branches | |
| **rale**<br>RĂL | Abnormal respiratory sound heard on auscultation, caused by exudates, spasms, hyperplasia, or when air enters moisture-filled alveoli; also called *crackle* | |
| **rhonchus**<br>RŎNG-kŭs | Adventitious breath sound that resembles snoring, commonly suggesting secretions in the larger airways | |
| **stridor**<br>STRĪ-dor | High-pitched, harsh adventitious breath sound caused by a spasm or swelling of the larynx or an obstruction in the upper airway<br>*The presence of stridor requires immediate intervention.* | |
| **sudden infant death syndrome (SIDS)** | Completely unexpected and unexplained death of an apparently normal and healthy infant, usually less than 12 months of age; also called *crib death*<br>*The rate of SIDS has declined more than 30% since parents have been instructed to place their baby on the back for sleeping rather than the stomach.* | |
| **wheeze**<br>HWĒZ | Whistling or sighing sound on auscultation that results from narrowing of the lumen of the respiratory passageway<br>*Wheezing is a characteristic of asthma, croup, hay fever, obstructive emphysema, and other obstructive respiratory conditions.* | |

 **It is time to review pathological, diagnostic, symptomatic, and related terms by completing Learning Activity 7–3.**

## Diagnostic and Therapeutic Procedures

This section introduces procedures used to diagnose and treat respiratory disorders. Descriptions are provided as well as pronunciations and word analyses for selected terms.

| Procedure | Description |
|---|---|
| **DIAGNOSTIC PROCEDURES** | |
| **Clinical** | |
| **Mantoux test**<br>măn-TŪ | Intradermal test to determine tuberculin sensitivity based on a positive reaction where the area around the test site becomes red and swollen<br><br>*A positive test suggests a past or present exposure to TB or past TB vaccination. However, the Mantoux test does not differentiate between active or inactive infection.* |
| **oximetry**<br>ŏk-SĬM-ă-trē<br><br>*ox/i:* oxygen<br>*-metry:* act of measuring | Noninvasive method of monitoring the percentage of hemoglobin (Hb) saturated with oxygen; also called *pulse oximetry*<br><br>*In oximetry, a probe is attached to the patient's finger or earlobe and linked to a computer that displays the percentage of hemoglobin saturated with oxygen and, in some units, provides an audible signal for each pulse beat.* |
| **polysomnography**<br>pŏl-ē-sŏm-NŎG-ră-fē<br><br>*poly-:* many, much<br>*somn/o:* sleep<br>*-graphy:* process of recording | Test of sleep cycles and stages using continuous recordings of brain waves (EEGs), electrical activity of muscles, eye movement (electro-oculogram), respiratory rate, blood pressure, blood oxygen saturation, heart rhythm and, sometimes, direct observation of the person during sleep using a video camera |
| **pulmonary function studies**<br><br>*pulmon:* lung<br>*-ary:* pertaining to, relating to | Multiple tests used to evaluate the ability of the lungs to take in and expel air as well as perform gas exchange across the alveolocapillary membrane |
| **spirometry**<br>spī-RŎM-ĕ-trē<br><br>*spir/o:* breathe<br>*-metry:* act of measuring | Measurement of ventilatory ability by assessing lung capacity and flow, including the time necessary for exhaling the total volume of inhaled air<br><br>*A spirometer produces a graphic record for placement in the patient's chart.* |
| **Endoscopic** | |
| **bronchoscopy**<br>brŏng-KŎS-kō-pē<br><br>*bronch/o:* bronchus<br>*-scopy:* visual examination | Visual examination of the bronchi using an endoscope (flexible fiberoptic or rigid) inserted through the mouth and trachea for direct viewing of structures or for projection on a monitor<br><br>*Bronchoscopy also allows suctioning, biopsy, removal of foreign bodies, and collection of fluid or sputum for examination and diagnosis.* |

*(Continued)*

| Procedure | Description | (Continued) |
|---|---|---|
| **laryngoscopy**<br>lăr-ĭn-GŎS-kō-pē<br><br>*laryng/o:* larynx (voice box)<br>*-scopy:* visual examination | Visual examination of the inside of the larynx to detect tumors, foreign bodies, nerve or structural injury, or other abnormalities | |
| **mediastinoscopy**<br>mē-dē-ăs-tĭ-NŎS-kō-pē<br><br>*mediastin/o:* mediastinum<br>*-scopy:* visual examination | Visual examination of the mediastinal structures including the heart, trachea, esophagus, bronchus, thymus, and lymph nodes<br><br>*The mediastinoscope is inserted through a very small incision made above the sternum. The attached camera projects images on a monitor. Additional incisions may be made if nodes are removed or other diagnostic or therapeutic procedures are performed.* | |

### Laboratory

| | | |
|---|---|---|
| **arterial blood gases (ABGs)** | Test that measures the partial pressure of oxygen ($PaO_2$), carbon dioxide ($PaCO_2$), pH (acidity or alkalinity), and bicarbonate level of an arterial blood sample<br><br>*This test evaluates pulmonary gas exchange and helps to guide treatment of acid-base imbalances.* | |
| **sputum culture**<br>SPŪ-tŭm | Microbial test used to identify disease-causing organisms of the lower respiratory tract, especially those that cause pneumonias | |
| **sweat test** | Measurement of the amount of salt (sodium chloride) in sweat<br><br>*This test is used almost exclusively in children to confirm cystic fibrosis.* | |
| **throat culture** | Test used to identify pathogens, especially group A streptococci<br><br>*Untreated streptococcal infections may lead to serious secondary complications, including kidney and heart disease.* | |

### Radiographic

| | | |
|---|---|---|
| **radiography**<br>rā-dē-ŎG-ră-fē<br><br>*radi/o:* radiation, x-ray; radius (lower arm bone on thumb side)<br>*-graphy:* process of recording | Producing images using an x-ray that is passed through the body or area and captured on a film | |
| **chest** | Images of the chest taken from anteroposterior (AP), posteroanterior (PA), or lateral projection, or a combination of these projections<br><br>*Radiography is used to diagnose rib fractures and lung diseases, including atelectasis, masses, pneumonia, and emphysema.* | |

| Procedure | Description |
|---|---|
| **scan** | Term used to describe a computed image by modality (such as CT scan, MRI scan, and nuclear scan) or structure (such as thyroid scan and bone scan) |
| **thoracic (CT)**<br>thō-RĂS-ĭk<br><br>*thorac:* chest<br>*-ic:* pertaining to, relating to | A cross-sectional view of the chest taken with or without an injected contrast medium to visualize injuries, tumors, fluid in the lungs, or other pathologies |
| **lung** | Nuclear scanning procedure commonly used to diagnose blood clots and pulmonary emboli |

## THERAPEUTIC PROCEDURES

### Clinical

| | |
|---|---|
| **aerosol therapy**<br>ĀR-ō-sŏl | Inhalation of microdrops of medication directly into the respiratory system via a nebulizer (liquid), metered-dose inhaler (gas), or dry-powder inhaler (solid) (See Figure 7–6.)<br><br>*In aerosol therapy, the medication is deposited directly into the respiratory system, thus allowing lower dosages, providing rapid action, and minimizing side effects and systemic toxicity.* |

**Figure 7–6**   Nebulizer.

| | |
|---|---|
| **lavage**<br>lă-VĂZH | Irrigating or washing out of an organ, stomach, bladder, bowel, or body cavity with a stream of water or other fluid |
| **antral**<br>ĂN-trăl | Irrigation of the paranasal sinuses usually performed to remove mucopurulent material in an immunosuppressed patient or one with known sinusitis that has failed medical management |
| **postural drainage**<br>PŎS-tū-răl | Positioning a patient so that gravity aids in the drainage of secretions from the bronchi and lobes of the lungs |

*(Continued)*

| Procedure | Description | (Continued) |
|---|---|---|
| **Surgical** | | |

| Procedure | Description |
|---|---|
| **rhinoplasty**<br>RĪ-nō-plăs-tē<br><br>*rhin/o:* nose<br>*-plasty:* surgical repair | Reconstructive surgery of the nose to correct deformities or for cosmetic purposes |
| **pleurectomy**<br>ploor-ĔK-tō-mē<br><br>*pleur:* pleura<br>*-ectomy:* excision, removal | Excision of part of the pleura, usually parietal<br><br>*Pleurectomy is performed to reduce pain caused by a tumor mass or to prevent the recurrence of pleural effusion but is generally ineffective in the treatment of malignancy of the pleura.* |
| **pneumectomy**<br>nūm-ĔK-tō-mē<br><br>*pneum:* air; lung<br>*-ectomy:* excision, removal | Excision of a lung or lobe (lobectomy) of the lung<br><br>*Other partial types of lung excisions include resection, segmental, and wedge.* |
| **septoplasty**<br>sĕp-tō-PLĂS-tē<br><br>*sept/o:* septum<br>*-plasty:* surgical repair | Surgical repair of a deviated nasal septum usually performed when the septum is encroaching on the breathing passages or nasal structures<br><br>*Common complications of a deviated septum include interference with breathing and a predisposition to sinus infections.* |
| **thoracentesis**<br>thō-ră-sĕn-TĒ-sĭs | Surgical puncture and drainage of the pleural cavity; also called *pleurocentesis* or *thoracocentesis* (See Figure 7–5.)<br><br>*Thoracentesis is performed as a diagnostic procedure to determine the nature and cause of an effusion or as a therapeutic procedure to relieve the discomfort caused by the effusion. The procedure is usually carried out at the bedside using local anesthetic.* |

 **Pharmacology**

In addition to antibiotics used to treat respiratory infections, there are several classes of drugs that treat pulmonary disorders. (See Table 7–1.) Bronchodilators are especially significant in the treatment of COPD and exercise-induced asthma. They relax smooth muscles of the bronchi, thus increasing airflow. Some bronchodilators are delivered as a fine mist directly to the airways via aerosol delivery devices, including nebulizers and metered-dose inhalers (MDIs). Another method of delivering medications directly to the lungs is dry-powder inhalers (DPIs) that dispense medications in the form of a powder. Steroidal and nonsteroidal anti-inflammatory drugs are important in the control and management of many pulmonary disorders.

## Table 7-1    DRUGS USED TO TREAT RESPIRATORY DISORDERS

This table lists common drug classifications used to treat respiratory disorders, their therapeutic actions, and selected generic and trade names.

| Classification | Therapeutic Action | Generic and Trade Names |
|---|---|---|
| antihistamines | Relieve nasal congestion and seasonal allergic rhinitis symptoms<br><br>*Antihistamines exert their therapeutic effect by blocking histamine receptors in the nose and throat. They dry up secretions, decrease mucous membrane swelling, and decrease redness and itching.* | **fexofenadine**<br>fĕks-ō-FĔN-ă-dēn<br>*Allegra*<br>**loratadine**<br>lor-ĂH-tă-dēn<br>*Claritin*<br>**diphenhydramine**<br>dī-fĕn-HĪ-dră-mēn<br>*Benadryl* |
| antitussives | Relieve or suppress coughing<br><br>*Antitussives are used to alleviate nonproductive dry coughs. Some antitussives contain narcotics, such as codeine and hydrocodone. Other over-the-counter antitussives contain the non-narcotic dextromethorphan or diphenhydramine.* | **hydrocodone**<br>hī-drō-KŌ-dŏn<br>*Hycodan*<br>**codeine**<br>KŌ-dēn<br>*no trade names except in combination*<br>**dextromethorphan**<br>dĕk-strō-MĔTH-or-făn<br>*Benylin DM, Sucrets, Vicks Formula 44* |
| bronchodilators | Relax smooth muscle surrounding the bronchi resulting in increased air flow<br><br>*Bronchodilators are used to treat chronic symptoms and to prevent acute attacks in respiratory diseases, such as asthma and COPD. The pharmacological agent may be delivered by an inhaler (as in Proventil, Ventolin, and Serevent), orally, or intravenously.* | **albuterol**<br>ăl-BŪ-tĕr-ăl<br>*Proventil, Ventolin*<br>**salmeterol**<br>săl-mē-TĔR-ŏl<br>*Serevent* |
| corticosteroids | Treat chronic lung disease (including asthma) by suppressing the immune response and decreasing inflammation<br><br>*Vanceril and Beclovent decrease the frequency and intensity of asthma attacks, thereby preventing pulmonary damage associated with chronic asthma.* | **beclomethasone dipropionate**<br>bĕ-klō-MĔTH-ă-sōn<br>di-PRŌ-pē-ō-nāt<br>*Vanceril, Beclovent*<br>**triamcinolone**<br>trī-ăm-SĬN-ō-lōn<br>*Azmacort* |
| decongestants | Decrease mucous membrane swelling to alleviate nasal stuffiness<br><br>*Decongestants are commonly prescribed for allergies and colds and are usually combined with antihistamines in cold remedies. They can be administered orally or topically as nasal sprays and nasal drops.* | **oxymetazoline**<br>ŏks-ē-mĕt-ĂZ-ō-lēn<br>*Afrin, Dristan, Sinex*<br>**pseudoephedrine**<br>soo-dō-ĕ-FĔD-rin<br>*Drixoral, Sudafed* |
| expectorants | Reduce the thickness or viscosity of sputum<br><br>*Reducing the viscosity of secretions aids the patient's ability to cough up sputum. Expectorants are prescribed only for productive coughs.* | **guaifenesin**<br>gwī-FĔN-ĕ-sĭn<br>*Robitussin*<br>**iodinated glycerol**<br>ī-Ō-dĭn-ā-tĭd<br>GLĬS-ĕr-ŏl<br>*Organidin* |

## Abbreviations

This section introduces respiratory-related abbreviations and their meanings.

| Abbreviation | Meaning |
| --- | --- |
| ABGs | arterial blood gases |
| AFB | acid-fast bacillus (TB organism) |
| AP | anteroposterior |
| ARDS | acute respiratory distress syndrome |
| $CO_2$ | carbon dioxide |
| COPD | chronic obstructive pulmonary disease |
| CPR | cardiopulmonary resuscitation |
| CT scan | computed tomography scan |
| CXR | chest x-ray, chest radiograph |
| FVC | forced vital capacity |
| HMD | hyaline membrane disease |
| IPPB | intermittent positive-pressure breathing |
| IRDS | infant respiratory distress syndrome |
| MRI scan | magnetic resonance imaging scan |
| NMTs | nebulized mist treatments |
| $O_2$ | oxygen |

| Abbreviation | Meaning |
|---|---|
| PA | posteroanterior; pernicious anemia |
| $P_{CO_2}$ | partial pressure of carbon dioxide |
| PCP | *Pneumocystis carinii* pneumonia |
| PFT | pulmonary function tests |
| pH | symbol for degree of acidity or alkalinity |
| PND | paroxysmal nocturnal dyspnea |
| $P_{O_2}$ | partial pressure of oxygen |
| RD | respiratory distress |
| RDS | respiratory distress syndrome |
| $Sa_{O_2}$ | arterial oxygen saturation |
| SIDS | sudden infant death syndrome |
| SOB | shortness of breath |
| T & A | tonsillectomy and adenoidectomy |
| TB | tuberculosis |
| TPR | temperature, pulse, and respiration |
| URI | upper respiratory infection |
| VC | vital capacity |

 **It is time to review procedures, pharmacology, and abbreviations by completing Learning Activity 7–4.**

# LEARNING ACTIVITIES

The following activities provide review of the respiratory system terms introduced in this chapter. Complete each activity and review your answers to evaluate your understanding of the chapter.

## Learning Activity 7–1

### Identifying respiratory structures

*Label the illustration on page 177 using the terms listed below.*

| | | |
|---|---|---|
| adenoids | larynx | parietal pleura |
| alveoli | left lung | pleural cavity |
| bronchi | mediastinum | pulmonary capillaries |
| bronchiole | nasal cavity | right lung |
| diaphragm | nasopharynx | trachea |
| epiglottis | oropharynx | visceral pleura |
| laryngopharynx | palatine tonsils | |

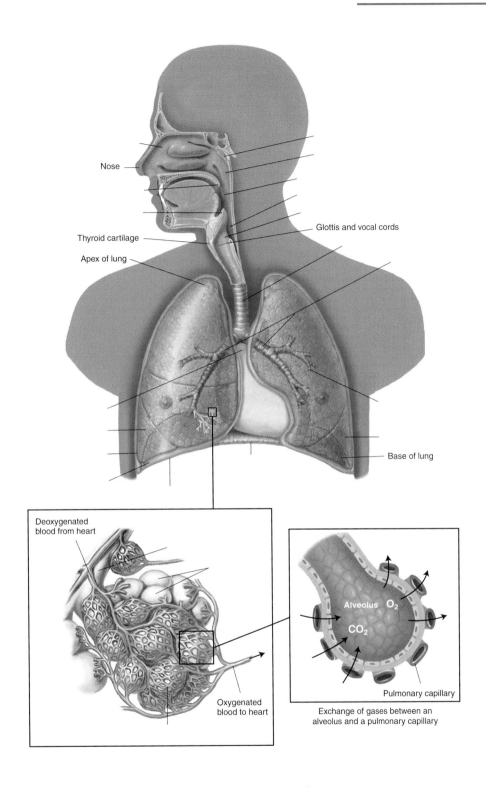

Nose

Glottis and vocal cords

Thyroid cartilage

Apex of lung

Base of lung

Deoxygenated
blood from heart

Oxygenated
blood to heart

Alveolus  O₂

CO₂

Pulmonary capillary

Exchange of gases between an
alveolus and a pulmonary capillary

 Check your answers by referring to Figure 7–1 on page 154. Review material that you did not answer correctly.

Learning Activity 7–2

## Building medical words

*Use **rhin/o** (nose) to build words that mean:*

1. discharge from the nose _____

2. inflammation of the (mucous membranes of the) nose _____

*Use **laryng/o** (larynx [voice box]) to build words that mean:*

3. visual examination of the larynx _____

4. inflammation of the larynx _____

5. stricture or narrowing of the larynx _____

*Use **bronch/o** or **bronchi/o** (bronchus) to build words that mean:*

6. dilation or expansion of the bronchus _____

7. disease of the bronchus _____

8. spasm of the bronchus _____

*Use **pneumon/o** or **pneum/o** (air; lung) to build words that mean:*

9. air in the chest (pleural space) _____

10. inflammation of the lungs _____

*Use **pulmon/o** (lung) to build words that mean:*

11. specialist in lung (diseases) _____

12. pertaining to the lung _____

*Use **-pnea** (breathing) to build words that mean:*

13. difficult breathing _____

14. slow breathing _____

15. rapid breathing _____

16. absence of breathing _____

*Build surgical words that mean:*

17. surgical repair of the nose _____

18. surgical puncture of the chest _____

19. removal of a lung _____

20. forming an opening (mouth) in the trachea _____

Check your answers in Appendix A. Review material that you did not answer correctly.

**CORRECT ANSWERS** _____ × 5 = _____ **% SCORE**

Learning Activity 7-3

## Matching pathological, diagnostic, symptomatic, and related terms

*Match the following terms with the definitions in the numbered list.*

| | | |
|---|---|---|
| anosmia | deviated nasal septum | pneumoconiosis |
| apnea | emphysema | pulmonary edema |
| ascites | empyema | rale, crackle |
| atelectasis | epistaxis | stridor |
| compliance | hypoxemia | surfactant |
| consolidation | pertussis | tubercles |
| coryza | pleurisy | |

1. _____ collapsed or airless lung
2. _____ pus in the pleural cavity
3. _____ phospholipid that allows the lungs to expand with ease
4. _____ solidification of the lungs
5. _____ accumulation of fluid in the abdominal or pleural cavities
6. _____ absence or decrease in the sense of smell
7. _____ deficiency of oxygen in the blood; also called *anoxemia*
8. _____ granulomas associated with tuberculosis
9. _____ temporary loss of breathing
10. _____ disease characterized by decrease in alveolar elasticity
11. _____ ease with which lung tissue can be stretched
12. _____ nosebleed; nasal hemorrhage
13. _____ excessive fluid in the lungs that induces cough and dyspnea
14. _____ abnormal respiratory sound associated with exudates, spasms, or hyperplasia
15. _____ displacement of the cartilage dividing the nostrils
16. _____ head cold; upper respiratory infection
17. _____ condition in which dust particles are found in the lungs
18. _____ inflammation of the pleural membrane
19. _____ abnormal sound caused by spasms or swelling of larynx
20. _____ whooping cough

Check your answers in Appendix A. Review any material that you did not answer correctly.

**CORRECT ANSWERS** _____ × 5 = _____ **% SCORE**

Learning Activity 7–4

## Matching procedures, pharmacology, and abbreviations

*Match the following terms with the definitions in the numbered list.*

| | | |
|---|---|---|
| *ABGs* | *expectorants* | *pulmonary function studies* |
| *aerosol therapy* | *laryngoscopy* | *resection of lung* |
| *AFB* | *lung scan* | *rhinoplasty* |
| *antihistamines* | *Mantoux test* | *septoplasty* |
| *antitussives* | *oximetry* | *sweat test* |
| *antral lavage* | *pneumectomy* | *throat culture* |
| *decongestants* | *polysomnography* | |

1. _____ imaging procedure that uses radionuclide to evaluate blood flow in the lungs

2. _____ test of sleep cycles and stages

3. _____ excision of a portion of the lung

4. _____ washing or irrigating sinuses

5. _____ relieve nasal congestion and seasonal allergic rhinitis symptoms

6. _____ relieve or suppress coughing

7. _____ test used primarily in children to confirm cystic fibrosis

8. _____ noninvasive test used to monitor percentage of hemoglobin saturated with oxygen

9. _____ TB organism

10. _____ inhalation of medication directly into the respiratory system via a nebulizer

11. _____ decrease mucous membrane swelling to alleviate nasal stuffiness

12. _____ intradermal test to determine presence of TB infections

13. _____ laboratory tests to assess gases and pH of arterial blood

14. _____ reduces the viscosity of sputum to facilitate productive coughing

15. _____ used to identify pathogens, especially group A streptococci

16. _____ multiple tests used to determine the ability of lungs and capillary membranes to exchange oxygen

17. _____ visual examination of the voice box to detect tumors and other abnormalities

18. _____ surgery to correct a deviated nasal septum

19. _____ excision of the entire lung

20. _____ reconstructive surgery of the nose, commonly for cosmetic purposes

Check your answers in Appendix A. Review any material that you did not answer correctly.

**CORRECT ANSWERS** _____ × 5 = _____ **% SCORE**

# MEDICAL RECORD ACTIVITIES

The two medical records included in the activities that follow use common clinical scenarios to show how medical terminology is used to document patient care. Complete the terminology and analysis sections for each activity to help you recognize and understand terms related to the respiratory system.

## Medical Record Activity 7–1

### Respiratory evaluation

#### Terminology

The terms listed in the chart come from the medical record *Respiratory Evaluation* that follows. Use a medical dictionary such as *Taber's Cyclopedic Medical Dictionary*, the appendices of this book, or other resources to define each term. Then review the pronunciations for each term and practice by reading the medical record aloud.

| Term | Definition |
|------|------------|
| **anteriorly**<br>ăn-TĒR-ē-or-lē | |
| **bilateral**<br>bī-LĂT-ĕr-ăl | |
| **COPD** | |
| **exacerbation**<br>ĕks-ăs-ĕr-BĀ-shŭn | |
| **heart failure**<br>hărt FĀL-yĕr | |
| **Hx** | |
| **hypertension**<br>hī-pĕr-TĔN-shŭn | |
| **interstitial**<br>ĭn-tĕr-STĬSH-ăl | |
| **PE** | |
| **peripheral vascular disease**<br>pĕr-ĬF-ĕr-ăl VĂS-kū-lăr dĭ-ZĒZ | |
| **pleural**<br>PLOO-răl | |

| Term | Definition |
|------|------------|
| **posteriorly** pŏs-TĒR-ē-or-lē | |
| **rhonchi** RŎNG-kī | |
| **SOB** | |
| **wheezes** HWĒZ-ĕz | |

## Respiratory Evaluation

**HISTORY OF PRESENT ILLNESS:** This 49-year-old man with known history of COPD is admitted because of exacerbation of SOB over the past few days. Patient was a heavy smoker and states that he quit smoking for a short while but now smokes three to four cigarettes a day. He has a Hx of difficult breathing, high blood pressure, COPD, and peripheral vascular disease. He underwent triple bypass surgery in 19xx. PE indicates scattered bilateral wheezes and rhonchi heard anteriorly and posteriorly.

Compared with a portable chest film from 4/17/xx, deterioration since the previous study is noted that most likely indicates interstitial vascular congestion. Some superimposed inflammatory change cannot be excluded. There may also be some pleural reactive change.

**DIAGNOSIS:**

1. Acute exacerbation of chronic pulmonary disease
2. Heart failure
3. Peripheral vascular disease

## Analysis

**Review the medical record *Respiratory Evaluation* to answer the following questions.**

1. What symptom caused the patient to seek medical help?

_____

2. What was the patient's previous history?

_____

3. What were the findings of the physical examination?

_____

4. What changes were noted from the previous film?

_____

5. What is the present Dx?

_____

6. What new diagnosis was made that did not appear in the previous medical history?

_____

## Chronic interstitial lung disease

### Terminology

The terms listed in the chart come from the medical record *Chronic Interstitial Lung Disease* that follows. Use a medical dictionary such as *Taber's Cyclopedic Medical Dictionary*, the appendices of this book, or other resources to define each term. Then review the pronunciations for each term and practice by reading the medical record aloud.

| Term | Definition |
| --- | --- |
| ABGs | |
| adenopathy<br>ăd-ĕ-NŎP-ă-thē | |
| basilar crackles<br>BĂS-ĭ-lăr  KRĂK-ĕlz | |
| cardiomyopathy<br>kăr-dē-ō-mī-ŎP-ă-thē | |
| chronic<br>KRŎN-ĭk | |
| diuresis<br>dī-ū-RĒ-sĭs | |
| dyspnea<br>dĭsp-NĒ-ă | |
| fibrosis<br>fī-BRŌ-sĭs | |
| interstitial<br>ĭn-tĕr-STĬSH-ăl | |
| kyphosis<br>kī-FŌ-sĭs | |
| Lasix<br>LĀ-sĭks | |
| neuropathy<br>nū-RŎP-ă-thē | |
| Pco$_2$ | |
| pedal edema<br>PĔD-l  ĕ-DĒ-mă | |

| Term | Definition |
|---|---|
| **pH** | |
| **Po$_2$** | |
| **pulmonary fibrosis**<br>PŬL-mō-nĕ-rē fĭ-BRŌ-sĭs | |
| **renal insufficiency**<br>RĒ-năl ĭn-sŭ-FĬSH-ĕn-sē | |
| **rhonchi**<br>RŎNG-kī | |
| **silicosis**<br>sĭl-ĭ-KŌ-sĭs | |
| **thyromegaly**<br>thī-rō-MĔG-ă-lē | |

## CHRONIC INTERSTITIAL LUNG DISEASE

**CHIEF COMPLAINT**: Dyspnea with activity; pedal edema

**HISTORY OF PRESENT ILLNESS**: The patient is an 84-year-old male who carries the diagnosis of cardiomyopathy, renal insufficiency, COPD, and pulmonary fibrosis. He also has peripheral neuropathy, which has improved with Elavil therapy.

**ASSESSMENT**: BP: 140/70. Pulse: 76. Neck is supple without thyromegaly or adenopathy. Mild kyphosis without scoliosis is present. Chest reveals basilar crackles without wheezing or rhonchi. Cardiac examination shows trace edema without clubbing or murmur. Abdomen is soft and nontender. ABGs on room air demonstrate a Po$_2$ of 55, Pco$_2$ of 45, and pH of 7.42.

**IMPRESSION**: Chronic interstitial lung disease, likely a combination of pulmonary fibrosis and heart failure. We do believe he would benefit from further diuresis, which was implemented by Dr. Lu. Should there continue to be concerns about his volume status or lack of response to Lasix therapy, then he might benefit from right heart catheterization.

**PLAN**: Supplemental oxygen will be continued. We plan no change in his pulmonary medication at this time and will see him in return visit in 4 months. He has been told to contact us should he worsen in the interim.

## Analysis

**Review the medical record *Chronic Interstitial Lung Disease* to answer the following questions.**

1. When did the patient notice SOB?

   _____

2. Other than the respiratory system, what other body systems are identified in the history of present illness?

   _____

3. What were the findings regarding the neck?

_____

4. What was the finding regarding the spine?

_____

5. What appears to be the likely cause of the chronic interstitial lung disease?

_____

6. Define the following abbreviations: ABGs, $P_{O_2}$, $P_{CO_2}$, and pH.

_____

7. What is the therapeutic action of Lasix?

_____

# Chapter

# 8

# Cardiovascular System

## OBJECTIVES

*Upon completion of this chapter, you will be able to:*

- Locate and describe the structures of the cardiovascular system.
- Recognize, pronounce, spell, and build words related to the cardiovascular system.
- Describe pathological conditions, diagnostic and therapeutic procedures, and other terms related to the cardiovascular system.
- Explain pharmacology related to the treatment of cardiovascular disorders.
- Demonstrate your knowledge of this chapter by completing the learning and medical record activities.

187

## Key Terms

This section introduces important cardiovascular system terms and their definitions. Word analyses are also provided.

| Term | Definition |
|------|-----------|
| **diaphoresis**<br>dī-ă-fō-RĒ-sĭs<br><br>*dia-:* through, across<br>*-phoresis:* carrying, transmission | Profuse sweating |
| **incompetent**<br>ĭn-KŎM-pĕ-tĕnt | Inability to adequately perform a given function or action |
| **leaflet** | Thin, flattened structure; term used to describe the leaf-shaped structures that compose a heart valve |
| **lumen**<br>LŪ-mĕn | Tubular space or channel within any organ or structure of the body; space within an artery, vein, intestine, or tube |
| **malaise**<br>mă-LĀZ | Vague, uneasy feeling of body weakness, distress, or discomfort, commonly marking the onset of and persisting throughout a disease |
| **occlusion**<br>ŏ-KLOO-zhŭn | Blockage in a canal, vessel, or passage of the body; the state of being closed |
| **patent**<br>PĂT-ĕnt | Open and unblocked, such as a patent artery |
| **prophylaxis**<br>prō-fĭ-LĂK-sĭs<br><br>*pro-:* before, in front of<br>*-phylaxis:* protection | Preventive measure or technique commonly involving the use of a biologic, chemical, or mechanical agent to destroy or prevent the entry of infectious organisms |
| **viscosity**<br>vĭs-KŎS-ĭ-tē | State of being sticky or gummy<br>*A solution that has high viscosity is relatively thick and flows slowly.* |

## Anatomy and Physiology

The cardiovascular system is composed of the heart and blood vessels. The heart is a hollow muscular organ lying in the mediastinum, the center of the thoracic cavity between the lungs. The pumping action of the heart propels blood containing oxygen, nutrients, and other vital products to body cells through a vast network of blood vessels called *arteries*. Blood returns to the heart through blood vessels called *veins* to begin the cycle again. On its return trip to the heart, blood picks up waste products from the body cells to deliver them to the organs of excretion. The trillions of body cells rely on the cardiovascular system for their survival. When this transportation system fails, life at the cellular level is not possible and, ultimately, the organism will die.

## Vascular System

Three major types of vessels—(1) **artery,** (2) **capillary,** and (3) **vein**—carry blood throughout the body. (See Figure 8–1.) Each type of vessel differs in structure, depending on its function.

**Figure 8–1**   Vascular structures.

### Arteries

Arteries carry blood from the heart to trillions of body cells that make up an organism. Because blood is propelled thorough the arteries by the pumping action of the heart, the walls of the arteries must be able to withstand the surge of blood that results from each contraction of the heart.

The walls of the large arteries have three layers to provide the necessary strength and flexibility. The (4) **tunica externa** is a tough, outer coat of connective tissue that provides strength. The (5) **tunica media** is a layer of smooth muscular tissue. Depending on the needs of the body, it can cause *vasoconstriction* (reduction of the lumen diameter caused by smooth muscle contraction) or *vasodilation* (widening of the lumen caused by smooth muscle relaxation). The (6) **tunica intima** is a thin, inner lining composed of endothelial cells that provides a smooth surface so blood can flow easily through its (7) **lumen.**

The surge of blood felt in the arteries when blood is pumped from the heart is referred to as a *pulse*. Because of the pressure against arterial walls associated with the pumping action of the heart, a cut or severed artery may lead to profuse bleeding.

Arterial blood (except for that found in the pulmonary artery) contains a high concentration of oxygen. It appears bright red and is said to be *oxygenated*. Oxygenated blood travels to smaller arteries called (8) **arterioles** and finally to the smallest vessels, the capillaries.

## Capillaries

Capillaries are microscopic vessels that join the arterial system with the venous system. Although seemingly the most insignificant of the three vessel types because of their microscopic size, they are actually the most important because of their function. At the capillary level, nutrients and oxygen in the blood are exchanged for waste products formed by the surrounding cells. Because capillary walls are composed of a single layer of endothelial cells, they are very thin. This thinness enables the exchange of water, macromolecules, metabolites, and wastes. Because there are vast numbers of capillaries branching from arterioles, blood flows slowly through them, providing sufficient time for exchange of necessary substances.

Blood flow through the highly branched capillary system is regulated by the contraction of smooth muscle precapillary sphincters that lead into the capillary bed. When tissues require more blood, these sphincters open; when less blood is required, they close. Once the exchange of products is complete, blood enters the venous system for its return cycle to the heart.

## Veins

Veins return blood to the heart. They are formed from smaller vessels called (9) **venules** that develop from the union of capillaries. Because the extensive network of capillaries absorbs the propelling pressure exerted by the heart, veins use other methods to propel blood to the heart, including:

- skeletal muscle contraction
- gravity
- respiratory activity
- valves

The (10) **valves** are small structures within veins that prevent the backflow of blood. Valves are found predominantly in the extremities and are especially important for returning blood from the legs to the heart because blood must travel a long distance against the force of gravity to reach the heart. Large veins such as those found in the abdomen contain smooth muscle that contract peristaltically to propel blood toward the heart against gravity.

Blood carried in the veins (except for the blood in the pulmonary veins) contains a low concentration of oxygen (**deoxygenated**) with a corresponding high concentration of carbon dioxide. Deoxygenated blood takes on a characteristic purple color. Blood continuously circulates to the lungs so that carbon dioxide can be exchanged for oxygen.

## Heart

The heart is contained in a sac called the **pericardium** and has three distinct tissue layers:

1. The **endocardium** is a serous membrane that lines the four chambers of the heart and its valves and is continuous with the endothelium of the arteries and veins.
2. The **myocardium** is the muscular layer of the heart.
3. The **epicardium** is the outermost layer of the heart.

The heart is a four-chambered muscular pump supplied with an electrical conduction system whose function is to propel blood throughout the body through a closed vascular system. (See Figures 8–2A and 8–2B.) The heart is divided into four chambers. The two upper

A.

Left subclavian artery

Left internal jugular vein

Left common carotid artery

Brachiocephalic trunk

Aortic arch

(5) Superior vena cava

(9) Right pulmonary artery

(8) Left pulmonary artery

(11) Right pulmonary veins

(12) Left pulmonary veins

(2) Left atrium

(17) Left coronary artery

(1) Right atrium

(19) Circumflex artery

(16) Right coronary artery

Left coronary vein

(6) Inferior vena cava

(4) Left ventricle

(3) Right ventricle

Apex

(14) Aorta

(18) Left anterior descending artery

Brachiocephalic trunk

Left common carotid artery

Left subclavian artery

Aortic arch

(14) Aorta

(8) Left pulmonary artery

(5) Superior vena cava

B.   (11) Right pulmonary veins

(12) Left pulmonary veins

(10) Pulmonic valve

(2) Left atrium

(1) Right atrium

(15) Aortic semilunar valve

(7) Tricuspid valve

(13) Mitral (bicuspid) valve

Chordae tendineae

(6) Inferior vena cava

(4) Left ventricle

Apex

Papillary muscles

(3) Right ventricle

Interventricular septum

**Figure 8–2**   Structures of the heart.  (A) Anterior view of the heart. (B) Frontal section of the heart.

chambers, the atria, are composed of the (1) **right atrium** and (2) **left atrium** and collect blood. The two lower chambers, the ventricles, are composed of the (3) **right ventricle** and (4) **left ventricle** and pump blood from the heart. The right side of the heart pumps blood to the lungs (pulmonary circulation) for oxygenation, and the left side of the heart pumps oxygenated blood to all body systems (systemic circulation).

Deoxygenated blood from the body returns to the heart by way of two large veins: the (5) **superior vena cava,** which collects and carries blood from the upper part of the body; and the (6) **inferior vena cava,** which collects and carries blood from the lower part of the body. The superior and inferior venae cavae deposit deoxygenated blood into the upper right chamber of the heart, the right atrium. From the right atrium, blood passes through the (7) **tricuspid valve** to the right ventricle. When the heart contracts, blood leaves the right ventricle by way of the (8) **left pulmonary artery** and (9) **right pulmonary artery** and travels to the lungs. During contraction of the ventricle, the tricuspid valve closes to prevent a backflow of blood to the right atrium. The (10) **pulmonic valve** (or *pulmonary semilunar valve*) prevents a backflow of blood into the right ventricle. In the lungs, the pulmonary artery branches into millions of capillaries, each lying close to an alveolus. Here, carbon dioxide in the blood is exchanged for oxygen that has been drawn into the lungs during inhalation.

Pulmonary capillaries unite to form four pulmonary veins—two (11) **right pulmonary veins** and two (12) **left pulmonary veins**—which are the vessels that carry oxygenated blood back to the heart. Pulmonary veins deposit blood in the left atrium. From here, blood passes through the (13) **mitral (bicuspid) valve** to the left ventricle. Upon contraction of the ventricles, the oxygenated blood leaves the left ventricle through the largest artery of the body, the (14) **aorta.** The aorta contains the (15) **aortic semilunar valve** (or *aortic valve*) that permits blood to flow in only one direction—from the left ventricle to the aorta. The aorta branches into many smaller arteries that carry blood to all parts of the body. Some arteries derive their names from the organs or areas of the body they vascularize. For example, the splenic artery vascularizes the spleen and the renal arteries vascularize the kidneys.

It is important to understand that oxygen, present in the blood passing through the chambers of the heart, cannot be used by the myocardium as a source of oxygen and nutrients. Instead, an arterial system composed of the coronary arteries branches from the aorta and provides the heart with its own blood supply. These arteries lie over the top of the heart much as a crown fits over a head, hence the name **coronary** (pertaining to a crown). The artery vascularizing the right side of the heart is the (16) **right coronary artery.** The artery vascularizing the left side of the heart is the (17) **left coronary artery.** The left coronary artery divides into the (18) **left anterior descending artery** and the (19) **circumflex artery.** If blood flow in the coronary arteries is diminished, myocardial damage may result. When severe damage occurs, part of the heart muscle may die.

## Conduction System of the Heart

Within the heart, a specialized cardiac tissue known as *conductive tissue* has the sole function of initiating and spreading contraction impulses. (See Figure 8–3.) This tissue consists of four masses of highly specialized cells:

1. **sinoatrial (SA) node**
2. **atrioventricular (AV) node**
3. **bundle of His (AV bundle)**
4. **Purkinje fibers.**

The SA node, located in the upper portion of the right atrium, possesses its own intrinsic rhythm. Without being stimulated by external nerves, it has the ability to initiate and propagate each heartbeat, thereby setting the basic pace for the cardiac rate. For this reason, the SA node is commonly known as the *pacemaker* of the heart. Cardiac rate may be altered by

**Figure 8–3**  Conduction system.

impulses from the autonomic nervous system. Such an arrangement allows outside influences to accelerate or decelerate the heart rate. For example, the heart beats faster during physical exertion and slower during rest.

Each electrical impulse discharged by the SA node is transmitted to the AV node, causing the atria to contract. The AV node is located at the base of the right atrium. From this point, a tract of conduction fibers called the bundle of His, composed of a right and left branch, relays the impulse to the Purkinje fibers. These fibers extend up the ventricle walls. The Purkinje fibers transmit the impulse to both the right and left ventricles, causing them to contract. Blood is now forced from the heart through the pulmonary artery and aorta.

In summary, the sequence of the four structures responsible for conduction of a contraction impulse is as follows:

**SA node ⟶ AV node ⟶ bundle of His ⟶ Purkinje fibers**

Impulse transmission through the conduction system generates weak electrical currents that can be detected on the surface of the body. These electrical impulses can be recorded on an instrument called an *electrocardiograph*. The needle deflection of the electrocardiograph produces waves or peaks designated by the letters P, Q, R, S, and T, each of which is associated with a specific electrical event:

- The *P wave* is the depolarization (contraction) of the atria.
- The *QRS complex* is the depolarization (contraction) of the ventricles.
- The *T wave*, which appears a short time later, is the repolarization (recovery) of the ventricles.

## Blood Pressure

Blood pressure measures the force exerted by blood against the arterial walls during two phases of a heartbeat: the contraction phase, called *systole*, when the blood is forced out of the heart, and the relaxation phase, called *diastole*, when the ventricles are filling with blood. Systole is the maximum force exerted by blood against the arterial walls; diastole, the weakest. These measurements are recorded as two figures separated by a diagonal line; the systolic pressure is given first, followed by the diastolic pressure. For instance, blood pressure may be recorded as 120/80 mm Hg; in this example, 120 is the systolic pressure, 80 the diastolic pressure. A consistently elevated blood pressure is called **hypertension;** decreased blood pressure is called *hypotension*.

Several factors influence blood pressure:

- resistance of blood flow in blood vessels
- pumping action of the heart
- **viscosity,** or thickness, of blood
- elasticity of arteries
- quantity of blood in the vascular system

## Fetal Circulation

Blood circulation through a fetus is, by necessity, different from that of a newborn infant. Respiration, the procurement of nutrients, and the elimination of metabolic wastes occur through the maternal blood instead of the organs of the fetus. The capillary exchange between the maternal and fetal circulation occurs within the placenta during pregnancy. This remarkable structure includes part of the mother's uterus and is discharged following delivery.

There are several major structures involved in fetal circulation. (See Figure 8–4.) The (1) **umbilical cord,** containing (2) two **arteries,** carries deoxygenated blood from the fetus to the (3) **placenta.** After oxygenation in the placenta, blood returns to the fetus via the (4) **umbilical vein.** Most of the blood in the umbilical vein enters the (5) **inferior vena cava** through the (6) **ductus venosus,** where it is delivered to the (7) **right atrium.** Some of this blood passes to the (8) **right ventricle;** however, most of it passes to the (9) **left atrium** through a small opening in the atrial septum called the (10) **foramen ovale,** which closes shortly after birth. From the left atrium, blood enters the (11) **left ventricle** and finally exits the heart through the aorta, where it is sent to the head and upper extremities. Because fetal lungs are nonfunctional, most of the blood in the pulmonary arteries is shunted through a connecting vessel called the (12) **ductus arteriosus** to the aorta. Immediately after birth, the ductus arteriosus withers and closes off. As circulation increases in the neonate, the increase of blood flow to the right atrium forces the foramen ovale to close. Normal circulation is now fully established.

**Figure 8–4** Fetal circulation.

 **It is time to review cardiovascular structures by completing Learning Activity 8–1.**

**Medical Word Elements**

This section introduces combining forms, suffixes, and prefixes related to the cardiovascular system. Word analyses are also provided.

| Element | Meaning | Word Analysis |
|---------|---------|---------------|
| **COMBINING FORMS** | | |
| **aneurysm/o** | a widening, a widened blood vessel | aneurysm/o/rrhaphy (ăn-ū-rĭz-MOR-ă-fē): surgical closure of an aneurysm sac<br>*-rrhaphy:* suture |
| **angi/o** | vessel (usually blood or lymph) | angi/o/plasty (ĂN-jē-ō-plăs-tē): any endovascular procedure that reopens narrowed blood vessels and restores blood flow<br>*-plasty:* surgical repair<br>*The blocked vessel is usually opened by balloon dilation.* |
| **vascul/o** | | vascul/itis (văs-kū-LĪ-tĭs): inflammation of blood vessels<br>*-itis:* inflammation |
| **aort/o** | aorta | aort/o/stenosis (ā-or-tō-stĕ-NŌ-sĭs): narrowing of the aorta<br>*-stenosis:* narrowing, stricture |
| **arteri/o** | artery | arteri/o/rrhexis (ăr-tē-rē-ō-RĔK-sĭs): rupture of an artery<br>*-rrhexis:* rupture |
| **arteriol/o** | arteriole | arteriol/itis (ăr-tēr-ē-ō-LĪ-tĭs): inflammation of the wall of an arteriole<br>*-itis:* inflammation |
| **atri/o** | atrium | atri/o/megaly (ā-trē-ō-MĔG-ă-lē): enlargement of the atrium<br>*-megaly:* enlargement |
| **ather/o** | fatty plaque | ather/oma (ăth-ĕr-Ō-mă): abnormal condition of fatty-plaque buildup on the inner lining of arterial walls<br>*-oma:* tumor<br>*Atheroma is the most common cause of hardening of the arteries.* |
| **cardi/o** | heart | cardi/o/megaly (kăr-dē-ō-MĔG-ă-lē): enlargement of the heart<br>*-megaly:* enlargement |
| **electr/o** | electricity | electr/o/cardi/o/gram (ē-lĕk-trō-KĂR-dē-ō-grăm): graphic recording of the electrical impulses of the heart<br>*cardi/o:* heart<br>*-gram:* record, recording<br>*Electrocardiogram is commonly used to diagnose abnormalities of the heart.* |

| Element | Meaning | Word Analysis |
|---|---|---|
| **embol/o** | plug | embol/ectomy (ĕm-bō-LĔK-tō-mē): removal of an embolus through a surgical procedure or treatment with enzymes<br>*-ectomy:* excision, removal |
| **hemangi/o** | blood vessel | hemangi/oma (hē-măn-jē-Ō-mă): benign tumor of dilated blood vessels<br>*-oma:* tumor |
| **my/o** | muscle | my/o/cardi/al (mī-ō-KĂR-dē-ăl): pertaining to heart muscle<br>*cardi:* heart<br>*-al:* pertaining to, relating to |
| **phleb/o** | vein | phleb/ectasis (flĕ-BĔK-tă-sĭs): dilation of a vein; varicosity<br>*-ectasis:* dilation, expansion |
| **ven/o** | | ven/o/stasis (vē-nō-STĀ-sĭs): abnormally slow flow of blood in the veins, usually with distension of the vessel; also called *phlebostasis*<br>*-stasis:* standing still |
| **scler/o** | hardening; sclera (white of eye) | arteri/o/scler/osis (ăr-tē-rē-ō-sklĕ-RŌ-sĭs): thickening, hardening, and loss of elasticity of arterial walls<br>*arteri/o:* artery<br>*-osis:* abnormal condition; increase (used primarily with blood cells)<br>*Arteriosclerosis results in decreased blood supply that primarily affects the heart, cerebrum, and lower extremities.* |
| **sept/o** | septum | sept/o/stomy (sĕp-TŎS-tō-mē): surgical formation of an opening in a septum<br>*-stomy:* forming an opening (mouth)<br>*Septostomy is performed to treat congenital heart defects that affect the aorta and pulmonary arteries.* |
| **sphygm/o** | pulse | sphygm/oid (SFĬG-moyd): resembling a pulse<br>*-oid:* resembling |
| **sten/o** | narrowing, stricture | sten/o/tic (stĕ-NŎT-ĭk): pertaining to a narrowing or stricture<br>*-tic:* pertaining to, relating to |
| **thromb/o** | blood clot | thromb/o/lysis (thrŏm-BŎL-ĭ-sĭs): destruction of a blood clot<br>*-lysis:* separation; destruction; loosening<br>*In thrombolysis, enzymes that destroy the blood clot are infused into the vessel.* |
| **ventricul/o** | ventricle (of the heart or brain) | ventricul/ar (vĕn-TRĬK-ū-lăr): pertaining to a ventricle (chamber of the heart or brain)<br>*-ar:* pertaining to, relating to |

*(Continued)*

| Element | Meaning | Word Analysis | (Continued) |
|---|---|---|---|
| **SUFFIXES** | | | |
| **-gram** | record, writing | arteri/o/gram (ăr-TĒ-rē-ō-grăm): radiograph of an artery after injection of a radiopaque contrast medium, usually directly into the artery or near its origin<br>    *arteri/o:* artery<br>*An arteriogram is used to visualize almost any artery, including those of the heart, head, kidneys, lungs, and other organs.* | |
| **-graph** | instrument for recording | electr/o/cardi/o/graph (ē-lĕk-trō-KĂR-dē-ō-grăf): device used to record changes in the electrical activity produced by the action of the heart muscles<br>    *electr/o:* electricity<br>    *cardi/o:* heart | |
| **-graphy** | process of recording | angi/o/graphy (ăn-jē-ŎG-ră-fē): visualization of the internal anatomy of the heart and blood vessels after introduction of a radiopaque contrast medium<br>    *angi/o:* vessel (usually blood or lymph)<br>*Angiography is commonly used to identify atherosclerosis and diagnose heart and peripheral vascular disease.* | |
| **-sphyxia** | pulse | a/sphyxia (ăs-FĬK-sē-ă): deficiency of oxygen and excess of carbon dioxide in the blood and body tissues; also called *suffocation*<br>    *a-:* without, not | |
| **-stenosis** | narrowing, stricture | aort/o/stenosis (ā-or-tō-stĕ-NŌ-sĭs): narrowing of the aorta<br>    *aort/o:* aorta | |
| **PREFIXES** | | | |
| **brady-** | slow | brady/cardia (brăd-ē-KĂR-dē-ă): abnormally slow heart rate<br>    *-cardia:* heart condition | |
| **endo-** | in, within | endo/vascul/ar (ĕn-dō-VĂS-kū-lăr): relating to the inside of a vessel<br>    *vascul:* vessel<br>    *-ar:* pertaining to, relating to | |
| **extra-** | outside | extra/vascul/ar (ĕks-tră-VĂS-kū-lăr): relating to the outside of a vessel<br>    *vascul:* vessel<br>    *-ar:* pertaining to, relating to | |

| Element | Meaning | Word Analysis |
|---|---|---|
| **peri-** | around | peri/cardi/o/tomy (pĕr-ĭ-kăr-dē-ŎT-ō-mē): incision of the pericardium, usually performed to drain a pericardial effusion<br><br>*cardi/o:* heart<br>*-tomy:* incision |
| **tachy-** | rapid | tachy/cardia (tăk-ē-KĂR-dē-ă): abnormally rapid heart rate<br><br>*-cardia:* heart condition |
| **trans-** | across | trans/sept/al (trăns-SĔP-tăl): across the septum<br>*sept:* septum<br>*-al:* pertaining to, relating to |

 It is time to review medical word elements by completing Learning Activity 8–2.

# Pathology

Many cardiac disorders, especially coronary artery disease, and valvular disorders are associated with a genetic predisposition. Thus, a complete history as well as a physical examination is essential in the diagnosis of cardiovascular disease. Although some of the most serious cardiovascular diseases have few signs and symptoms, when they occur they may include pain, palpitations, dyspnea, and syncope. The pain's location, duration, pattern of radiation, and severity are important qualities in differentiating the various forms of cardiovascular disease and are sometimes characteristic of specific disorders. Because of the general nature of the signs and symptoms of CV disorders, both invasive and noninvasive tests are usually required to confirm or rule out a suspected disease.

For diagnosis, treatment, and management of cardiovascular disorders, the medical services of a specialist may be warranted. *Cardiology* is the medical specialty concerned with disorders of the cardiovascular system. The physician who treats these disorders is called a *cardiologist.*

## Arteriosclerosis

Arteriosclerosis is a hardening of arterial walls that causes them to become thickened and brittle. It commonly results from an accumulation of a plaquelike substance composed of cholesterol, lipids, and cellular debris (**atheroma**) that builds up on the innermost lining (**tunica intima**) of the arterial walls. Over time, the plaque hardens (**atherosclerosis**) causing a loss of vascular elasticity. The vascular channel (**lumen**) narrows as the plaque enlarges. Eventually, it becomes difficult for blood to pass through the occluded areas, and tissue distal to the occlusion becomes ischemic. Commonly, blood hemorrhages into the plaque and forms a clot (**thrombus**) that may dislodge. When a thrombus travels though the vascular system it is called an *embolus.* Emboli that travel in venous circulation may cause death. Emboli that travel in arterial circulation frequently lodge in a capillary bed and cause a localized infarct. Plaque sometimes weakens the vessel wall to such an extent that it forms a bulge (**aneurysm**) that may rupture. (See Figure 8–5.)

**Figure 8–5**    Aneurysms.

Arteriosclerosis usually affects large- or medium-sized arteries, including the abdominal aorta, the coronary, cerebral, and renal arteries, and major arteries of the legs **(femoral arteries).** One of the major risk factors for developing arteriosclerosis is an elevated cholesterol level **(hypercholesterolemia).** Other major risk factors include age, family history, smoking, hypertension, and diabetes.

Treatment for arthrosclerosis varies depending on the location and symptoms. In one method, especially in the carotid or femoral arteries, the innermost layer of the artery is surgically removed **(endarterectomy).** Other, less invasive methods include using a catheter with a balloon at its tip and inserting it into the affected area. The balloon is inflated to stretch the narrowed artery **(angioplasty).** After the procedure, the balloon is deflated and removed. A hollow, thin mesh tube **(stent)** is usually placed on the balloon and positioned against the artery wall. It remains in place after the balloon catheter is removed and acts as scaffolding to hold the artery open.

## Coronary Artery Disease

Any disease that interferes with the ability of coronary arteries to deliver sufficient blood to the myocardium is referred to as **coronary artery disease (CAD).** The major cause of CAD is arteriosclerosis. About 20% of the total cardiac output is needed to meet the oxygen requirements of the heart muscle. When coronary arteries are unable to deliver sufficient oxygen, localized areas of the heart experience oxygen deprivation **(ischemia)** and, with total lack of oxygen, the affected area of the heart muscle dies **(myocardial infarction [MI]).** (See Figure 8–6.) The clin-

Plaque reduces blood flow

Area of ischemia

Blood flow is blocked

Area of infarct

**Figure 8–6**    Occlusions. (A) Partial occlusion. (B) Total occlusion.

ical signs and symptoms of an MI include intense chest pain **(angina),** diaphoresis, paleness **(pallor),** and dyspnea. An arrhythmic heartbeat with tachycardia or bradycardia may also accompany MI.

As the heart muscle undergoes necrotic changes, several highly specific cardiac enzymes, including troponin T, troponin I, and creatinine kinase (CK-MB), are released. The rapid elevation of these enzymes at predictable times following MI helps differentiate MI from pericarditis, aortic aneurysm, and acute pulmonary embolism.

When angina cannot be controlled with medication, surgical repair of the vessel **(angioplasty)** may be necessary. In one method of treatment, a deflated balloon is passed through a small incision in the skin and into the diseased blood vessel **(percutaneous transluminal coronary angioplasty [PTCA]).** When it is inflated, the balloon presses the occluding material against the lumen walls to increase their diameter. (See Figure 8–7.) A more invasive procedure involves rerouting blood around the occluded area using a small graft of a vein to bypass the obstruction **(coronary artery bypass graft [CABG]).** One end of the graft vessel is sutured to the aorta and the other end is sutured to the coronary artery below the blocked area. This re-establishes blood flow to the heart muscle. (See Figure 8–8.)

## Endocarditis

Endocarditis is an inflammation of the inner lining of the heart and its valves. It may be noninfective in nature, caused by thrombi formation, or infective, caused by various microorganisms. Although the infecting organism can be viral or fungal, the usual culprit is a bacterium.

**Figure 8–7**  Balloon angioplasty.

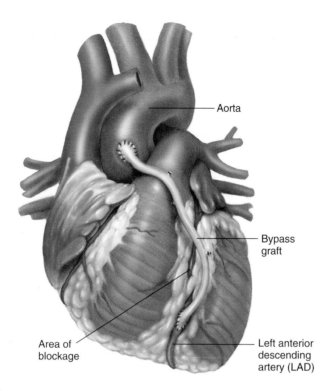

Aorta

Bypass
graft

Area of
blockage

Left anterior
descending
artery (LAD)

**Figure 8–8**   Coronary artery bypass graft.

Congenital valvular defects, scarlet fever, rheumatic fever, bicuspid or calcific aortic valves, mitral valve prolapse, and prosthetic valves are predisposing factors. Bacteria, traveling in the bloodstream **(bacteremia),** lodge in the weakened heart tissue and form small masses called *vegetations* composed of fibrin and platelets. Vegetations frequently collect on the leaflets of the valves and their cords, causing a backflow of blood **(regurgitation).** With valve scarring, there may be a narrowing of the valves **(stenosis)** or an inability of the valves to close properly **(insufficiency).** Some may dislodge and travel as emboli to the brain, lungs, kidneys, or spleen. Although medications may prove helpful, if heart failure develops as a result of damaged heart valves, surgery may be the only recourse. Whenever possible, the original valve is repaired. When the damage is extensive, a mechanical or bioprosthetic valve may be used.

Patients who are susceptible to endocarditis are given antibiotic treatment to protect against infection prior to invasive procedures **(prophylactic treatment).** Because many of the bacteria that are normally found in the mouth are also responsible for endocarditis, prophylactic treatment is warranted for tooth removal, root canal procedures, and even routine cleaning.

## Varicose Veins

Varicose veins are enlarged, twisted, superficial veins. They develop when the valves of the veins do not function properly **(incompetent)** and fail to prevent the backflow of blood in the vein. Blood accumulates and the vein appears engorged and distended. Excess fluid eventually seeps from the vein, causing swelling in surrounding tissues **(edema).** Varicose veins may develop in almost any part of the body, but occur most commonly in the lower legs, involving the greater and lesser saphenous veins. Types of varicose veins include reticular veins, which appear as small blue veins seen through the skin, and "spider" veins, which look like short, fine lines, starburst clusters, or a weblike maze.

Varicose veins of the legs are not typically painful but may be unsightly in appearance. However, if open lesions or pain is present, treatment includes laser ablation, microphlebectomies, ligation, stripping, and sclerotherapy. The same methods are used as an elective procedure to enhance the appearance of the legs. Treatment of mild cases of varicose veins includes use of elastic stockings and rest periods during which the legs are elevated.

## Oncology

Although rare, the most common primary tumor of the heart is composed of mucous connective tissue **(myxoma)**; however, these tumors tend to be benign. Although some myxomas originate in the endocardium of the heart chambers, most arise in the left atrium. Occasionally, they interfere with mitral valve function and cause a decrease in exercise tolerance, dyspnea, fluid in the lungs **(pulmonary edema),** and systemic disturbances, including joint pain **(arthralgia), malaise,** and anemia. These tumors are usually identified and located by two-dimensional echocardiography. The tumor should be excised surgically.

Most malignant tumors of the heart are the result of a malignancy originating in another area of the body **(primary tumor)** that has spread **(metastasized)** to the heart. The type usually found originates as a darkly pigmented mole or tumor **(malignant melanoma)** of the skin. Other primary sites of malignancy that metastasize to the heart are bone marrow and lymphatic tissue. Treatment of the metastatic tumor of the heart involves treating the primary tumor.

## Diagnostic, Symptomatic, and Related Terms

This section introduces diagnostic, symptomatic, and related terms and their meanings. Word analyses for selected terms are also provided.

| Term | Definition |
| --- | --- |
| **aneurysm**<br>ĂN-ū-rĭzm | Localized abnormal dilation of a vessel, usually an artery (See Figure 8–5.) |
| **arrest**<br>ă-RĔST | Condition of being stopped or bringing to a stop |
|   **cardiac**<br>  KĂR-dē-ăk<br><br>    *cardi:* heart<br>    *-ac:* pertaining to,<br>    relating to | Loss of effective cardiac function, which results in cessation of circulation<br>*Cardiac arrest may be due to ventricular fibrillation or asystole in which there is no observable myocardial activity.* |
|   **circulatory**<br>  SĔR-kū-lă-tor-ē | Cessation of the circulation of blood due to ventricular standstill or fibrillation |

*(Continued)*

| Term | Definition | (Continued) |
|------|------------|-------------|
| **arrhythmia**<br>ă-RĬTH-mē-ă | Inability of the heart to maintain a steady rhythm, possibly including a rapid or slow beat or "skipping" a beat | |
| **bruit**<br>brwē, broot | Soft blowing sound heard on auscultation, possibly due to vibrations associated with the movement of blood, valvular action, or both; also called *murmur* | |
| **cardiomyopathy**<br>kăr-dē-ō-mi-ŎP-ă-thē<br><br>*cardi/o:* heart<br>*my/o:* muscle<br>*-pathy:* disease | Any disease of heart muscle that diminishes cardiac function<br><br>*Cardiomyopathy may be caused by viral infections, metabolic disorders, or general systemic disease.* | |
| **catheter**<br>KĂTH-ĕ-tĕr | Thin, flexible, hollow plastic tube that is small enough to be threaded through a vein, artery, or tubular structure | |
| **coarctation**<br>kō-ărk-TĀ-shŭn | Narrowing of a vessel, especially the aorta | |
| **heart failure**<br>hărt FĀL-yĕr | Failure of the heart to supply an adequate amount of blood to tissues and organs<br><br>*Heart failure is commonly caused by impaired coronary blood flow, cardiomyopathies, and heart valve disease. The term* heart failure *is currently replacing the term* congestive heart failure (CHF). | |
| **embolus**<br>ĔM-bō-lŭs<br><br>*embol:* plug<br>*-us:* condition, structure | Mass of undissolved matter (foreign object, air, gas, tissue, thrombus) circulating in blood or lymphatic channels until it becomes lodged in a vessel | |
| **fibrillation**<br>fĭ-brĭl-Ā-shŭn | Quivering or spontaneous muscle contractions, especially of the heart, causing ineffectual contractions<br><br>*Fibrillation is commonly corrected with a* defibrillator. | |
| **hemostasis**<br>hē-mō-STĀ-sĭs<br><br>*hem/o:* blood<br>*-stasis:* standing still | Arrest of bleeding or circulation | |
| **hyperlipidemia**<br>hī-pĕr-lip-ĭ-DĒ-mē-ă<br><br>*hyper-:* excessive, above normal<br>*lipid:* fat<br>*-emia:* blood condition | Excessive amounts of lipids (cholesterol, phospholipids, and triglycerides) in the blood | |

| Term | Definition |
|------|------------|
| **hypertension**<br>hi-pĕr-TĔN-shŭn<br><br>*hyper-:* excessive, above normal<br>*-tension:* to stretch | Common disorder characterized by elevated blood pressure persistently exceeding 140 mm Hg systolic or 90 mm Hg diastolic |
| **primary** | Hypertension in which there is no identifiable cause; also called *essential hypertension*<br><br>*Primary hypertension is the most common form of hypertension and is associated with obesity, a high serum sodium level, hypercholesterolemia, or family history.* |
| **secondary** | Hypertension that results from an underlying, identifiable, commonly correctable cause |
| **hypertensive heart disease**<br>hi-pĕr-TĔN-sĭv | Any heart disorder caused by prolonged hypertension, including left ventricular hypertrophy, coronary artery disease, cardiac arrhythmias, and heart failure |
| **implantable cardioverter-defibrillator (ICD)**<br>ĭm-PLĂN-tă-băl<br>KĂR-dē-ō-vĕr-tĕr-dē-FĬB-rĭ-lā-tor | Implantable battery-powered device that monitors and, if necessary, corrects an irregular heart rhythm by sending impulses to the heart<br><br>*ICD is a therapeutic device that automatically terminates ventricular arrhythmias.* |
| **infarct**<br>ĭn-FĂRCT | Area of tissue that undergoes necrosis following cessation of blood supply |
| **ischemia**<br>ĭs-KĒ-mē-ă | Local and temporary deficiency of blood supply due to circulatory obstruction |
| **mitral valve prolapse (M V P)**<br>MĪ-trăl,<br>PRŌ-lăps | Common and occasionally serious condition in which the leaflets of the mitral valve prolapse into the left atrium during systole causing a characteristic murmur heard on auscultation<br><br>*Common signs and symptoms of MVP include palpitations of the heart and, occasionally, panic attacks with pounding heartbeat. Because of the possibility of valve infection, prophylactic treatment with antibiotics is suggested before undergoing invasive procedures such as dental work.* |
| **radioisotope**<br>rā-dē-ō-Ī-sō-tōp | Chemical radioactive substance used as a tracer to follow a substance through the body or a structure |
| **palpitation**<br>păl-pĭ-TĀ-shŭn | Sensation that the heart is not beating normally, possibly including "thumping," "fluttering," "skipped beats," or a pounding feeling in the chest<br><br>*Although most palpitations are harmless, those caused by arrhythmias may be serious. Medical attention should be sought if palpitations are accompanied by pain, dizziness, overall weakness, or shortness of breath.* |
| **patent ductus arteriosus**<br>PĂT-ĕnt  DŬK-tŭs<br>ăr-tē-rē-Ō-sŭs | Failure of the ductus arteriosus to close after birth, allowing blood to flow from the aorta into the pulmonary (lung) artery |
| **perfusion**<br>pĕr-FŪ-zhŭn | Circulation of blood through tissues or the passage of fluids through vessels of an organ |

*(Continued)*

| Term | Definition | (Continued) |
|------|------------|-------------|
| **tetralogy of Fallot**<br>tĕ-TRĂL-ō-jē,<br>făl-Ō | Congenital anomaly consisting of four elements: (1) pulmonary artery stenosis; (2) interventricular septal defect; (3) transposition of the aorta, so that both ventricles empty into the aorta; (4) right ventricular hypertrophy caused by increased workload of the right ventricle | |
| **stent**<br>STĔNT | Slender or threadlike device used to hold open vessels, tubes, or an obstructed artery<br>*Stents are used to support tubular structures that are being anastomosed or to induce or maintain patency within these tubular structures.* | |
| **Stokes-Adams syndrome**<br>stōks-ĂD-ăms<br>SĬN-drōm | Altered state of consciousness or fainting due to decreased blood flow to the brain caused by prolonged asystole (absence of muscular contraction of the heart) | |
| **thrombus**<br>THRŎM-bŭs<br><br>  *thromb:* blood clot<br>  *-us:* condition; structure | Blood clot that obstructs a vessel | |

 It is time to review pathological, diagnostic, symptomatic, and related terms by completing Learning Activity 8–3.

## Diagnostic and Therapeutic Procedures

This section introduces procedures used to diagnose and treat cardiovascular disorders. Descriptions are provided as well as pronunciations and word analyses for selected terms.

| Procedure | Description |
|-----------|-------------|
| **DIAGNOSTIC PROCEDURES** | |
| **Clinical** | |
| **cardiac catheterization**<br>KĂR-dē-ăk kăth-<br>ĕ-tĕr-ĭ-ZĀ-shŭn<br><br>  *cardi:* heart<br>  *-ac:* pertaining to, relating to | Passage of a catheter into the heart through a vein or artery to provide a comprehensive evaluation of the heart<br>*Cardiac catheterization gathers information about the heart, such as blood supply through the coronary arteries and blood flow and pressure in the chambers of the heart as well as enabling blood sample collection and x-rays of the heart.* |

| Procedure | Description |
|---|---|
| **electrocardiogram (ECG, EKG)**<br>ē-lĕk-trō-KĂR-dē-ō-grăm<br><br>*electr/o:* electricity<br>*cardi/o:* heart<br>*-gram:* record, writing | Graphic line recording that shows the spread of electrical excitation to different parts of the heart using small metal electrodes applied to the chest, arms, and legs<br><br>*ECGs help diagnose abnormal heart rhythms and myocardial damage.* |
| **Holter monitor test**<br>HŎL-tĕr  MŎN-ĭ-tor | Electrocardiogram (ECG) taken with a small portable recording system capable of storing up to 24 hours of ECG tracings<br><br>*Holter monitoring is particularly useful in obtaining a cardiac arrhythmia record that would be missed during an ECG of only a few minutes' duration.* |
| **stress test**<br><br><br><br>**nuclear** | ECG taken under controlled exercise stress conditions<br><br>*A stress test may show abnormal ECG tracings that do not appear during an ECG taken when the patient is resting*<br><br>Utilizes a radioisotope to evaluate coronary blood flow<br><br>*In a nuclear stress test, the radioisotope is injected at the height of exercise. The area not receiving sufficient oxygen is visualized by decreased uptake of the isotope.* |

## Laboratory

| | |
|---|---|
| **cardiac enzyme studies**<br>KĂR-dē-ăk  ĔN-zīm | Blood test that measures troponin T, troponin I, and creatinine kinase (CK-MB)<br><br>*Cardiac enzymes are most specific to cardiac injury and are released into the bloodstream from damaged heart muscle. Along with other less specific enzymes, these enzymes are used as a diagnostic marker for myocardial injury.* |
| **lipid panel**<br>LĬP-ĭd | Series of tests (total cholesterol, high density lipoprotein, low density lipoprotein, and triglycerides) used to assess risk factors of ischemic heart disease |

## Radiographic

| | |
|---|---|
| **aortography**<br>ā-or-TŎG-ră-fē<br><br>*aort/o:* aorta<br>*-graphy:* process of recording | Radiological examination of the aorta and its branches following the injection of a contrast medium via a catheter |
| **coronary angiography**<br>KOR-ō-nă-rē  ăn-jē-ŎG-ră-fē<br><br>*angi/o:* vessel (usually blood or lymph)<br>*-graphy:* process of recording | Radiological examination of the blood vessels of and around the heart |

*(Continued)*

| Procedure | Description | (Continued) |
|---|---|---|

**echocardiography**
ĕk-ō-kăr-dē-
ŎG-ră-fē

   *echo-:* a repeated sound
   *cardi/o:* heart
   *-graphy:* process of recording

Noninvasive diagnostic method that uses ultrasound to visualize internal cardiac structures and produce images of the heart

*A transducer is placed on the chest to direct ultra-high-frequency sound waves toward cardiac structures. Reflected echoes are then converted to electrical impulses and displayed on a screen.*

   **Doppler ultrasound**
   DŎP-lĕr

Noninvasive adaptation of ultrasound technology in which blood flow velocity is assessed in different areas of the heart

*Sound waves strike moving red blood cells and are reflected back to a recording device that graphically records blood flow.*

**magnetic resonance imaging (MRI)**
măg-NĔT-ĭc RĔZ-
ĕn-ăns

Noninvasive imaging technique that uses radiowaves and a strong magnetic field rather than an x-ray beam to produce multiplanar cross-sectional images

**magnetic resonance angiography (MRA)**
măg-NĔT-ĭc RĔZ-ĕn-
ăns ăn-jē-ŎG-ră-fē

   *angi/o:* vessel (usually blood or lymph)
   *-graphy:* process of recording

Magnetic resonance imaging technique used to visualize vascular structures

*MRA is used to diagnose such vascular disorders as aneurysms, occlusions, atherosclerotic plaque, vascular rupture, and stenosis.*

**phonocardiography**
fō-nō-kăr-dē-
ŎG-ră-fē

   *phon/o:* voice, sound
   *cardi/o:* heart
   *-graphy:* process of recording

Imaging technique that provides a graphic display of heart sounds and murmurs during the cardiac cycle

*In phonocardiography, a transducer sends ultrasonic pulses through the chest wall and the echoes are converted into images on a monitor to assess overall cardiac performance. An electrocardiograph is simultaneously displayed to provide a reference point for each of the sounds and their duration.*

**subtraction angiography**
sŭb-TRĂK-shĕn
ăn-jē-ŎG-ră-fē

   *angi/o:* vessel (usually blood or lymph)
   *-graphy:* process of recording

Imaging technique used to display soft tissue structures such as blood vessels without the confusing overlay of bone images

*In subtraction angiography, two images are obtained—the first before a contrast medium is administered and the second, after the contrast. A computer "subtracts" the first image from the second image, leaving only the contrasted image with all other structures removed.*

**scintigraphy**
sĭn-TĬG-ră-fē

Injection and subsequent detection of radioactive isotopes to create images of body parts and identify body functions and diseases

*In scintigraphy, abnormal uptake of the radioactive isotope indicates abnormality.*

   **thallium study (resting)**
   THĂL-ē-ŭm

Scintigraphy procedure that identifies infarcted or scarred areas of the heart that show up as "cold spots" (areas of reduced radioactivity), taken when the patient is at rest

*In a thallium study, radioactive thallium is injected and the uptake of the isotope is recorded by a gamma camera to produce the image. A stress thallium study is commonly performed at the same time as a resting study, and the two images are compared to further identify abnormalities.*

| Procedure | Description |
|---|---|
| **venography**<br>vē-NŎG-ră-fē<br><br>*ven/o:* vein<br>*-graphy:* process of recording | Radiography of a vein after injection of a contrast medium; incomplete filling of a vein indicates obstruction |

## THERAPEUTIC PROCEDURES

### Clinical

| Procedure | Description |
|---|---|
| **cardioversion**<br>KĂR-dē-ō-vĕr-zhŭn<br><br>*cardi/o:* heart<br>*-version:* turning | Process of restoring the normal rhythm of the heart by applying a controlled electrical shock to the exterior of the chest |
| **embolization**<br>ĕm-bō-lĭ-ZĀ-shŭn<br><br>*embol:* plug<br>*-izaton:* process (of) | Technique used to block blood flow to a site by passing a catheter to the area and injecting a synthetic material or medication specially designed to occlude the blood vessel<br><br>*Embolization may serve to eliminate an abnormal communication between an artery and a vein, stop bleeding, or close vessels that are supporting tumor growth.* |

### Surgical

| Procedure | Description |
|---|---|
| **angioplasty**<br>ĂN-jē-ō-plăs-tē<br><br>*angi/o:* vessel (usually blood or lymph)<br>*-plasty:* surgical repair | Procedure that alters a vessel through surgery or dilation of the vessel using a balloon catheter |
| **coronary artery bypass graft (CABG)**<br>KOR-ō-nă-rē ĂR-tĕr-ē | Surgical procedure that uses a vessel graft from another part of the body to bypass the blocked part of a coronary artery and restore blood supply to the heart muscle |
| **percutaneous transluminal coronary angioplasty (PTCA)**<br>pĕr-kū-TĀ-nē-ŭs<br>trăns-LŪ-mĭ-năl<br>KOR-ō-nă-rē<br><br>*per-:* through<br>*cutane:* skin<br>*-ous:* pertaining to, relating to | Dilation of an occluded vessel using a balloon catheter under fluoroscopic guidance<br><br>*In PTCA, the catheter is inserted transcutaneously and the balloon is inflated, thereby dilating the narrowed vessel. A stent is commonly positioned to hold the vessel open.* |
| **atherectomy**<br>ăth-ĕr-ĔK-tō-mē<br><br>*ather:* fatty plaque<br>*-ectomy:* excision, removal | Removal of material from an occluded vessel using a specially designed catheter fitted with a cutting or grinding device |
| **biopsy**<br>BĪ-ŏp-sē | Removal and examination of a small piece of tissue for diagnostic purposes |
| **arterial**<br>ăr-TĒ-rē-ăl<br><br>*arteri:* artery<br>*-al:* pertaining to, relating to | Removal and examination of a segment of an arterial vessel wall to confirm inflammation of the wall or arteritis, a type of vasculitis |

*(Continued)*

| Procedure | Description | (Continued) |
|---|---|---|
| **catheter ablation**<br>KĂTH-ě-těr<br>ăb-LĀ-shŭn | Destruction of conductive tissue of the heart to interrupt abnormal contractions, thus allowing normal heart rhythm to resume<br>*Catheter ablation is usually performed under fluoroscopic guidance.* | |
| **commissurotomy**<br>kŏm-ĭ-shūr-ŎT-ō-mē | Surgical separation of the leaflets of the mitral valve, which have fused together at their "commissures" (points of touching)<br>*Many candidates for commissurotomy are now treated with balloon mitral valvuloplasty.* | |
| **laser ablation** | Procedure used to remove or treat varicose veins<br>*In laser ablation, the laser's heat coagulates blood inside the vessel, causing it to collapse and seal. Later, the vessels dissolve within the body, becoming less visible, or disappear altogether.* | |
| **ligation and stripping**<br>lĭ-GĀ-shŭn,<br>STRĬP-ĭng | Tying a varicose vein (ligation) followed by removal (stripping) of the affected segment<br>*Ligation and stripping are being replaced by laser ablation, in combination with microphlebectomies and sclerotherapy.* | |
| **open heart surgery** | Surgical procedure performed on or within the exposed heart, usually with the assistance of a heart-lung machine<br>*During the operation, the heart-lung machine takes over circulation to allow surgery on the resting (nonbeating) heart. After the heart has been restarted and is beating, the patient is disconnected from the heart-lung machine. Types of open heart surgery include coronary artery bypass graft, valve replacement, and heart transplant.* | |
| **pericardiocentesis**<br>pěr-ĭ-kăr-dē-ō-sĕn-TĒ-sĭs<br><br>*peri-:* around<br>*cardi/o:* heart<br>*-centesis:* surgical puncture | Puncturing of the pericardium to remove fluid to test for protein, sugar, and enzymes or determine the causative organism of pericarditis | |
| **phlebotomy**<br>flē-BŎT-ō-mē<br><br>*phleb/o:* vein<br>*-tomy:* incision | Incision or puncture of a vein to remove blood or introduce fluids or medications | |
| **thrombolysis**<br>thrŏm-BŎL-ĭ-sĭs<br><br>*thromb/o:* blood clot<br>*-lysis:* separation; destruction; loosening | Destruction of a blood clot using anticlotting agents called "clot-busters" such as tissue plasminogen activator<br>*Prompt thrombolysis can restore blood flow to tissue before serious irreversible damage occurs. However, many thrombolytic agents also pose the risk of hemorrhage.* | |
| **intravascular**<br>ĭn-tră-VĂS-kū-lăr<br><br>*intra-:* in, within<br>*vascul/o:* vessel<br>*-ar:* pertaining to, relating to | Infusion of a thrombolytic agent into a vessel to dissolve a blood clot | |

| Procedure | Description |
|---|---|
| **valvotomy**<br>văl-VŎT-ō-mē<br><br>*valv/o:* valve<br>*-tomy:* incision | Incision of a valve to increase the size of the opening; used in treating mitral stenosis |
| **venipuncture**<br>VĔN-ĭ-pŭnk-chŭr | Puncture of a vein by a needle attached to a syringe or catheter to withdraw a specimen of blood, perform a phlebotomy, instill a medication, start an intravenous infusion, or inject a radiopaque substance for radiological examination |

## Pharmacology

A healthy, functional cardiovascular system is needed to ensure adequate blood circulation and efficient delivery of oxygen and nutrients to all parts of the body. When any part of the cardiovascular system malfunctions or becomes diseased, drug therapy plays an integral role in establishing and maintaining perfusion and homeostasis.

Medications are used to treat a variety of cardiovascular conditions, including angina pectoris, myocardial infarction, heart failure (HF), arrhythmias, hypertension, hyperlipidemia, and vascular disorders. (See Table 8–1.) Many of the cardiovascular drugs treat multiple problems simultaneously.

## Table 8–1  DRUGS USED TO TREAT CARDIOVASCULAR DISORDERS

This table lists common drug classifications used to treat cardiovascular disorders, their therapeutic actions, and selected generic and trade names.

| Classification | Therapeutic Action | Generic and Trade Names |
|---|---|---|
| **angiotensin converting enzyme (ACE) inhibitors** | Decrease blood pressure<br><br>*ACE inhibitors lower blood pressure by dilating arterial blood vessels and inhibiting the conversion of angiotensin I (an inactive enzyme) to angiotensin II (a potent vasoconstrictor).* | **benazepril**<br>bĕn-Ā-ză-prĭl<br>*Lotensin*<br>**captopril**<br>KĂP-tō-prĭl<br>*Capoten*<br>**quinapril**<br>KWĬN-ă-prĭl<br>*Accupril* |
| **antiarrhythmics** | Help establish a regular heartbeat<br><br>*Most antiarrhythmic drugs exert a therapeutic effect by stabilizing the electrical cycle of the heart. These drugs are used to treat atrial and ventricular arrhythmias.* | **flecainide**<br>flă-KĀ-nĭd<br>*Tambocor*<br>**ibutilide**<br>ĭ-BŪ-tĭ-lĭd<br>*Corvert* |

*(Continued)*

| Table 8-1 | DRUGS USED TO TREAT CARDIOVASCULAR DISORDERS *(Continued)* |
|---|---|

| Classification | Therapeutic Action | Generic and Trade Names |
|---|---|---|
| **beta blockers** | Treat and manage angina, hypertension, and ventricular arrhythmias<br><br>*Beta blockers control heart rate to prevent tachycardia, which helps control hypertension and arrhythmias. They also dilate coronary blood vessels to increase blood flow to the myocardium and, thus, may relieve angina.* | **atenolol**<br>ă-TĔN-ō-lŏl<br>*Tenormin*<br>**metoprolol**<br>mĕ-TŌ-prō-lŏl<br>*Lopressor, Toprol*<br>**propranolol**<br>prō-PRĂN-ō-lŏl<br>*Inderal* |
| **calcium channel blockers** | Treat and manage angina, hypertension, and arrhythmias<br><br>*Calcium channel blockers block the movement of calcium in and out of the SA node and cause the heart to beat less forcefully and less frequently. They also dilate the coronary arteries and prevent coronary artery spasm, which can trigger angina.* | **amlodipine**<br>ăm-LŌ-dĭ-pēn<br>*Norvasc*<br>**diltiazem**<br>dĭl-TĪ-ă-zĕm<br>*Cardizem*<br>**nifedipine**<br>nĭ-FĔD-ĭ-pēn<br>*Adalat, Procardia* |
| **diuretics** | Manage edema associated with heart failure and treat hypertension<br><br>*Diuretics increase the excretion of water and sodium by the kidneys to reduce peripheral edema, a common symptom of heart failure. They also reduce total blood volume to treat certain types of hypertension.* | **furosemide**<br>fū-RŌ-sĕ-mĭd<br>*Lasix* |
| **statins** | Reduce low density lipoprotein (LDL) cholesterol in blood and possibly slightly increase high density lipoprotein (HDL) cholesterol<br><br>*LDL has been implicated in cardiovascular disease; HDL appears to have a beneficial cardiovascular effect.* | **atorvastatin**<br>ăh-tŏr-vă-STĂ-tĭn<br>*Lipitor*<br>**simvastatin**<br>SĬM-vă-stă-tĭn<br>*Zocor* |
| **nitrates** | Treat angina pectoris<br><br>*Nitrates act as vasodilators to increase the amount of oxygen delivered to the myocardium. Nitrates can be administered in several ways: sublingually as a spray or tablet, orally as a tablet, transdermally as a patch, topically as an ointment, or intravenously in an emergency setting.* | **nitroglycerin**<br>nĭ-trō-GLĬS-ĕr-ĭn<br>*Nitro-Dur, Nitrolingual, Nitrogard, Nitrostat* |
| **peripheral vasodilators** | Increase peripheral blood flow to treat peripheral vascular diseases, diabetic peripheral vascular insufficiency, and Raynaud disease<br><br>*Peripheral vasodilators selectively act to dilate arteries in skeletal muscles, thus improving peripheral blood flow.* | **cyclandelate**<br>sĭ-KLĂN-dĕ-lāt<br>*Cyclan*<br>**isoxsuprine**<br>ĭ-SŎK-sū-prēn<br>*Vasodilan* |

**Abbreviations**

This section introduces cardiovascular-related abbreviations and their meanings.

| Abbreviation | Meaning |
| --- | --- |
| AAA | abdominal aortic aneurysm |
| AF | atrial fibrillation |
| AS | aortic stenosis |
| ASD | atrial septal defect |
| ASHD | arteriosclerotic heart disease |
| AST | angiotensin sensitivity test; aspartate aminotransferase (cardiac enzyme, formerly called *SGOT*) |
| AV | atrioventricular, arteriovenous |
| BBB | bundle branch block |
| BP | blood pressure |
| CA | cancer; chronological age; cardiac arrest |
| CABG | coronary artery bypass graft |
| CAD | coronary artery disease |
| CC | cardiac catheterization |
| CCU | coronary care unit |
| CHD | coronary heart disease |
| Chol | cholesterol |
| CK | creatine kinase (cardiac enzyme) |
| CPR | cardiopulmonary resuscitation |
| CV | cardiovascular |
| DOE | dyspnea on exertion |
| DSA | digital subtraction angiography |
| DVT | deep vein thrombosis |
| ECG, EKG | electrocardiogram |

*(Continued)*

| Abbreviation | Meaning | *(Continued)* |
|---|---|---|
| **ECHO** | echocardiogram; echoencephalogram | |
| **HDL** | high-density lipoprotein | |
| **HF** | heart failure | |
| **I.V., IV** | intravenous | |
| **LD** | lactate dehydrogenase; lactic acid dehydrogenase (cardiac enzyme) | |
| **LDL** | low-density lipoprotein | |
| **MI** | myocardial infarction | |
| **MS** | musculoskeletal; multiple sclerosis; mental status; mitral stenosis | |
| **MVP** | mitral valve prolapse | |
| **PAC** | premature atrial contraction | |
| **PAT** | paroxysmal atrial tachycardia | |
| **PTCA** | percutaneous transluminal coronary angioplasty | |
| **PVC** | premature ventricular contraction | |
| **RV** | residual volume; right ventricle | |
| **SA** | sinoatrial | |
| **VSD** | ventricular septal defect | |
| **VT** | ventricular tachycardia | |

**It is time to review procedures, pharmacology, and abbreviations by completing Learning Activity 8–4.**

# LEARNING ACTIVITIES

The following activities provide review of the cardiovascular system terms introduced in this chapter. Complete each activity and review your answers to evaluate your understanding of the chapter.

## Learning Activity 8–1

### Identifying cardiovascular structures

*Label the following illustration using the terms listed below.*

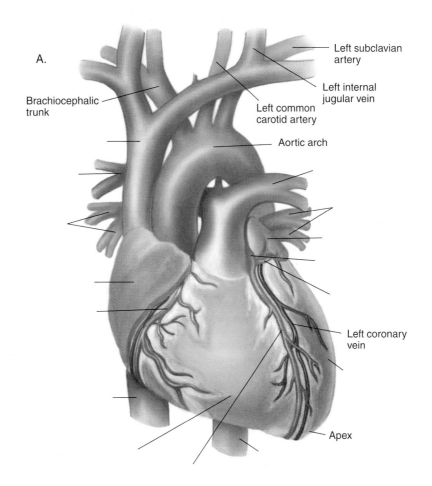

A.

Brachiocephalic trunk

Left subclavian artery

Left internal jugular vein

Left common carotid artery

Aortic arch

Left coronary vein

Apex

| | | |
|---|---|---|
| *aorta* | *left coronary artery* | *right coronary artery* |
| *circumflex artery* | *left pulmonary artery* | *right pulmonary artery* |
| *inferior vena cava* | *left pulmonary veins* | *right pulmonary veins* |
| *left anterior descending artery* | *left ventricle* | *right ventricle* |
| *left atrium* | *right atrium* | *superior vena cava* |

*Label the following illustration using the terms listed below.*

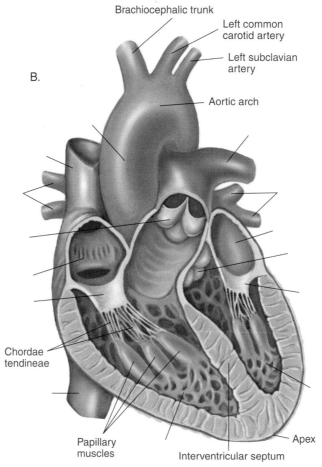

Brachiocephalic trunk

Left common
carotid artery

Left subclavian
artery

B.

Aortic arch

Chordae
tendineae

Papillary
muscles

Apex

Interventricular septum

| | | |
|---|---|---|
| *aorta* | *left pulmonary veins* | *right pulmonary veins* |
| *aortic semilunar valve* | *left ventricle* | *right ventricle* |
| *inferior vena cava* | *mitral (bicuspid) valve* | *superior vena cava* |
| *left atrium* | *pulmonic valve* | *tricuspid valve* |
| *left pulmonary artery* | *right atrium* | |

Check your answers by referring to Figures 8–2A and 8–2B on page 191. Review material that you did not answer correctly.

## Learning Activity 8–2

## Building medical words

---

*Use **ather/o** (fatty plaque) to build words that mean:*

1. tumor of fatty plaque _____
2. hardening of fatty plaque _____

*Use **phleb/o** (vein) to build words that mean:*

3. inflammation of a vein (wall) _____
4. abnormal condition of a blood clot in a vein _____

*Use **ven/o** (vein) to build words that mean:*

5. pertaining to or relating to a vein _____
6. spasm of a vein _____

*Use **cardi/o** (heart) to build words that mean:*

7. specialist in the study of the heart _____
8. rupture of the heart _____
9. poisonous to the heart _____
10. enlargement of the heart _____

*Use **angi/o** (vessel) to build words that mean:*

11. softening of a vessel (wall) _____
12. tumor of a vessel _____

*Use **thromb/o** (blood clot) to build words that mean:*

13. beginning or formation of a blood clot _____
14. abnormal condition of a blood clot _____

*Use **aort/o** (heart) to build words that mean:*

15. abnormal condition of narrowing or stricture of the aorta _____
16. process of recording the aorta _____

*Build surgical words that mean:*

17. puncture of the heart _____
18. suture of an artery _____
19. removal of an embolus _____
20. separation, destruction, or loosening of a blood clot _____

---

Check your answers in Appendix A. Review material that you did not answer correctly.

**CORRECT ANSWERS** _____ × 5 = _____ **% SCORE**

Learning Activity 8–3

## Matching pathological, diagnostic, symptomatic, and related terms

*Match the following terms with the definitions in the numbered list.*

| | | | |
|---|---|---|---|
| *aneurysm* | *catheter* | *infarct* | *secondary* |
| *angina* | *embolus* | *lumen* | *stent* |
| *arrest* | *hyperlipidemia* | *palpitation* | *thrombolysis* |
| *arrhythmia* | *hypertension* | *perfusion* | *varices* |
| *bruit* | *incompetent* | *primary* | *vegetations* |

1. _____ area of tissue that undergoes necrosis
2. _____ chest pain
3. _____ inability of a valve to close completely
4. _____ small masses of inflammatory material found on the leaflets of valves
5. _____ varicose veins of the esophagus
6. _____ soft, blowing sound heard on auscultation; murmur
7. _____ thin, flexible, hollow tube that can be inserted into a vessel or cavity (vein or artery) of the body
8. _____ sensation of the heart not beating normally
9. _____ vascular channel
10. _____ localized abnormal dilation of a vessel
11. _____ mass of undissolved matter circulating in blood or lymph channels
12. _____ inability of the heart to maintain a steady beat
13. _____ condition of being stopped or bringing to a stop
14. _____ destruction of a blood clot using anticlotting agents
15. _____ slender or threadlike device used to support tubular structures or hold arteries open during and after angioplasty
16. _____ common disorder characterized by persistent elevated blood pressure
17. _____ excessive amounts of lipids in the blood
18. _____ hypertension without an identifiable cause
19. _____ hypertension due to an underlying, identifiable cause
20. _____ circulation of blood through tissues

Check your answers in Appendix A. Review any material that you did not answer correctly.

**CORRECT ANSWERS** _____ × 5 = _____ **% SCORE**

# Learning Activity 8-4

## Matching procedures, pharmacology, and abbreviations

*Match the following terms with the definitions in the numbered list.*

| | | | |
|---|---|---|---|
| angioplasty | catheter ablation | embolization | scintigraphy |
| arterial biopsy | commissurotomy | Holter monitor test | statins |
| atherectomy | coronary angiography | ligation and stripping | stress test |
| CABG | diuretics | nitrates | thrombolysis |
| cardiac enzyme studies | echocardiography | PTCA | venipuncture |

1. _____ 24-hour ECG tracing taken with a small, portable recording system

2. _____ noninvasive ultrasound diagnostic test used to visualize internal cardiac structures

3. _____ radiological examination of the blood vessels of and around the heart

4. _____ agents used to treat angina pectoris

5. _____ drugs that have powerful lipid-lowering properties

6. _____ management of edema associated with heart failure and hypertension

7. _____ includes troponin T, troponin I, and creatinine kinase

8. _____ injection and detection of radioactive isotopes to create images and identify function and disease

9. _____ ECG taken under controlled exercise stress conditions

10. _____ tying of a varicose vein and subsequent removal

11. _____ surgical separation of the leaflets of the mitral valve

12. _____ removal of a small segment of an artery for diagnostic purposes

13. _____ destruction of conductive tissue of the heart to interrupt abnormal contractions

14. _____ technique used to block flow to a site by injecting an occluding agent

15. _____ procedure that alters a vessel through surgery or dilation

16. _____ dilation of an occluded vessel using a balloon catheter

17. _____ surgery that creates a bypass around a blocked segment of a coronary artery

18. _____ removal of occluding material using a cutting or grinding device

19. _____ incision or puncture of a vein to remove blood or introduce fluids

20. _____ destruction of a blood clot

Check your answers in Appendix A. Review any material that you did not answer correctly.

**CORRECT ANSWERS** _____ × 5 = _____ **% SCORE**

# MEDICAL RECORD ACTIVITIES

The two medical records included in the activities that follow use common clinical scenarios to show how medical terminology is used to document patient care. Complete the terminology and analysis sections for each activity to help you recognize and understand terms related to the cardiovascular system.

## Medical Record Activity 8–1

### Acute myocardial infarction

#### Terminology

The terms listed in the chart come from the medical record *Acute Myocardial Infarction* that follows. Use a medical dictionary such as *Taber's Cyclopedic Medical Dictionary*, the appendices of this book, or other resources to define each term. Then review the pronunciations for each term and practice by reading the medical record aloud.

| Term | Definition |
|---|---|
| **acute**<br>ă-KŪT | |
| **cardiac enzymes**<br>KĂR-dē-ăk  ĔN-zīmz | |
| **CCU** | |
| **ECG** | |
| **heparin**<br>HĔP-ă-rĭn | |
| **infarction**<br>ĭn-FĂRK-shŭn | |
| **inferior**<br>ĭn-FĒ-rē-or | |
| **ischemia**<br>ĭs-KĒ-mē-ă | |
| **lateral**<br>LĂT-ĕr-ăl | |
| **MI** | |
| **myocardial**<br>mī-ō-KĂR-dē-ăl | |

| Term | Definition |
|------|------------|
| **partial thromboplastin time**<br>thrŏm-bō-PLĂS-tĭn | |
| **streptokinase**<br>strĕp-tō-KĪ-nās | |
| **substernal**<br>sŭb-STĔR-năl | |

## ACUTE MYOCARDIAL INFARCTION

**HISTORY OF PRESENT ILLNESS:** The patient is a 68-year-old woman hospitalized for acute anterior myocardial infarction. She has a history of sudden onset of chest pain. Approximately 2 hours before hospitalization, she had severe substernal pain with radiation to the back. ECG showed evidence of abnormalities. She was given streptokinase and treated with heparin at 800 units/hr. She will be evaluated with a partial thromboplastin time and cardiac enzymes in the morning.

The patient had been seen in 20xx, with a history of an inferior MI in approximately 19xx or 19xx, but she was stable and underwent a treadmill test, the results of which showed no ischemia and she had no chest pain. Her records confirmed an MI with enzyme elevation and evidence of a previous inferior MI.

At this time the patient is stable, is in the CCU, and will be given appropriate follow-up and supportive care.

**IMPRESSION:** Acute lateral anterior MI and old, healed inferior MI

## Analysis

**Review the medical record *Acute Myocardial Infarction* to answer the following questions.**

1. How long had the patient experienced chest pain before she was seen in the hospital?

   _____

2. Did the patient have a previous history of chest pain?

   _____

3. What are the cardiac enzymes that are tested to confirm the diagnosis of MI?

   _____

4. Initially, what medications were administered to stabilize the patient?

   _____

5. During the current admission, what part of the heart was damaged?

   _____

6. Was the location of damage to the heart for this admission the same as for the initial MI?

   _____

# Medical Record Activity 8-2

## Operative report: Rule out temporal arteritis

### Terminology

The terms listed in the chart come from the medical record *Operative Report: Rule Out Temporal Arteritis* that follows. Use a medical dictionary such as *Taber's Cyclopedic Medical Dictionary*, the appendices of this book, or other resources to define each term. Then review the pronunciations for each term and practice by reading the medical record aloud.

| Term | Definition |
|------|------------|
| **arteritis**<br>ăr-tĕ-RĪ-tĭs | |
| **Betadine**<br>BĀ-tă-dĭn | |
| **biopsy**<br>BĪ-ŏp-sē | |
| **dissected**<br>dĭ-SĔKT-ĕd | |
| **distally**<br>DĬS-tă-lē | |
| **incised**<br>ĭn-SĪZD | |
| **IV** | |
| **ligated**<br>LĪ-gā-tĕd | |
| **palpable**<br>PĂL-pă-b'l | |
| **preauricular**<br>prē-aw-RĬK-ū-lăr | |
| **proximally**<br>PRŎK-sĭ-mă-lē | |
| **superficial fascia**<br>soo-pĕr-FĬSH-ăl<br>FĂSH-ē-ă | |
| **supine**<br>sū-PĪN | |
| **temporal**<br>TĔM-por-ăl | |
| **Xylocaine**<br>ZĪ-lō-kān | |

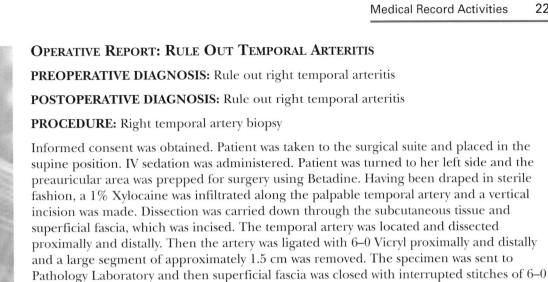

### OPERATIVE REPORT: RULE OUT TEMPORAL ARTERITIS

**PREOPERATIVE DIAGNOSIS:** Rule out right temporal arteritis

**POSTOPERATIVE DIAGNOSIS:** Rule out right temporal arteritis

**PROCEDURE:** Right temporal artery biopsy

Informed consent was obtained. Patient was taken to the surgical suite and placed in the supine position. IV sedation was administered. Patient was turned to her left side and the preauricular area was prepped for surgery using Betadine. Having been draped in sterile fashion, a 1% Xylocaine was infiltrated along the palpable temporal artery and a vertical incision was made. Dissection was carried down through the subcutaneous tissue and superficial fascia, which was incised. The temporal artery was located and dissected proximally and distally. Then the artery was ligated with 6–0 Vicryl proximally and distally and a large segment of approximately 1.5 cm was removed. The specimen was sent to Pathology Laboratory and then superficial fascia was closed with interrupted stitches of 6–0 Vicryl and skin was closed with interrupted stitches of 6–0 Prolene. A sterile dressing was applied. Patient tolerated the procedure well. There were no apparent complications.

## Analysis

**Review the medical record *Operative Report: Rule Out Temporal Arteritis* to answer the following questions.**

1. Why was the right temporal artery biopsied?

   _____

2. In what position was the patient placed?

   _____

3. What was the incision area?

   _____

4. How was the temporal artery described in the report?

   _____

5. How was the dissection carried out?

   _____

6. What was the size of the specimen?

   _____

# Chapter

# 9

# Blood, Lymph, and Immune Systems

## CHAPTER OUTLINE

## OBJECTIVES

*Upon completion of this chapter, you will be able to:*

- Identify and describe the components of blood.
- Locate and identify the structures associated with the lymphatic system.
- Identify the cells associated with the acquired immune response and describe their function.

225

- Recognize, pronounce, spell, and build words related to the blood, lymph, and immune systems.
- Describe pathological conditions, diagnostic and therapeutic procedures, and other terms related to the blood, lymph, and immune systems.
- Explain pharmacology related to the treatment of blood, lymph, and immune disorders.
- Demonstrate your knowledge of this chapter by completing the learning and medical record activities.

## Key Terms

This section introduces important blood, lymph, and immune system terms and their definitions. Word analyses are also provided.

| Term | Definition |
|---|---|
| **anaphylaxis** <br> ăn-ă-fĭ-LĂK-sĭs <br><br> *ana-:* against; up; back <br> *-phylaxis:* protection | Exaggerated, life-threatening hypersensitivity reaction to a previously encountered antigen |
| **antibody** <br> ĂN-tĭ-bŏd-ē | Protective protein produced by B lymphocytes in response to the presence of a foreign substance called an *antigen,* which the immune system regards as harmful to the host |
| **antigen** <br> ĂN-tĭ-jĕn | Substance that is recognized as harmful to the host and stimulates the formation of antibodies in an immunocompetent individual |
| **cellular immunity** <br> SĔL-ū-lăr ĭ-MŪ-nĭ-tē | Acquired specific resistance, mediated by T cells, that produces reactive substances or directly exerts a cytotoxic effect on a cell that is identified as harmful |
| **host** | Organism in or on which another, usually parasitic, organism is nourished and harbored |
| **humoral immunity** <br> HŪ-mor-ăl ĭ-MŪ-nĭ-tē | Acquired specific resistance, mediated by B cells, that produces antibodies that bind to and dispose of antigens |
| **immunocompetent** <br> ĭm-ū-nō-KŎM-pĕ-tĕnt | Able to develop an immune response; able to recognize antigens and respond to them |
| **immunopathology** <br> ĭm-ū-nō-pă-THŎL-ō-jē <br><br> *immun/o:* immune, immunity, safe <br> *path/o:* disease <br> *-logy:* study of | Study of disease states associated with overreactivity or underreactivity of the immune response |

| Term | Definition |
|------|-----------|
| **opportunistic infection**<br>ŏp-or-too-NĬS-tĭk | Infection occurring in a person with a weakened immune system and caused by a microorganism that, under normal conditions, would not bring about disease |
| **palliative treatment**<br>PĂL-ē-ā-tĭv | Treatment that provides relief, but not a cure |
| **serum**<br>SĒ-rŭm | Liquid portion of blood that remains after the removal of fibrinogen<br><br>*Blood collected without an anticoagulant yields a serum sample.*<br>*Blood collected with an anticoagulant yields a plasma sample.* |

## Anatomy and Physiology

The blood, lymph, and immune systems share common cells, structures, and functions. Blood is the source of certain immune cells that locate, identify, and destroy disease-causing agents. These immune cells either actively engage in the destruction of the invading agent or produce proteins that seek out and tag it for destruction. Immune cells rely on lymph vessels and blood vessels to deliver their protective benefits to the entire body. Furthermore, immune cells use lymph structures (the spleen and nodes) to provide permanent or temporary lodging sites where they monitor the extracellular fluid of the body. When disease-causing agents are identified, the immune cells destroy them before irreparable damage occurs in the **host.** The lymph system operates in close association with blood, returning lymph and immune substances back to the circulatory system for redelivery to the entire body. Although these three systems are discussed separately, they commonly function as a single entity to keep the body healthy.

**Figure 9–1**  Blood composition.

## Blood

Blood is connective tissue composed of a liquid medium called *plasma* in which solid components are suspended. These solid components are *erythrocytes* **(red blood cells),** *leukocytes* **(white blood cells),** and cell fragments called *thrombocytes* **(platelets).** (See Figure 9–1.) In adults, blood cells are formed in the bone marrow (myelogenic) tissue of the skull, ribs, sternum, vertebrae, and pelvis as well as at the ends of the long bones of the arms and legs. Blood cells develop from an undifferentiated cell called a *stem cell.* The development and maturation of blood cells is called *hematopoiesis* or *hemopoiesis.* (See Figure 9–2.) Red blood cell (RBC) development is called *erythropoiesis;* white blood cell development, *leukopoiesis;* and platelet development, *thrombopoiesis.* When blood cells are mature, they enter the circulatory system.

Red blood cells transport oxygen and carbon dioxide; white blood cells provide defenses against invasion by foreign substances and aid in tissue repair; and platelets provide mechanisms for blood coagulation, in case the blood vessels become severed. Although it makes up only about 8% of all body tissues, blood is essential to life.

**Figure 9–2**  Hematopoiesis.

## Erythrocytes

Erythrocytes, or RBCs, are the most numerous of the circulating blood cells. In their mature form, they resemble a biconcave disk. During erythropoiesis, erythrocytes develop a specialized iron-containing compound called *hemoglobin* that gives them their red color. Hemoglobin carries oxygen to body tissues, and exchanges it for carbon dioxide. The millions of hemoglobin molecules in each of the billions of RBCs attest to the magnitude of the job they perform. During development, RBCs decrease in size and, just before maturity, the nucleus is extruded from the cell, leaving behind a small fragment of nuclear material that resembles a fine, lacy net, giving this cell its name, *reticulocyte*. Although a few reticulocytes are found in circulation, most erythrocytes lose their nuclear material prior to entering the circulatory system.

Red blood cells live about 120 days and then rupture, releasing hemoglobin and cell fragments. Hemoglobin breaks down into *hemosiderin* (an iron compound) and several bile pigments. Most hemosiderin returns to the bone marrow and is reused to manufacture new blood cells. The liver eventually excretes the bile pigments.

## Leukocytes

The chief functions of leukocytes (WBCs) include protecting the body against invasion by bacteria and foreign substances, removing debris from injured tissue, and aiding in the healing process. Whereas RBCs remain in the bloodstream, WBCs are able to migrate through the endothelial walls of capillaries and venules and enter tissue spaces through a process called *diapedesis*. (See Figure 9–3.) There they can initiate inflammatory or immune responses at sites of injury or infection. Leukocytes are divided into two groups: **granulocytes** and **agranulocytes**.

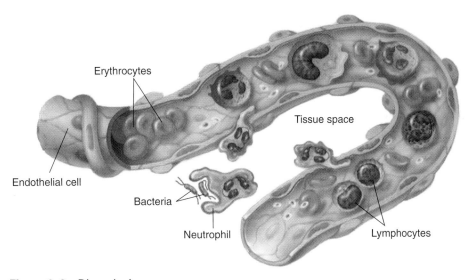

**Figure 9–3**  Diapedesis.

**Granulocytes.** **Granulocytes** are the most abundant type of leukocyte. They contain granules in their cytoplasm and, in their mature form, exhibit a multilobed nucleus (**polymorphonuclear**). The three types of granulocytes are **neutrophils,** *eosinophils,* and *basophils.* These names are derived from the type of dye that stains their cytoplasmic granules when a blood smear is stained in the laboratory.

- *Neutrophils* are the most numerous circulating type of leukocyte. They are very motile and highly phagocytic, permitting them to ingest and devour bacteria and other particulate matter. They are the first cell to appear at a site of injury or infection to begin the work of phagocytizing foreign material. (See Figure 9–4.) Their importance in body protection cannot be underestimated. Someone with a serious deficiency of this blood cell type will die, despite protective attempts by other body defenses.

**Figure 9–4**   Phagocytosis.

- *Eosinophils* protect the body by releasing many substances capable of neutralizing toxic compounds, especially of a chemical nature. Eosinophils increase in number during allergic reactions and animal parasite infestations.
- *Basophils* release histamines and heparin when tissue is damaged. Histamines initiate inflammation, leading to increased blood flow. This brings additional blood cells to injured areas to help in damage containment and tissue repair. Heparin acts to prevent blood from clotting.

**Agranulocytes.**  *Agranulocytes* arise in the bone marrow from stem cells. Because their nuclei do not form lobes, they are frequently called *mononuclear leukocytes.* Agranulocytes include monocytes and lymphocytes:

- *Monocytes* are mildly phagocytic when found within blood vessels. However, they remain there only a short time. When they exit the vascular system, they transform into **macrophages,** voracious phagocytes capable of ingesting pathogens, dead cells, and debris found at sites of inflammation. Macrophages play a chief role in many activities associated with specific immunity.
- *Lymphocytes* include B cells, T cells, and natural killer cells. B cells and T cells provide a specialized type of defense called the **specific immune response.** This mode of

protection is custom-made and aimed at a specific antigen. Its dual response includes **humoral immunity** and **cellular immunity.** Natural killer cells are highly effective against cancer cells and other infected cells. They release potent chemicals that destroy these aberrant cells. (See Table 9–1.)

## Table 9–1    PROTECTIVE ACTIONS OF WHITE BLOOD CELLS

This chart lists the two main categories of white blood cells: granulocytes and agranulocytes along with their subcategories and the protective actions of each.

| Cell Type | Protective Action |
|---|---|
| **Granulocytes** | |
| Neutrophils | Phagocytosis |
| Eosinophils | Allergy, animal parasites |
| Basophils | Inflammation mediators, immediate allergic reactions |
| **Agranulocytes** | |
| Monocytes | Phagocytosis |
| Lymphocytes<br>  B cells<br>  T cells<br>  Natural killer | <br>Humoral immunity<br>Cellular immunity<br>Destruction without specificity |

## Platelets

The smallest formed elements found in blood are platelets. Although they are sometimes called *thrombocytes,* they are not true cells, as this term erroneously suggests, but merely fragments of cells. Platelets initiate blood clotting **(homeostasis)** when injury occurs.

Blood clotting is not a single reaction but, rather, a chain of interlinked reactions that can be summarized as follows:

* Thromboplastin is released by traumatized tissue or ruptured platelets.
* Thromboplastin and other blood clotting factors combine with calcium ions to form prothrombin activator.
* Prothrombin activator reacts with prothrombin and calcium ions to form thrombin.
* Thrombin converts the soluble blood protein, fibrinogen, to fibrin, an insoluble protein that forms a "protein net" entangling blood cells and platelets. This jellylike mass of fibrin, blood cells, and platelets is known as a blood clot.

## Plasma

Plasma is the liquid portion of the blood in which blood cells are suspended. When blood cells are absent, plasma is a thin, almost colorless fluid. It is composed of about 92% water and contains proteins (albumins, globulins, and fibrinogen), gases, nutrients, salts, hormones, and excretory products. Plasma makes possible the chemical communication between all body cells by transporting these products to all parts of the body.

Blood **serum** is a product of blood plasma. It differs from plasma in that the clotting elements have been removed. When a blood sample is placed in a test tube and permitted to clot, the resulting clear fluid that remains after the clot is removed is serum, because fibrinogen and other clotting elements are used to form the clot.

## Blood Groups

Human blood is divided into four groups based on the presence or absence of specific antigens on the surface of RBCs. (See Table 9–2.) Four blood groups, A, B, AB, and O, are identified by the presence or absence of these antigens. In each of these four blood groups, the plasma does not contain the antibody against the antigen that is present on the RBCs. Rather, the plasma contains the opposite antibodies. These antibodies occur naturally; that is, they are present or develop shortly after birth even though there has been no previous exposure to the antigen.

In addition to antigens to the four blood groups, there are numerous other antigens that may be present on RBCs. One such antigen group includes the Rh blood factor. This particular factor is implicated in hemolytic disease of the newborn (HDN) caused by an incompatibility between maternal and fetal blood.

Blood groups are medically important in transfusions, transplants, and maternal-fetal incompatibilities. Although hematologists have identified more than 300 different blood antigens, most of these are not of medical concern.

## Table 9–2   ABO SYSTEM

The table below lists the four blood types along with their respective antigens and antibodies and the percentage of the population that have each type.

| Blood Type | Antigen (RBC) | Antibody (plasma) | % Population |
|------------|---------------|-------------------|-------------|
| A | A | anti-B | 41 |
| B | B | anti-A | 10 |
| AB | A and B | none | 4 |
| O | none | anti-A and anti-B | 45 |

## Lymph System

The lymph system consists of a fluid called lymph (in which lymphocytes and monocytes are suspended), a network of transporting vessels called *lymph vessels,* and a multiplicity of other structures, including nodes, spleen, thymus, and tonsils. Lymph vessels are a one-way transport system that begin as capillaries within tissues, which gradually increase in size as they transport lymph to the bloodstream. Along the journey, lymph passes through lymph nodes and other lymphoid tissue. Functions of the lymph system include:

- maintaining the fluid balance of the body by draining extracellular fluid from tissue spaces and returning it to the blood
- transporting lipids away from the digestive organs for use by body tissues
- filtering and removing unwanted or infectious products in lymph nodes.

Lymph vessels begin as closed-ended capillaries in tissue spaces and terminate at the right lymphatic duct and the thoracic duct in the chest cavity. (See Figure 9–5.) As whole blood circulates, a small amount of plasma seeps out of (1) **blood capillaries.** This fluid, now called *extracellular* fluid **(interstitial or tissue fluid),** resembles plasma but contains slightly less protein. Extracellular fluid carries needed products to tissue cells while removing their wastes. As extracellular fluid moves through tissues, it also collects cellular debris, bacteria, and particulate matter. Eventually, extracellular fluid returns to blood capillaries or enters (2) **lymph capillaries.** If it enters a lymph capillary, it is called **lymph.** Lymph passes into larger and larger vessels on its return trip to the bloodstream. Before it reaches its destination, it first enters (3) **lymph nodes.** These nodes serve as depositories for cellular debris. In the node, macrophages phagocytize bacteria and other harmful material while T cells and B cells exert their protective influence. When a local infection exists, the number of bacteria entering a node is so great and their destruction so powerful that the node frequently enlarges and becomes tender.

Lymph vessels from the right chest and arm join the (4) **right lymphatic duct.** This duct drains into the (5) **right subclavian vein,** a major vessel in the cardiovascular system. Lymph from all other parts of the body enters the (6) **thoracic duct** and drains into the (7) **left subclavian vein.** Lymph is redeposited into the circulating blood and becomes plasma. This cycle continually repeats itself.

The three organs associated with the lymphatic system are the (8) **spleen,** (9) **thymus,** and (10) **tonsils:**

- Like lymph nodes, the *spleen* acts as a filter. Phagocytic cells within the spleen lining remove cellular debris, bacteria, parasites, and other infectious agents. The spleen also destroys old RBCs and serves as a repository for healthy blood cells that are placed into circulation when needed.
- The *thymus* gland is located in the upper part of the chest **(mediastinum).** It partially controls the immune system by transforming lymphocytes into T cells, the cell responsible for cellular immunity.
- *Tonsils* are masses of lymphatic tissue located in the pharynx. They act as a filter to protect the upper respiratory structures from invasion by pathogens.

## Immune System

Although exposed to a vast number of harmful substances, most people suffer relatively few diseases throughout their lives. Numerous body defenses called resistance work together to protect against disease. Resistance includes physical barriers (skin, mucous membranes), and chemical and cellular barriers (tears, saliva, gastric juices, and neutrophils). These barriers are present at birth. Another form of resistance called *acquired immune response* develops after birth. This form of resistance is, by far, the most complex in both structure and function. It develops throughout life as a result of exposure to one disease after another. With each exposure, the immune system identifies the invader (antigen), musters a unique response to destroy it, and then retreats with a memory of both the invader and the method of destruction. In the event of a second encounter by the same invader, the immune system is armed and ready to destroy it before it can cause disease. The WBCs responsible for the specific immune response include monocytes and lymphocytes.

### Monocytes

After a brief stay in the vascular system, monocytes enter tissue spaces and become highly phagocytic *macrophages.* In this form, they consume large numbers of bacteria and other antigens. They process these substances and place their antigenic property on their cell surface, thus becoming antigen-presenting cells **(APCs).** The APC awaits an encounter with an immunocompetent lymphocyte (one capable of responding to that specific antigen) to initiate the specific immune response.

Area drained by
right lymphatic duct

Area drained by
thoracic duct

(10) Tonsil
Submandibular node
(5) Right
subclavian vein
Cervical node
(4) Right
lymphatic duct
(6) Thoracic duct
(7) Left subclavian vein
(9) Thymus
Axillary node
(8) Spleen
Aggregated lymphatic
follicle (Peyer's patch)
(6) Thoracic duct
Small
intestine
Cysterna chyli
Intestinal node
Large intestine
Inguinal node
Iliac node
Red bone
marrow
Lymphatic vessel

Lymph
(2) Lymph capillary
Venule
Arteriole
A
(1) Blood capillary    Extracellular
fluid

B cells
T cells
Valves
Afferent
vessels
Arteriole
Venule
Cortex
Capsule
Densely packed
B and T cells,
macrophages,
and plasma cells
Valve
Vein    Efferent
Artery    vessel
(3) Lymph node
B

**Figure 9–5** Lymph system. (A) Capillary. (B) Lymph node.

## Lymphocytes

Two types of lymphocytes, T cells and B cells, are the active cells in the acquired immune response. Each cell type mediates a specific response: humoral or cellular immunity.

- **Humoral immunity** protects primarily against extracellular antigens, such as bacteria and viruses, that have not yet entered a cell. It is mediated by B cells, which originate and mature in the bone marrow. During maturation, these B cells develop receptors for a specific antigen. Upon an encounter with their specific antigen, B cells produce a clone of cells called *plasma cells*. Plasma cells produce proteins called **antibodies.** Antibodies enter the circulatory system and travel throughout the body in plasma, tissue fluid, and lymph. When antibodies encounter their specific antigen, they form an antigen-antibody complex that inactivates, neutralizes, or tags the antigen for destruction. All such reactions are highly specific; that is, the antibody reacts only against the specific antigen that caused its formation, a characteristic called *specificity*. After the encounter, B memory cells migrate to lymph tissue and are available for immediate recall, should the antigen be encountered again.

- **Cellular immunity** protects primarily against intracellular antigens such as viruses and also has the ability to destroy cancer cells. It is mediated by T cells, which originate in the bone marrow but migrate and mature in thymus. Four types of T cells include the cytotoxic T cell ($T_C$), helper T cell ($T_H$), suppressor T cell ($T_S$), and memory T cell ($T_M$). $T_C$ is the cell that actually destroys the invading antigen. It determines its specific weakness and uses this weakness as a point of attack to destroy the antigen. The $T_H$ is essential to the proper functioning of both humoral and cellular immunity. It activates other cells of the immune system using chemical messengers called *cytokines*. If the $T_H$ cell is unavailable, the immune system essentially shuts down and the patient becomes a victim of even the most harmless organisms and eventually dies. The $T_S$ monitors the progression of the infection. When the infection is resolved, the $T_S$ suppresses, or "shuts down," the immune system until the next encounter with an antigen. Finally, like the humoral response, the cellular response also produces memory cells. These $T_M$ cells find their way to the lymph system and remain there long after the encounter with the antigen. (See Table 9–3.)

## Table 9–3    LYMPHOCYTES AND IMMUNE RESPONSE

The chart below lists the lymphocytes involved in humoral and cellular immunity along with their specific functions and their sites of origin and maturation in the blood and lymph systems.

| Lymphocyte | Function | Origin | Maturation |
|---|---|---|---|
| **Humoral immunity** | | | |
| *B lymphocytes* | | Bone | Bone marrow |
| • Plasma cells | • Antibody formation for destruction of extracellular antigens | | |
| • Memory cells | • Provides active immunity | | |
| **Cellular immunity** | | | |
| *T lymphocytes* | | Bone marrow | Thymus |
| • Cytotoxic T cell ($T_C$) | • Destruction of infected cells and cancer cells | | |
| • Helper T cell ($T_H$) | • Assistance for B cells and cytotoxic T cells ($T_C$) | | |
| • Suppressor T cell ($T_S$) | • Suppression (shutting down) of humoral and cellular response when infection resolves | | |
| • Memory T cell ($T_M$) | • Provides active immunity | | |

The memory component is unique to the acquired immune system. These memory cells are able to "recall" how the B cells and T cells previously disposed of the antigen and are able to repeat the process. The repeat performance is immediate, powerful, and sustained. Disposing of the antigen during the second and all subsequent exposures is extremely rapid and much more effective than it was during the first exposure.

Finally, a unique type of lymphocyte called the *natural killer (NK) cell*, works independently of the specific immune response. It will attack any cell that appears abnormal, and does not require the specificity needed by T cells and B cells. Although NK cells have the ability to kill over and over again, they do not have a memory component like B cells and T cells.

 **It is time to review lymph structures by completing Learning Activity 9–1.**

 ## Medical Word Elements

This section introduces combining forms, suffixes, and prefixes related to the blood, lymph, and immune systems. Word analyses are also provided.

| Element | Meaning | Word Analysis |
|---|---|---|
| **COMBINING FORMS** | | |
| **aden/o** | gland | aden/oid (ĂD-ĕ-noyd): having the appearance or resembling a gland<br>*-oid:* resembling |
| **agglutin/o** | clumping, gluing | agglutin/ation (ă-gloo-tĭ-NĀ-shŭn): process of clumping<br>*-ation:* process (of) |
| **bas/o** | base (alkaline, opposite of acid) | bas/o/phil (BĀ-sō-fĭl): granulocytic white blood cell whose granules have an attraction for alkaline dyes<br>*-phil:* attraction for<br>*The granules of the basophil appear dark blue when stained with methylene blue, an alkaline dye used in hematology.* |
| **blast/o** | embryonic cell | erythr/o/blast/osis (ĕ-rith-rō-blăs-TŌ-sĭs): abnormal condition marked by embryonic red cells in circulating blood<br>*erythr/o:* red (cell)<br>*-osis:* abnormal condition; increase (used primarily with blood cells) |
| **chrom/o** | color | hypo/chrom/ic (hī-pō-KRŌM-ĭk): refers to red blood cells with less color (paler) than normal and, therefore, containing less hemoglobin than normal<br>*hypo-:* under, below<br>*-ic:* pertaining to, relating to<br>*Hypochromic cells are commonly associated with iron-deficiency anemia.* |

| Element | Meaning | Word Analysis |
|---------|---------|---------------|
| **eosin/o** | dawn (rose-colored) | eosin/o/phil (ē-ō-SĬN-ō-fĭl): granulocytic leukocyte whose granules have an attraction for eosin<br><br>*-phil:* attraction for<br><br>*The granules of an eosinophil appear red when stained with eosin, a dye used in hematology.* |
| **erythr/o** | red | erythr/o/cyte (ĕ-RĬTH-rō-sīt): red blood cell<br><br>*-cyte:* cell |
| **granul/o** | granule | granul/o/cyte (GRĂN-ū-lō-sĭt): group of leukocytes that have cytoplasmic granules<br><br>*-cyte:* cell<br><br>*The three types of granulocytes include neutrophils, basophils, and eosinophils.* |
| **hem/o**<br><br>**hemat/o** | blood | hem/o/phobia (hē-mō-FŌ-bē-ă): an aversion to seeing blood<br><br>*-phobia:* fear<br><br>hemat/oma (hē-mă-TŌ-mă): mass of extravasated, usually clotted blood; caused by a break or leak in a blood vessel<br><br>*-oma:* tumor<br><br>*A hematoma may be found in organs, tissues, or spaces within the body.* |
| **immun/o** | immune, immunity, safe | immun/o/logy (ĭm-ū-NŎL-ō-jē): study of the components and function of the immune system<br><br>*-logy:* study of |
| **kary/o**<br><br>**nucle/o** | nucleus | kary/o/lysis (kăr-ē-ŎL-ĭ-sĭs): destruction of the nucleus of a cell resulting in cell death<br><br>*-lysis:* separation; destruction; loosening<br><br>mono/nucle/ar (mŏn-ō-NŪ-klē-ăr): pertaining to cells that have a single nucleus<br><br>*mono-:* one<br>*-ar:* pertaining to, relating to<br><br>*The two mononuclear leukocytes are monocytes and lymphocytes.* |
| **leuk/o** | white | leuk/emia (loo-KĒ-mē-ă): any of several types of malignancy that affect white blood cells<br><br>*-emia:* blood condition<br><br>*Leukemia involves a profoundly elevated white blood cell count and a very low red blood cell count.* |

*(Continued)*

| Element | Meaning | Word Analysis | (Continued) |
|---|---|---|---|
| **lymphaden/o** | lymph gland (node) | lymphaden/o/pathy (lĭm-făd-ĕ-NŎP-ă-thē): any disease of lymph nodes<br><br>*-pathy:* disease<br><br>*Lymphadenopathy is characterized by changes in size, consistency, or number of lymph nodes.* | |
| **lymph/o** | lymph | lymph/oid (LĬM-foyd): resembling lymph or lymph tissue<br><br>*-oid:* resembling | |
| **lymphangi/o** | lymph vessel | lymphangi/oma (lĭm-făn-jē-Ō-mă): benign tumor composed of a mass of dilated lymph vessels<br><br>*-oma:* tumor | |
| **morph/o** | form, shape, structure | morph/o/logy (mor-FŎL-ō-jē): study of form, shape, and structure<br><br>*-logy:* study of | |
| **myel/o** | bone marrow, spinal cord | myel/o/gen/ic (mī-ĕ-lō-JĔN-ĭk): relating to or having origin in bone marrow<br><br>*gen:* forming, producing, origin<br>*-ic:* pertaining to, relating to<br><br>*All blood cells are formed in the bone marrow and are thus considered myelogenic.* | |
| **neutr/o** | neutral, neither | neutr/o/phil/ic (nū-trō-FĬL-ĭk): pertaining to a neutrophil, a granular leukocyte that stains easily with neutral dyes<br><br>*-phil:* attraction for<br>*-ic:* pertaining to, relating to | |
| **phag/o** | swallowing, eating | phag/o/cyte (FĂG-ō-sīt): cell that surrounds, engulfs, and digests microorganisms and cellular debris<br><br>*-cyte:* cell | |
| **plas/o** | formation, growth | a/plas/tic (ā-PLĂS-tĭk): failure of a tissue or organ to develop or grow normally<br><br>*a-:* without, not<br>*-tic:* pertaining to, relating to | |
| **poikil/o** | varied, irregular | poikil/o/cyt/osis (poy-kĭl-ō-sī-TŌ-sĭs): abnormal increase in red blood cells that are irregular in shape<br><br>*cyt:* cell<br>*-osis:* abnormal condition; increase (used primarily with blood cells) | |
| **reticul/o** | net, mesh | reticul/o/cyte (rĕ-TĬK-ū-lō-sīt): immature erythrocyte characterized by a meshlike pattern of threads and particles at the former site of the nucleus<br><br>*-cyte:* cell | |

| Element | Meaning | Word Analysis |
|---|---|---|
| **sider/o** | iron | sider/o/penia (sĭd-ĕr-ō-PĒ-nē-ă): deficiency of iron in the blood<br><br>*-penia:* decrease, deficiency |
| **ser/o** | serum | ser/o/logy (sē-RŎL-ō-jē): study of the serum components of blood, especially antigens and antibodies<br><br>*-logy:* study of<br><br>*Serology also includes the study of antigens and antibodies from sources other than serum.* |
| **splen/o** | spleen | splen/o/rrhagia (splē-nō-RĀ-jē-ă): hemorrhaging from a ruptured spleen<br><br>*-rrhagia:* bursting forth |
| **thromb/o** | blood clot | thromb/o/cyt/osis (thrŏm-bō-sī-TŌ-sĭs): abnormal increase in the number of platelets in the blood<br><br>*cyt:* cell<br>*-osis:* abnormal condition; increase (used primarily with blood cells) |
| **thym/o** | thymus gland | thym/o/pathy (thī-MŎP-ă-thē): any disease of the thymus gland<br><br>*-pathy:* disease |
| **xen/o** | foreign, strange | xen/o/graft (ZĔN-ō-grăft): transplantation of tissues from one species to another; also called *heterograft*<br><br>*-graft:* transplantation<br><br>*Xenograft is used as a temporary measure when there is insufficient tissue available from the patient or other human donors.* |
| **SUFFIXES** | | |
| **-blast** | embryonic cell | erythr/o/blast (ĕ-RĬTH-rō-blăst): embryonic red blood cell<br><br>*erythr/o:* red |
| **-emia** | blood condition | an/emia (ă-NĒ-mē-ă): blood condition characterized by a reduction in the number of red blood cells or a deficiency in their hemoglobin<br><br>*an-:* without, not |
| **-globin** | protein | hem/o/globin (HĒ-mō-glō-bĭn): blood protein found in erythrocytes<br><br>*hem/o:* blood<br><br>*Hemoglobin contains iron, gives blood its red color, and transports oxygen.* |

*(Continued)*

| Element | Meaning | Word Analysis | (Continued) |
|---|---|---|---|
| **-graft** | transplantation | auto/graft (AW-tō-grăft): surgical transplantation of tissue from one part of the body to another location in the same individual<br>*auto-:* self, own | |
| **-osis** | abnormal condition; increase (used primarily with blood cells) | leuk/o/cyt/osis (loo-kō-si-TŌ-sĭs): abnormal increase in white blood cells<br>*leuk/o:* white<br>*cyt/o:* cell | |
| **-penia** | decrease, deficiency | erythr/o/penia (ĕ-rĭth-rō-PĒ-nē-ă): abnormal decrease in red blood cells<br>*erythr/o:* red | |
| **-phil** | attraction for | neutr/o/phil (NŪ-trō-fĭl): leukocyte whose granules have an attraction for a neutral dye<br>*neutr/o:* neutral, neither<br>*Neutrophils are the most numerous type of leukocyte. They provide phagocytic protection for the body.* | |
| **-phoresis** | carrying, transmission | electr/o/phoresis (ē-lĕk-trō-fō-RĒ-sĭs): laboratory technique that uses an electric current to separate various plasma proteins<br>*electr/o:* electricity | |
| **-phylaxis** | protection | ana/phylaxis (ăn-ă-fĭ-LĂK-sĭs): exaggerated, life-threatening hypersensitivity reaction to a previously encountered antigen<br>*ana-:* against | |
| **-poiesis** | formation, production | hem/o/poiesis (hē-mō-poy-Ē-sĭs): production of blood cells, normally within the bone marrow<br>*hem/o:* blood | |
| **-stasis** | standing still | hem/o/stasis (hē-mō-STĀ-sĭs): termination of bleeding by mechanical or chemical means or by coagulation<br>*hem/o:* blood | |
| PREFIXES | | | |
| **a-** | without, not | a/morph/ic (ā-MOR-fĭk): lacking a definite form<br>*morph:* form, shape, structure<br>*ic:* pertaining to, relating to | |
| **allo-** | other, differing from the normal | allo/graft (ĂL-ō-grăft): graft transplanted between genetically nonidentical individuals of the same species; also called *homograft*<br>*-graft:* transplantation<br>*An allograft is a transplant between two individuals who are not identical twins.* | |

| Element | Meaning | Word Analysis |
|---------|---------|---------------|
| **aniso-** | unequal, dissimilar | aniso/cyt/osis (ăn-ĭ-sō-sĭ-TŌ-sĭs): condition of the blood characterized by red blood cells of variable and abnormal size<br><br>*cyt:* cell<br>*-osis:* abnormal condition; increase (used primarily with blood cells) |
| **iso-** | same, equal | iso/chrom/ic (ī-sō-KRŌM-ĭk): having the same color<br><br>*chrom:* color<br>*ic:* pertaining to, relating to |
| **macro-** | large | macro/cyte (MĂK-rō-sīt): abnormally large erythrocyte<br><br>*-cyte:* cell |
| **micro-** | small | micro/cyte (MĪ-krō-sīt): abnormally small erythrocyte<br><br>*-cyte:* cell |
| **mono-** | one | mono/nucle/osis (mŏn-ō-nū-klē-Ō-sĭs): presence of an abnormally high number of mononuclear leukocytes in the blood<br><br>*nucle:* nucleus<br>*-osis:* abnormal condition; increase (used primarily with blood cells) |
| **poly-** | many, much | poly/morph/ic (pŏl-ē-MOR-fĭk): occurring in more than one form<br><br>*morph:* form, shape, structure<br>*ic:* pertaining to, relating to |

**It is time to review medical word elements by completing Learning Activity 9–2.**

## Pathology

Pathology associated with blood includes anemias, leukemias, and coagulation disorders. These three disorders typically share common signs and symptoms that generally include paleness, weakness, shortness of breath, and heart palpitations.

Lymphatic disorders are commonly associated with edema and lymphadenopathy. In these disorders, tissues are swollen with enlarged, tender nodes.

Immunopathies include either abnormally heightened immune responses to antigens (allergies, hypersensitivities, and autoimmune disorders) or abnormally depressed responses (immunodeficiencies and cancers). Many immunologic disorders are manifested in other body systems. For example, asthma and hay fever are immunologic disorders that affect the respiratory system; atopic dermatitis and eczema are immunologic disorders that affect the integumentary system. Some of the most devastating diseases, such as rheumatoid arthritis, cancer, and AIDS, are caused by disordered immunity.

For diagnosis, treatment, and management of diseases that affect blood and blood-forming organs, the medical services of a specialist may be warranted. *Hematology* is the branch of medicine that studies blood cells, blood-clotting mechanisms, bone marrow, and lymph nodes. The physician who specializes in this branch of medicine is called a *hematologist*. *Allergy and immunology* is the branch of medicine involving disorders of the immune system, including asthma and anaphylaxis, adverse reactions to drugs, autoimmune diseases, organ transplantations, and malignancies of the immune system. The physician who specializes in this combined branch of medicine is called an *allergist and immunologist*.

## Anemias

Anemia is any condition in which the oxygen-carrying capacity of blood is less than that required by the body. It is not a disease but rather a symptom of various diseases. Some of the causes of anemias include excessive blood loss, excessive blood-cell destruction, decreased blood formation, and faulty hemoglobin production. It results from a decrease in the number of circulating RBCs (erythropenia), amount of hemoglobin (hypochromasia) within them, or volume of packed erythrocytes (hematocrit).

Anemia commonly causes changes in the appearance of RBCs when observed microscopically. In healthy individuals, RBCs fall within a normal range for size (**normocytic**) and amount of hemoglobin (**normochromic**). Variations in these normal values include RBCs that are excessively large (**macrocytic**), are excessively small (**microcytic**), or have decreased amounts of hemoglobin (**hypochromic**). The signs and symptoms associated with most anemias include difficulty breathing (**dyspnea**), weakness, rapid heartbeat (**tachycardia**), paleness (**pallor**), low blood pressure (**hypotension**) and, commonly, a slight fever. (See Table 9–4.)

## Table 9–4    COMMON ANEMIAS

This chart lists various types of anemia along with descriptions and causes for each.

| Type of Anemia | Description | Causes |
|---|---|---|
| **Aplastic (hypoplastic)** | • Associated with bone marrow failure<br>• Diminished numbers of white blood cells and platelets due to bone marrow suppression<br>• Serious form of anemia that may be fatal | Commonly caused by exposure to cytotoxic agents, radiation, hepatitis virus, and certain medications |
| **Folic-acid deficiency anemia** | • Normal levels achieved by increasing folic acid in the diet or eliminating contributing causes | Caused by insufficient folic acid intake, due to poor diet, impaired absorption, prolonged drug therapy, or increased requirements (pregnancy or rapid growth as seen in children) |
| **Hemolytic** | • Associated with premature destruction of red blood cells<br>• Usually accompanied by jaundice | Caused by the excessive destruction of red blood cells or such disorders as erythroblastosis and sickle cell anemia |
| **Hemorrhagic** | • Associated with loss of blood volume<br>• Normal levels achieved with correction of underlying disorder | Commonly caused by acute blood loss (as in trauma), childbirth, or chronic blood loss (as in bleeding ulcers) |

**Table 9-4** **COMMON ANEMIAS**

| Type of Anemia | Description | Causes |
|---|---|---|
| **Iron-deficiency anemia** | • Most common type of anemia worldwide | Caused by a greater demand on stored iron than can be supplied, commonly as a result of inadequate dietary iron intake or malabsorption of iron |
| **Pernicious anemia** | • Chronic, progressive disorder found mostly in people older than age 50<br>• Treated with $B_{12}$ injections | Caused by low levels of vitamin $B_{12}$ in peripheral red blood cells that may be the result of a lack of "intrinsic factor" in the stomach, which then inhibits absorption of vitamin $B_{12}$ |
| **Sickle cell anemia** | • Most common genetic disorder in people of African descent<br>• Characterized by red blood cells that change from their normal shape to crescents and other irregular shapes that cannot enter capillaries when oxygen levels are low, resulting in severe pain and internal bleeding<br>• Manifest only in patients with both genes for the trait, not those with only one gene for the trait, who are merely carriers of the disease | Caused by a defect in the gene responsible for hemoglobin synthesis |

## Acquired Immunodeficiency Syndrome (AIDS)

AIDS is a transmissible infectious disease caused by the human immunodeficiency virus (HIV), which slowly destroys the immune system. Eventually the immune system becomes so weak (**immunocompromised**) that, in the final stage of the disease, the patient falls victim to infections that usually do not affect healthy individuals (**opportunistic infections**). Gradually, the patient begins to display the symptoms of AIDS: swollen lymph glands (**lymphadenopathy**), malaise, fever, night sweats, and weight loss. Kaposi sarcoma, a neoplastic disorder, and *Pneumocystic carinii* pneumonia (PCP) are two diseases closely associated with AIDS.

Transmission of HIV occurs primarily through body fluids—mostly blood, semen, and vaginal secretions. The virus attacks the most important cell in the immune system, the $T_H$ cell. Once infected by HIV, the $T_H$ cell becomes a "mini-factory" for the replication of the virus. More importantly, the virus destroys the $T_H$, which is essential to both the humoral and cellular arms of the immune system. Without this cell, the entire acquired immune system completely closes down and the patient ultimately dies.

Although there is no cure for HIV, there are highly effective treatments available that can significantly slow the progression of both the virus and the disease. However, many of the medications have serious adverse effects, and once the decision for medical management is made, the patient should not discontinue treatment, as this causes the virus to become resistant.

## Allergy

An allergy is an acquired abnormal immune response. It requires initial exposure to an allergen (**antigen**) that causes an allergic response (**sensitization**). Subsequent exposures to the allergen produce increasing allergic reactions that cause a broad range of inflammatory changes. One common manifestation is hives **(urticaria).** Other manifestations include eczema, allergic rhinitis, coryza, asthma and, in the extreme, anaphylactic shock, a life-threatening condition.

The offending allergens are identified by allergy sensitivity tests. Usually small scratches are made on the patient's back and a liquid suspension of the allergen is introduced into the scratch. If antibodies to the allergen are present in the patient, the scratch becomes red, swollen, and hardened **(indurated).**

Desensitization involves repeated injections of a dilute solution containing the allergen. The initial concentration of the solution is too weak to cause symptoms. Additional exposure to higher concentrations promotes tolerance of the allergen.

## Autoimmune Disease

Failure of the body to distinguish accurately between "self" and "nonself" leads to a phenomenon called autoimmunity. In this abnormal response, the immune system attacks the antigens found on its own cells to such an extent that tissue injury results. Types of autoimmune disorders range from those that affect only a single organ to those that affect many organs and tissues **(multisystemic).**

Myasthenia gravis is an autoimmune disorder that affects the neuromuscular junction. Muscles of the limbs and eyes and those affecting speech and swallowing are usually involved. Other autoimmune diseases include rheumatoid arthritis, idiopathic thrombocytopenic purpura (ITP), vasculitis, and systemic lupus erythematosus (SLE).

Treatment consists of attempting to reach a balance between suppressing the immune response to avoid tissue damage while still maintaining the immune mechanism sufficiently to protect against disease. Most autoimmune diseases have periods of flare-up **(exacerbations)** and latency **(remissions).** Autoimmune diseases are commonly chronic, requiring lifelong care and monitoring, even when the person may look or feel well. Currently, few autoimmune diseases can be cured; however, with treatment, those afflicted can live relatively normal lives.

## Edema

*Edema* is an abnormal accumulation of fluids in the intercellular spaces of the body. One of the major conditions that cause edema is a decrease in the blood protein level **(hypoproteinemia),** especially albumin, which controls the amount of plasma leaving the vascular system. Other causes of edema include poor lymph drainage, high sodium intake, increased capillary permeability, and heart failure.

Edema limited to a specific area **(localized)** may be relieved by elevation of that body part and application of cold packs. Systemic edema may be treated with medications that promote urination **(diuretics).**

Closely associated with edema is a condition called *ascites,* in which fluid collects within the peritoneal or pleural cavity. The chief causes of ascites are interference in venous return during cardiac disease, obstruction of lymphatic flow, disturbances in electrolyte balance, and liver disease.

## Hemophilia

*Hemophilia* is a hereditary disorder in which the blood clotting mechanism is impaired. There are two types of hemophilia: hemophilia A, a deficiency in clotting factor VIII, and hemophilia B, a deficiency in clotting factor IX. The degree of deficiency varies from mild to severe. The disease is sex-linked and found most commonly in men. Women are the carriers of the trait but generally do not have symptoms of the disease.

Mild symptoms include nosebleeds, easy bruising, and bleeding from the gums. Severe symptoms produce areas of blood seepage (**hematomas**) deep within muscles. If blood enters joints (**hemarthrosis**), it is associated with pain and, possibly, permanent deformity. Uncontrolled bleeding anyplace in the body may lead to shock and death. Treatment involves a simple I.V. injection of the deficient factor directly into the individual's vein. The amount of factor replaced varies for a minor and major bleed.

## Infectious Mononucleosis

One of the acute infections caused by the Epstein-Barr virus (EBV) is infectious mononucleosis. It is found mostly in young adults and appears in greater frequency in early spring and early fall. Saliva and respiratory secretions have been implicated as significant infectious agents, hence the name "kissing disease." Sore throat, fever, and enlarged cervical lymph nodes characterize this disease. Other signs and symptoms include gum infection (**gingivitis**), headache, tiredness, loss of appetite (**anorexia**), and general malaise. In most cases, the disease resolves spontaneously and without complications. In some cases, however, the liver and spleen enlarge (**hepatomegaly** and **splenomegaly**). Less common clinical findings include hemolytic anemia with jaundice and thrombocytopenia. Recovery usually ensures a lasting immunity.

## Oncology

Oncological disorders associated with the blood, lymph, and immune systems include leukemia, Hodgkin disease, and Kaposi sarcoma.

### Leukemia

Leukemia is an oncological disorder of the blood-forming organs characterized by an overgrowth (**proliferation**) of blood cells. With this condition, malignant cells replace healthy bone marrow cells. The disease is generally categorized by the type of leukocyte population affected: granulocytic (**myelogenous**) or lymphocytic.

The various types of leukemia may be further classified as either chronic or acute. In acute form, the cells are highly embryonic (**blastic**) and lack mature forms resulting in severe anemia, infections, and bleeding disorders. This situation is commonly life threatening. Although there is a proliferation of blastic cells in the chronic forms of leukemia, there are usually a sufficient number of mature cells to carry on the functions of the various cells types.

Although the specific causes of leukemia are unknown, viruses, environmental conditions, high-dose radiation, and genetic factors have been implicated. Bone marrow aspiration and bone marrow biopsy are used to diagnose leukemia. Treatment methods include one or more of the following: chemotherapy with one or more of the anticancer drugs, radiation, biologic therapy, and bone marrow transplant. Left untreated, leukemias are fatal.

### Hodgkin Disease

*Hodgkin disease* (Hodgkin lymphoma) is a malignant disease that affects the lymphatic system, primarily the lymph nodes. Although it usually remains only in neighboring nodes, it may spread to the spleen, GI tract, liver, or bone marrow.

Hodgkin disease usually begins with a painless enlargement of lymph nodes, typically on one side of the neck, chest, or underarm. Other symptoms include extreme itching (**pruritus**), weight loss, progressive anemia, and fever. If nodes in the neck become excessively large, they may press on the trachea, causing difficulty in breathing (**dyspnea**), or on the esophagus, causing difficulty in swallowing (**dysphagia**).

Radiation and chemotherapy are important methods of controlling the disease. Newer methods of treatment include bone marrow transplants. Treatment is highly effective.

## Kaposi Sarcoma

*Kaposi sarcoma* is a malignancy of connective tissue including bone, fat, muscle, and fibrous tissue. It is closely associated with AIDS and is commonly fatal because the tumors readily metastasize to various organs. Its close association with HIV has resulted in this disorder being classified as one of several "AIDS-defining conditions." The lesions emerge as purplish-brown macules and develop into plaques and nodules. The lesions initially appear over the lower extremities and tend to spread symmetrically over the upper body, particularly the face and oral mucosa. Treatment for AIDS-related Kaposi sarcoma is usually palliative, relieving the pain and discomfort that accompany the lesions, but there is little evidence that it prolongs life.

 **Diagnostic, Symptomatic, and Related Terms**

This section introduces diagnostic, symptomatic, and related terms and their meanings. Word analyses for selected terms are also provided.

| Term | Definition |
|------|-----------|
| **anisocytosis**<br>ăn-ĭ-sō-sǐ-TŌ-sǐs<br><br>*an-:* without, not<br>*iso-:* same, equal<br>*cyt:* cell<br>*-osis:* abnormal condition, increase (used primarily with blood cells) | Condition of marked variation in the size of erythrocytes, when observed on a blood smear<br><br>*With anisocytosis, the blood smear will show macrocytes (large RBCs) and microcytes (small RBCs) as well as normocytes (RBCs that are normal in size).* |
| **ascites**<br>ă-SĪ-tēz | Accumulation of serous fluid in the peritoneal or pleural cavity |
| **bacteremia**<br>băk-tĕr-Ē-mē-ă<br><br>*bacter:* bacteria<br>*-emia:* blood condition | Presence of viable bacteria circulating in the bloodstream, and considered as "travelers" rather than a blood infection |
| **graft rejection**<br>GRĂFT | Recipient's immune system attacks a transplanted organ or tissue resulting in its distruction |
| **graft-versus-host reaction (GVHR)**<br>GRĂFT | Condition that occurs following bone marrow transplants where the immune cells in the transplanted marrow produce antibodies against the host's tissues<br><br>*Bone marrow graft-vs.-host disease can be acute or chronic. The acute form appears within 2 months of the transplant; the chronic form usually appears within 3 months. The symptoms are similar to an autoimmune disease called scleroderma.* |
| **hematoma**<br>hēm-ă-TŌ-mă<br><br>*hemat:* blood<br>*-oma:* tumor | Localized accumulation of blood, usually clotted, in an organ, space, or tissue due to a break in or severing of a blood vessel |

| Term | Definition |
|---|---|
| **hemoglobinopathy**<br>hē-mō-glō-<br>bǐ-NŎP-ă-thē<br><br>*hem/o:* blood<br>*globin/o:* protein<br>*-pathy:* disease | Any disorder caused by abnormalities in the hemoglobin molecule<br><br>*One of the most common hemoglobinopathies is sickle cell anemia.* |
| **hemolysis**<br>hē-MŎL-ǐ-sǐs<br><br>*hem/o:* blood<br>*-lysis:* separation; destruction;<br>loosening | Destruction of RBCs with a release of hemoglobin that diffuses into the surrounding fluid |
| **hemostasis**<br>hē-mō-STĀ-sǐs<br><br>*hem/o:* blood<br>*-stasis:* standing still | Arrest of bleeding or circulation |
| **immunity**<br>ǐ-MŪ-nǐ-tē | State of being protected against infectious diseases |
| **active** | Immunity developed as a consequence of exposure to an antigen and the subsequent development of antibodies<br><br>*Active immunity is generally long-lived because memory cells are formed. Two forms of active immunity include* natural immunity *and* artificial immunity. *In the natural active immunity, the individual acquires a disease and subsequently recovers from it. In artificial active immunity, the individual receives a vaccination or immunizing injection.* |
| **passive** | Immunity in which antibodies or other immune substances formed in one individual are transferred to another individual to provide immediate, temporary immunity<br><br>*Passive immunity is short-lived because memory cells are not transferred to the recipient. Two forms of passive immunity include* natural passive immunity *and* artificial passive immunity. *In the natural form, medical intervention is not required (infant receiving antibodies through breast milk). In the artificial form, antibodies, antitoxins, or toxoids (generally produced in sheep or horses) are transfused or injected into the individual to provide immediate protection.* |
| **lymphadenopathy**<br>lǐm-fǎd-ě-NŎP-ă-thē<br><br>*lymph:* lymph<br>*aden/o:* gland<br>*-pathy:* disease | Any disease of the lymph nodes<br><br>*In lymphadenopathy, the number, consistency, or size of the lymph nodes varies from the normal. In localized lymphadenopathy, only one area of the body is affected. In systemic lymphadenopathy, two or more noncontiguous areas are affected.* |
| **lymphosarcoma**<br>lǐm-fō-sǎr-KŌ-mǎ<br><br>*lymph/o:* lymph<br>*sarc:* flesh (connective tissue)<br>*-oma:* tumor | Malignant neoplastic disorder of lymphatic tissue (not related to Hodgkin disease) |

*(Continued)*

| Term | Definition | (Continued) |
|------|------------|-------------|
| **septicemia**<br>sĕp-tĭ-SĒ-mē-ă | Systemic disease associated with the presence and persistence of pathogenic microorganisms or their toxins in the blood; also called *blood infection*<br><br>*Septicemia is characterized by chills and fever, purpuric pustules, and abscesses. If left untreated, it may lead to shock and death.* | |
| **serology**<br>sē-RŎL-ō-jē<br><br>*ser/o:* serum<br>*-logy:* study of | Blood test to detect the presence of antibodies, antigens, or immune substances | |
| **titer**<br>TĪ-tĕr | Blood test that measures the amount of antibodies in blood; commonly used as an indicator of immune status | |

 It is time to review pathological, diagnostic, symptomatic, and related terms by completing Learning Activity 9–3.

 **Diagnostic and Therapeutic Procedures**

This section introduces procedures used to diagnose and treat blood, lymph, and immune disorders. Descriptions are provided as well as pronunciations and word analyses for selected terms.

| Procedure | Description |
|-----------|-------------|
| **DIAGNOSTIC** | |
| Laboratory | |
| **activated partial thromboplastin time (APTT)**<br>thrŏm-bō-PLĂS-tĭn | Test that screens for deficiencies of some clotting factors; valuable for preoperative screening for bleeding tendencies |
| **blood culture** | Test to determine the presence of pathogens in the bloodstream |
| **complete blood count (CBC)** | Series of tests that includes hemoglobin; hematocrit; red blood cell (RBC), white blood cell (WBC), and platelet counts; differential WBC count; RBC indices; and RBC and WBC morphology |
| **differential count**<br>dĭf-ĕr-ĔN-shăl | Test that enumerates the distribution of WBCs in a stained blood smear by counting the different kinds of WBCs and reporting each as a percentage of the total examined<br><br>*Because differential values change considerably in pathology, this test is commonly used as a first step in diagnosing a disease.* |

| Procedure | Description |
|---|---|
| **erythrocyte sedimentation rate (ESR; sed rate)** ĕ-RĬTH-rō-sīt sĕd-i-mĕn-TĀ-shŭn *erythr/o:* red *-cyte:* cell | Measurement of the distance RBCs settle in 1 hour when whole blood is placed in a narrow tube *The sedimentation rate increases in inflammatory diseases, cancer, and pregnancy and decreases in liver disease.* |
| **hemoglobin (Hgb, Hb)** HĒ-mō-glō-bĭn *hem/o:* blood *-globin:* protein | Measurement of the amount of hemoglobin found in a whole blood sample *Hemoglobin values decrease in anemia and increase in dehydration, polycythemia vera, and thrombocytopenia purpura.* |
| **hematocrit (Hct)** hē-MĂT-ō-krĭt | Measurement of the percentage of packed RBCs in a whole blood sample; also called *crit* |
| **Monospot** | Serological test performed on a blood sample to detect the presence of a nonspecific antibody called the *heterophile antibody* that is present in the serum of patients with infectious mononucleosis |
| **prothrombin time (PT)** prō-THRŎM-bĭn | Test used to evaluate portions of the coagulation system and indirectly measure prothrombin; also called *pro time* *Prothrombin time is commonly used to manage patients undergoing anticoagulant therapy.* |
| **RBC indices** | Mathematical calculation of the size, volume, and concentration of hemoglobin for an average red blood cell |
| **Schilling test** | Test used to assess the absorption of radioactive vitamin $B_{12}$ by the GI system *Schilling test is the definitive test for diagnosing pernicious anemia because vitamin $B_{12}$ is not absorbed in this disorder and passes from the body by way of stool.* |

## Radiographic

| | |
|---|---|
| **lymphadenography** lĭm-făd-ĕ-NŎG-ră-fē *lymph:* lymph *aden/o:* gland *-graphy:* process of recording | Radiographic examination of lymph nodes after injection of a contrast medium |
| **lymphangiography** lĭm-făn-jē-ŎG-ră-fē *lymph:* lymph *angi/o:* vessel *-graphy:* process of recording | Radiographic examination of lymph nodes or tissues after injection of contrast medium in lymph vessels |

*(Continued)*

| Procedure | Description | (Continued) |
|---|---|---|

**Surgical**

| | |
|---|---|
| **aspiration**<br>ăs-pĭ-RĀ-shŭn | Draw in or out using suction |
| **bone marrow** | Procedure using a syringe with a thin aspirating needle that is inserted (usually in the sternum or pelvic bone) to withdraw a small sample of bone marrow fluid for microscopic evaluation. (See Figure 9–6.) |

**Figure 9–6**   Bone marrow aspiration.

| | |
|---|---|
| **biopsy**<br>BĪ-ŏp-sē | Representative tissue sample removed from a body site for microscopic examination, usually to establish a diagnosis |
| **bone marrow** | Removal of a small core sample of tissue from bone marrow for examination under a microscope and, possibly, for analysis using other tests |
| **sentinel node**<br>SĔNT-nĕl  NŌD | Removal of the first lymph node (also called the sentinel node) that receives drainage from cancer-containing areas and the one most likely to contain malignant cells<br><br>*If the sentinel node does not contain malignant cells, there may be no need to remove additional lymph nodes.* |

**THERAPEUTIC**

**Surgical**

| | |
|---|---|
| **lymphangiectomy**<br>lĭm-făn-jē-ĔK-tō-mē<br><br>*lymph:* lymph<br>*angi:* vessel<br>*-ectomy:* excision | Removal of a lymph vessel |

| Procedure | Description |
|---|---|
| **transfusion**<br>trăns-FŪ-zhŭn | Injecting of blood or blood components into the bloodstream |
| **autologous**<br>aw-TŎL-ō-gŭs | Transfusion prepared from the recipient's own blood |
| **homologous**<br>hō-MŎL-ō-gŭs | Transfusion prepared from another individual whose blood is compatible with that of the recipient |
| **transplantation** | Grafting of living tissue from its normal position to another site or from one person to another |
| **autologous bone marrow**<br>aw-TŎL-ō-gŭs | Harvesting, freezing (cryopreserving), and reinfusing the patient's own bone marrow; used to treat bone marrow hypoplasia following cancer therapy |
| **homologous bone marrow**<br>hō-MŎL-ō-gŭs | Transplantation of bone marrow from one individual to another; used for treating aplastic anemia and immunodeficiency disorders |

 **Pharmacology**

Various drugs are prescribed to treat blood, lymph, and immune systems disorders. (See Table 9–5.) These drugs act directly on individual components of each system. For example, anticoagulants are used to prevent clot formation but are ineffective in destroying formed clots. Instead, thrombolytics are used to dissolve clots that obstruct coronary, cerebral, or pulmonary arteries, and, conversely, hemostatics are used to prevent or control hemorrhage. In addition, chemotherapy and radiation are commonly used to treat diseases of the immune system. For example, antineoplastics prevent cellular replication to halt the spread of cancer in the body; antivirals prevent viral replication within cells and have been effective in slowing the progression of HIV and AIDS.

**Table 9–5    DRUGS USED TO TREAT BLOOD, LYMPH, AND IMMUNE DISORDERS**

This table lists common drug classifications used to treat blood, lymph, and immune disorders, their therapeutic actions, and selected generic and trade names.

| Classification | Therapeutic Action | Generic and Trade Names |
|---|---|---|
| **anticoagulants** | Prevent blood clot formation by inhibiting one or more clotting factors<br><br>*Anticoagulants are used to prevent deep venous thrombosis (DVT), prevent postoperative clot formation, and decrease the risk of stroke.* | **enoxaparin**<br>ē-nŏk-să-PĂR-ĭn<br>*Lovenox*<br>**heparin**<br>HĔP-ă-rĭn<br>*Hep-Lock, Hep-Lock U/P*<br>**warfarin**<br>WOR-făr-ĭn<br>*Coumadin* |

*(Continued)*

| Table 9–5 | DRUGS USED TO TREAT BLOOD, LYMPH, AND IMMUNE DISORDERS *(Continued)* |
| --- | --- |

| Classification | Therapeutic Action | Generic and Trade Names |
| --- | --- | --- |
| antineoplastics | Kill or damage rapidly metabolizing cells<br><br>*Antineoplastics are commonly used in combination with other treatment modalities and have been successful in the treatment of various cancers.* | **doxorubicin hydrochloride**<br>dŏk-sō-RŪ-bĭ-sĭn<br>  *Adriamycin PFS, Adriamycin RDF, Rubex*<br>**bleomycin**<br>blē-ō-MĪ-sĭn<br>  *Blenoxane* |
| antiprotozoals, antibiotics, and sulfa drugs (to treat PCP) | Treat *Pneumocystis carinii* pneumonia (PCP)<br><br>*Neutrexin is an antibiotic; Bactrim and Septra are sulfonamides, and NebuPent and Pentam-300 are antiprotozoals. Pneumocystis carinii shares characteristics of protozoa and fungi. It seldom causes symptoms in healthy individuals.* | **trimetrexate glucuronate**<br>trī-mě-TRĚK-sāt gloo-KŪ-rō-nāt<br>  *Neutrexin*<br>**trimethoprim, sulfamethoxazole**<br>trī-MĚTH-ō-prĭm, sŭl-fă-měth-ŎK-să-zōl<br>  *Bactrim, Septra*<br>**pentamidine**<br>pěn-TĂM-ĭ-dēn<br>  *NebuPent, Pentam-300* |
| antivirals (to treat HIV-AIDS) | Prevent the replication of viruses within host cells<br><br>*Combinations of antivirals are commonly given for treatment and management of HIV infection and AIDS.* | **nelfinavir**<br>něl-FĬN-ă-vēr<br>  *Viracept*<br>**lamivudine/zidovudine**<br>lă-MĬV-ŭ-dēn/zī-DŌ-vŭ-dēn<br>  *Combivir*<br>**zidovudine**<br>zī-DŌ-vŭ-dēn<br>  *AZT, Retrovir* |
| fat-soluble vitamins | Prevent and treat bleeding disorders resulting from a lack of prothrombin, which is commonly caused by vitamin K deficiency | **phytonadione**<br>fī-tō-nă-DĪ-ōn<br>  *Vitamin K₁, Mephyton* |
| hemostatics | Prevent or control bleeding<br><br>*Hemostatics are used to treat certain bleeding problems associated with surgery, blood disorders, and liver disease.* | **aminocaproic acid**<br>ă-mē-nō-kă-PRŌ-ĭk ĂS-ĭd<br>  *Amicar* |
| thrombolytics | Dissolve blood clots by destroying the fibrin strands that make up the clot<br><br>*Thrombolytics are used to break apart or lyse thrombi, especially those that obstruct coronary, pulmonary, and cerebral arteries.* | **alteplase**<br>ĂL-tě-plās<br>  *Activase, t-PA*<br>**streptokinase**<br>strěp-tō-KĪ-nās<br>  *Streptase*<br>**urokinase**<br>ū-rō-KĪ-nās<br>  *Abbokinase, Abbokinase Open-Cath* |

## Abbreviations

This section introduces blood, lymph, and immune system abbreviations and their meanings.

| Abbreviation | Meaning |
|---|---|
| AB, ab | abortion, antibodies |
| ABO | blood groups A, AB, B, and O |
| AIDS | acquired immunodeficiency syndrome |
| ALL | acute lymphocytic leukemia |
| AML | acute myelogenous leukemia |
| APTT | activated partial thromboplastin time |
| baso | basophil (type of white blood cell) |
| CBC | complete blood count |
| CLL | chronic lymphocytic leukemia |
| CML | chronic myelogenous leukemia |
| diff | differential count (white blood cells) |
| EBV | Epstein-Barr virus |
| eos | eosinophil (type of white blood cell) |
| ESR, sed rate | erythrocyte sedimentation rate; sedimentation rate |
| Hb, Hgb | hemoglobin |
| HCT, Hct | hematocrit |
| HDN | hemolytic disease of the newborn |
| HIV | human immunodeficiency virus |
| Igs | immunoglobulins |
| ITP | idiopathic thrombocytopenia purpura |
| I.V., IV | intravenous |
| lymphos | lymphocytes |

*(Continued)*

| Abbreviation | Meaning | (Continued) |
|---|---|---|
| MCH | mean corpuscular hemoglobin; mean cell hemoglobin (average amount of hemoglobin per cell) | |
| MCHC | mean cell hemoglobin concentration (average concentration of hemoglobin in a single red cell) | |
| MCV | mean cell volume (average volume or size of a single red blood cell; high MCV = macrocytic cells; low MCV = microcytic cells) | |
| mL, ml | milliliters | |
| PA | posteroanterior; pernicious anemia | |
| PCV | packed cell volume | |
| poly, PMN, PMNL | polymorphonuclear leukocyte | |
| PT | prothrombin time, physical therapy | |
| PTT | partial thromboplastin time | |
| RBC, rbc | red blood cell, red blood count | |
| segs | segmented neutrophils | |
| SLE | systemic lupus erythematosus | |
| WBC, wbc | white blood cell, white blood count | |

**It is time to review procedures, pharmacology, and abbreviations by completing Learning Activity 9–4.**

# LEARNING ACTIVITIES

The following activities provide review of the blood, lymph, and immune system terms introduced in this chapter. Complete each activity and review your answers to evaluate your understanding of the chapter.

## Learning Activity 9–1

### Identifying lymph structures

*Label the following illustration using the terms listed below.*

Area drained by right lymphatic duct

Area drained by thoracic duct

Submandibular node

Cervical node

Axillary node

Aggregated lymphatic follicle (Peyer's patch)

Small intestine

Cysterna chyli

Intestinal node

Large intestine

Inguinal node

Iliac node

Red bone marrow

Lymphatic vessel

Lymph

Venule

Arteriole

Extracellular fluid

A

B cells

T cells

Valves

Afferent vessels

Arteriole

Venule

Cortex

Capsule

Densely packed B and T cells, macrophages, and plasma cells

Valve

Vein

Artery

Efferent vessel

B

*blood capillary*                *right lymphatic duct*              *thoracic duct*

*left subclavian vein*           *right subclavian vein*            *thymus*

*lymph capillary*                *spleen*                          *tonsil*

*lymph node*

Check your answers by referring to Figure 9–5 on page 234. Review material that you did not answer correctly.

Learning Activity 9-2

## Building medical words

*Use* -osis *(abnormal condition, increase) to build words that mean:*

1. abnormal increase in RBCs _____
2. abnormal increase in WBCs _____
3. abnormal increase in lymphocytes _____
4. abnormal increase in reticulocytes _____

*Use* -penia *(deficiency, decrease) to build words that mean:*

5. decrease in RBCs _____
6. decrease in WBCs _____
7. decrease in platelets _____
8. decrease in lymphocytes _____

*Use* -poiesis *(formation, production) to build words that mean:*

9. production of blood _____
10. production of white cells _____
11. production of platelets _____

*Use* immun/o *(immune, immunity, safe) to build words that mean:*

12. specialist in the study of immunity _____
13. study of immunity _____

*Use* splen/o *(spleen) to build words that mean:*

14. herniation of the spleen _____
15. destruction of the spleen _____

*Build surgical words that mean:*

16. excision of the spleen _____
17. removal of the thymus _____
18. destruction of the thymus _____
19. incision of the spleen _____
20. fixation of (a displaced) spleen _____

Learning Activity 9–3

## Matching pathological, diagnostic, symptomatic, and related terms

*Match the following terms with the definitions in the numbered list.*

| | | |
|---|---|---|
| *active* | *hemoglobinopathy* | *lymphadenopathy* |
| *anisocytosis* | *hemolysis* | *myelogenous* |
| *artificial* | *hemophilia* | *normocytic* |
| *bacteremia* | *hemostasis* | *passive* |
| *exacerbations* | *immunocompromised* | *septicemia* |
| *graft rejection* | *infectious mononucleosis* | *titer* |
| *hematoma* | *Kaposi sarcoma* | |

1. _____ periods of flare-up
2. _____ any disorder due to abnormalities in the hemoglobin molecule
3. _____ presence of bacteria in blood, more as travelers, rather than a blood infection
4. _____ arrest of bleeding or circulation
5. _____ type of immunity where memory cells are formed
6. _____ malignancy of connective tissue commonly associated with HIV
7. _____ used to denote an erythrocyte that is normal in size
8. _____ swollen or diseased lymph glands
9. _____ term that denotes a weakened immune system
10. _____ blood clotting disorder
11. _____ common viral disorder caused by the Epstein-Barr virus
12. _____ leukemia that affects granulocytes
13. _____ type of immunity where memory cells are not transferred to the recipient
14. _____ immunity where medical intervention is required
15. _____ destruction of erythrocytes with the release of hemoglobin
16. _____ localized accumulation of blood in tissue; blood clot
17. _____ destruction of a transplanted organ or tissue by the recipient's immune system
18. _____ condition of marked variation in the size of erythrocytes
19. _____ blood test that measures the amount of antibodies in blood
20. _____ blood infection

Check your answers in Appendix A. Review any material that you did not answer correctly.

**CORRECT ANSWERS** _____ × 5 = _____ **% SCORE**

Learning Activity 9–4

## Matching procedures, pharmacology, and abbreviations

*Match the following terms with the definitions in the numbered list.*

| | | |
|---|---|---|
| anticoagulants | hemostatics | RBC |
| aspiration | homologous | RBC indices |
| autologous | lymphadenography | Shilling |
| differential | lymphangiectomy | thrombolytics |
| hematocrit | Monospot | WBC |

1. _____ drawing in or out by suction
2. _____ measurement of packed erythrocytes in a whole blood sample
3. _____ serologic test for infectious mononucleosis
4. _____ used to prevent blood clot formation
5. _____ leukocyte
6. _____ term used to describe a transplantation from another individual
7. _____ removal of a lymph vessel
8. _____ mathematical calculation of the size, volume, and concentration of hemoglobin for an average RBC
9. _____ definitive test for pernicious anemia
10. _____ radiographic examination of lymph nodes
11. _____ term used to describe a transfusion from the recipient's own blood
12. _____ used to prevent or control bleeding
13. _____ erythrocyte
14. _____ used to dissolve blood clots
15. _____ test to enumerate the distribution of WBCs in a stained blood smear

Check your answers in Appendix A. Review any material that you did not answer correctly.

**CORRECT ANSWERS** _____ × **6.67** = _____ **% SCORE**

# MEDICAL RECORD ACTIVITIES

The two medical records included in the activities that follow use common clinical scenarios to show how medical terminology is used to document patient care. Complete the terminology and analysis sections for each activity to help you recognize and understand terms related to the integumentary system.

## Medical Record Activity 9–1

### Discharge summary: Sickle cell crisis

#### Terminology

The terms listed in the chart come from the medical record *Discharge Summary: Sickle Cell Crisis* that follows. Use a medical dictionary such as *Taber's Cyclopedic Medical Dictionary*, the appendices of this book, or other resources to define each term. Then review the pronunciations for each term and practice by reading the medical record aloud.

| Term | Definition |
|---|---|
| **ambulating**<br>ĂM-bū-lāt-ĭng | |
| **analgesia**<br>ăn-ăl-JĒ-zē-ă | |
| **anemia**<br>ă-NĒ-mē-ă | |
| **crisis**<br>KRĪ-sĭs | |
| **CT scan** | |
| **hemoglobin**<br>HĒ-mō-glō-bĭn | |
| **ileus**<br>ĬL-ē-ŭs | |
| **infarction**<br>ĭn-FĂRK-shŭn | |
| **morphine**<br>MOR-fēn | |

*(Continued)*

| Term | Definition | (Continued) |
|---|---|---|
| **sickle cell**<br>SĬK-ăl SĔL | | |
| **splenectomy**<br>splē-NĔK-tō-mē | | |
| **Vicodin**<br>VĪ-kō-dĭn | | |

## DISCHARGE SUMMARY: SICKLE CELL CRISIS

### ADMITTING AND DISCHARGE DIAGNOSES:

(1) Sickle cell crisis
(2) Abdominal pain

**PROCEDURES:** Two units of packed red blood cells and CT scan of the abdomen

**REASON FOR ADMISSION:** This is a 46-year-old African-American man who reports a history of sickle cell anemia, which results in abdominal cramping when he is in crisis. His hemoglobin was 6 upon admission. He says his baseline runs 7 to 8. The patient states that he has not had a splenectomy. He describes the pain as midabdominal and cramplike. He denied any chills, fevers, or sweats.

**HOSPITAL COURSE BY PROBLEM:** (1) Sickle cell crisis. The patient was admitted to a Medical/Surgical bed, and placed on oxygen and IV fluids. He received morphine for analgesia, as well as Vicodin. At discharge his abdominal pain had resolved; however, he reported weakness. He was kept for an additional day for observation.

(2) A CT scan was performed on the belly and showed evidence of ileus in the small bowel with somewhat dilated small bowel loops and also an abnormal enhancement pattern in the kidney. The patient has had no nausea or vomiting. He is moving his bowels without any difficulty. He is ambulating. He even goes outside to smoke cigarettes, which he has been advised not to do. Certainly, we should obtain some information on his renal function and have his regular doctor assess this problem.

**DISCHARGE INSTRUCTIONS:** The patient has been advised to stop smoking and to see his regular doctor for follow-up on renal function.

## Analysis

**Review the medical record *Discharge Summary: Sickle Cell Crisis* to answer the following questions.**

1. What blood product was administered to the patient?

_____

2. Why was this blood product given to the patient?

_____

3. Why was a CT scan performed on the patient?

_____

4. What were the three findings of the CT scan?

_____

5. Why should the patient see his regular doctor?

_____

## Medical Record Activity 9–2

### Discharge summary: PCP and HIV

#### Terminology

The terms listed in the chart come from the medical record *Discharge Summary: PCP and HIV* that follows. Use a medical dictionary such as *Taber's Cyclopedic Medical Dictionary*, the appendices of this book, or other resources to define each term. Then review the pronunciations for each term and practice by reading the medical record aloud.

| Term | Definition |
|---|---|
| **alveolar lavage**<br>ăl-VĒ-ō-lăr  lă-VĂZH | |
| **Bactrim**<br>BĂK-trĭm | |
| **bronchoscopy**<br>brŏng-KŎS-kō-pē | |
| **diffuse**<br>dĭ-FŪS | |
| **HIV** | |
| **human immunodeficiency virus**<br>ĭm-ū-nō-dē-FĬSH-ĕn-sē | |
| **infiltrate**<br>ĬN-fĭl-trāt | |
| **Kaposi sarcoma**<br>KĂP-ō-sē  săr-KŌ-mă | |
| **leukoencephalopathy**<br>loo-kō-ĕn-sĕf-ă-LŎP-ă-thē | |
| **multifocal**<br>mŭl-tĭ-FŌ-kăl | |
| **PCP** | |
| **PMN** | |

*(Continued)*

| Term | Definition | (Continued) |
|---|---|---|

**_Pneumocystis carinii_ pneumonia**
nū-mō-SĬS-tĭs
kă-RĪ-nē-ī  nū-MŌ-nē-ă

**thrush**
THRŬSH

**vaginal candidiasis**
VĂJ-ĭn-ăl
kăn-dĭ-DĪ-ă-sĭs

## DISCHARGE SUMMARY: PCP AND HIV

### FINAL DIAGNOSES:

(1) *Pneumocystis carinii* pneumonia
(2) Human immunodeficiency virus infection
(3) Wasting

**SOCIAL HISTORY:** The patient's husband is deceased from AIDS 1 year ago with progressive multifocal leukoencephalopathy (PML) and Kaposi sarcoma. She denies any history of intravenous drug use, transfusion, and identifies three lifetime sexual partners.

**PAST MEDICAL HISTORY:** The patient's past medical history is significant for HIV and several episodes of diarrhea, sinusitis, thrush, and vaginal candidiasis. She gave a history of a 10-pound weight loss. The chest x-ray showed diffuse lower lobe infiltrates, and she was diagnosed with presumptive *Pneumocystis carinii* pneumonia and placed on Bactrim. She was admitted for a bronchoscopy with alveolar lavage to confirm the diagnosis. The antiretroviral treatment was reinitiated, and she was counseled as to the need to strictly adhere to her therapeutic regimen.

**DISCHARGE INSTRUCTIONS:** Complete medication regimen. Return to the care of Dr. Amid Shaheen.

## Analysis

**Review the medical record *Discharge Summary: PCP and HIV* to answer the following questions.**

1. How do you think the patient acquired the HIV infection?

_____

2. What were the two diagnoses of the husband?

_____

3. What four disorders in the medical history are significant for HIV?

_____

4. What was the x-ray finding?

_____

5. What two procedures are going to be performed to confirm the diagnosis of PCP pneumonia?

_____

# Chapter

## 10

# Musculoskeletal System

## CHAPTER OUTLINE

## OBJECTIVES

*Upon completion of this chapter, you will be able to:*

- Locate and describe the structures of the musculoskeletal system.
- Recognize, pronounce, spell, and build words related to the musculoskeletal system.
- Describe pathological conditions, diagnostic and therapeutic procedures, and other terms related to the musculoskeletal system.

■ Explain pharmacology related to the treatment of musculoskeletal disorders.

■ Demonstrate your knowledge of this chapter by completing the learning and medical record activities.

## Key Terms

This section introduces important musculoskeletal system terms and their definitions. Word analyses are also provided.

| Term | Definition |
|------|-----------|
| **appendage**<br>ă-PĔN-dĭj | Any body part attached to a main structure<br>*Examples of appendages include the arms and legs.* |
| **articulation**<br>ăr-tĭk-ū-LĀ-shŭn | Place of union between two or more bones; also called *joint* |
| **arthritis**<br>ăr-THRĪ-tĭs<br><br>*arthr:* joint<br>*-itis:* inflammation | Inflammation of a joint; usually accompanied by pain, swelling and, commonly, changes in structure<br>*Types of arthritis include osteoarthritis, rheumatoid arthritis, gouty arthritis, and ankylosing spondylitis.* |
| **cruciate ligaments**<br>KROO-shē-āt<br><br>*cruci:* cross | Ligaments that cross each other forming an X within the notch between the femoral condyles<br>*These ligaments help to prevent anterior-posterior displacement of the articular surfaces and to secure the articulating bones when standing.* |
| **hematopoiesis**<br>hĕm-ă-tō-poy-Ē-sĭs<br><br>*hemat/o:* blood<br>*-poiesis:* formation, production | Production and development of blood cells, normally in the bone marrow |
| **meatus**<br>mē-Ā-tŭs<br><br>*meat:* opening, meatus<br>*-us:* condition; structure | An opening or passage through any part of the body |

## Anatomy and Physiology

The musculoskeletal system includes muscles, bones, joints, and related structures, such as the tendons and connective tissue that function in the movement of body parts and organs.

## Muscles

Muscle tissue is composed of contractile cells or fibers that provide movement of an organ or body part. Muscles contribute to posture, produce body heat, and act as a protective covering for internal organs. Muscles make up the bulk of the body and have the ability to contract, to relax, to be excited by a stimulus, and to return to their original size and shape. Regardless if muscles are attached to bones or to internal organs and blood vessels, the primary responsibility of muscles is movement. Apparent motion includes walking and talking. Less apparent motions provided by muscles are the passage and elimination of food through the digestive system, propulsion of blood through the arteries, and contraction of the bladder to eliminate urine. Review Figure 10–1 to familiarize yourself with the names and locations of selected muscles. These terms will appear when pathological conditions of muscles are discussed in both the textbook and medical reports.

There are three types of muscle tissue in the body:

- *Skeletal muscles,* also called *voluntary* or *striated muscles,* are muscles whose action is under voluntary control. Some examples of voluntary muscles are the muscles that move the eyeballs, tongue, and bones. Except for cardiac muscle, all striated muscles are voluntary.

**Figure 10–1**  Selected muscles of the body.

- *Cardiac muscle,* found only in the heart, is unique for its branched interconnections, and it makes up most of the wall of the heart. It shares similarities with both skeletal and smooth muscles. Like skeletal muscle, it is striated, but it experiences rhythmic involuntary contractions like smooth muscle.
- *Smooth muscles (involuntary* or *visceral muscles)* are muscles whose action are involuntary. They are found principally in the visceral organs, the walls of arteries, the walls of respiratory passages, and in the urinary and reproductive ducts. The contraction of smooth muscle is controlled by the autonomic (involuntary) nervous system.

Figure 10–2 and Table 10–1 illustrate body movements produced by actions of muscles. Most are identified in pairs and provide opposing functions.

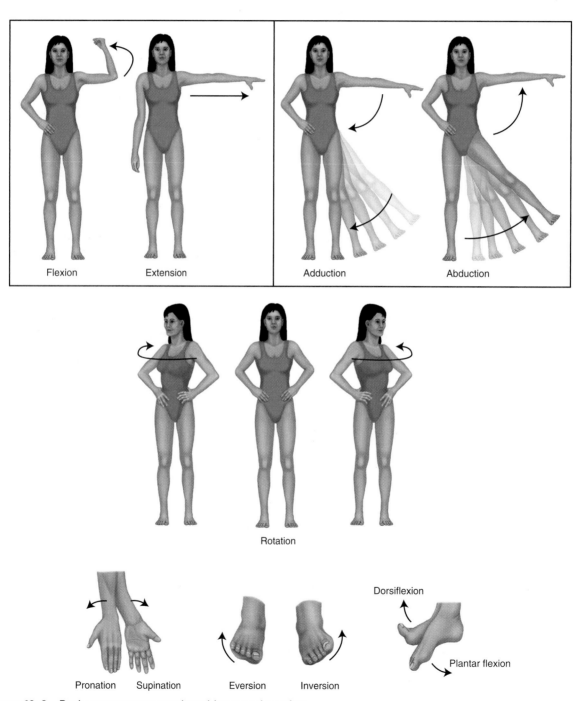

**Figure 10–2** • Body movements produced by muscle action.

## Table 10-1    BODY MOVEMENTS PRODUCED BY MUSCLE ACTION

This chart lists body movements and the muscles used to produce them. With the exception of rotation, these movements are grouped in pairs of opposing functions.

| Motion | Action |
|---|---|
| Adduction | Moves closer to the midline |
| Abduction | Moves away from the midline |
| Flexion | Decreases the angle of a joint |
| Extension | Increases the angle of a joint |
| Rotation | Moves a bone around its own axis |
| Pronation | Turns the palm down |
| Supination | Turns the palm up |
| Inversion | Moves the sole of the foot inward |
| Eversion | Moves the sole of the foot outward |
| Dorsiflexion | Elevates the foot |
| Plantar flexion | Lowers the foot (points the toes) |

### Attachments

Muscles attach to bones either by fleshy or fibrous attachments. In **fleshy attachments,** muscle fibers arise directly from bone. Although these fibers distribute force over wide areas, they are weaker than a fibrous attachment. In **fibrous attachments,** the connective tissue converges at the end of the muscle to become continuous and indistinguishable from the periosteum. When the fibrous attachment spans a large area of a particular bone, the attachment is called an *aponeurosis.* Such attachments are found in the lumbar region of the back. In some instances, this connective tissue penetrates the bone itself. When connective tissue fibers form a cord or strap, it is referred to as a *tendon.* This localizes a great deal of force in a small area of bone. Ligaments are composed of connective tissue and attach one bone to another.

 **It is time to review muscle structures by completing Learning Activity 10–1.**

### Bones

Bones provide the framework of the body, protect internal organs, store calcium and other minerals, and produce blood cells within bone marrow. Together with other soft tissue, most vital organs are enclosed and protected by bones. For example, the bones of the skull protect the brain; the rib cage protects the heart and lungs. In addition to support and protection, the skeletal system carries out a number of other important functions. Movement is possible because bones provide points of attachment for muscles, tendons, and ligaments. As muscles contract, tendons and ligaments pull on bones and cause skeletal movement. Bone marrow, found within the larger bones, is responsible for **hematopoiesis,** continuously producing millions of blood cells to replace those that have been destroyed. Bones serve as a storehouse for minerals, particularly phosphorus and calcium. When the body experiences a need for a certain mineral, such as calcium during pregnancy, and a sufficient dietary supply is not available, calcium is withdrawn from the bones.

## Bone Types

The four principal types of bones are short bones, flat bones, irregular bones, and long bones:

- *Short bones* are somewhat cube-shaped. They consist of a core of spongy bone, also known as *cancellous bone,* that is enclosed in a thin surface layer of compact bone. Examples of short bones include the bones of the ankles, wrists, and toes.
- *Irregular bones* include the bones that cannot be classified as short or long because of their complex shapes. Examples of irregular bones include vertebrae and the bones of the middle ear.
- *Flat bones* are exactly what their name suggests. They provide broad surfaces for muscular attachment or protection for internal organs. Examples of flat bones include bones of the skull, shoulder blades, and sternum.
- *Long bones* are found in the extremities of the body, such as the legs, arms, and fingers. (See Figure 10–3.) The parts of a long bone include:
  - The (1) **diaphysis** is the shaft or long, main portion of a bone.
  - The two ends of the bones, the (2) **distal epiphysis** and (3) **proximal epiphysis,** have a somewhat bulbous shape to provide space for muscle and ligament attachments near the joints. The epiphyses (singular, *epiphysis*) are made up largely of (4) **spongy bone** surrounded by a layer of compact bone. Red bone marrow is found within the porous chamber of spongy bone. This marrow is richly supplied with blood and

**Figure 10–3** Longitudinal structure of a long bone.

consists of immature and mature blood cells in various stages of development. In an adult, the production of red blood cells (**erythropoiesis**) occurs in red bone marrow. Red bone marrow is also responsible for the formation of white blood cells (**leukopoiesis**) and platelets. Both ends of the epiphysis are covered by (5) **articular cartilage,** a type of elastic connective tissue that provides a smooth surface for movement of joints.

- In long bones, the bone shaft, or diaphysis, consists of (6) **compact bone** forming a cylinder that surrounds a central canal called the (7) **medullary cavity.** This medullary cavity, or *marrow cavity,* contains fatty yellow marrow in adults and consists primarily of fat cells and a few scattered blood cells.
- The (8) **periosteum,** a dense, white, fibrous membrane, covers the remaining surface of the bone. It contains numerous blood and lymph vessels and nerves. In growing bones, the inner layer contains the bone-forming cells known as *osteoblasts.* Because blood vessels and osteoblasts are located here, the periosteum provides a means for bone repair and general bone nutrition. Bones that lose periosteum through injury or disease usually scale or die. The periosteum also serves as a point of attachment for muscles, ligaments, and tendons.

 **It is time to review bone structures by completing Learning Activity 10–2.**

## Surface Features of Bones

Surfaces of bones are rarely smooth. Rather, they consist of projections, depressions, and openings that provide sites for muscle and ligament attachment. They also provide pathways and openings for blood vessels, nerves, and ducts. Various types of projections are evident in bones, some of which serve as points of **articulation.** Surfaces of bones may be rounded, sharp, or narrow or have a large ridge. Depressions and openings are cavities and holes in a bone. The most common types of projections, depressions, and openings are summarized in Table 10–2.

| Table 10–2 | SURFACE FEATURES OF BONES |
|---|---|

This chart lists the most common types of projections, depressions, and openings along with the bones involved, descriptions, and examples for each. Becoming familiar with these terms will help you identify parts of individual bones described in medical reports related to orthopedics.

| Surface Type | Bone Marking | Description | Example |
|---|---|---|---|
| **Projections**<br>• Nonarticulating surfaces<br>• Sites of muscle and ligament attachment | • Trochanter<br><br>• Tubercle<br>• Tuberosity | • Very large, irregularly shaped process found only on the femur<br>• Small, rounded process<br>• Large, rounded process | • Greater trochanter of the femur<br><br>• Tubercle of the femur<br>• Tuberosity of the humerus |
| **Articulating surfaces**<br>• Projections that form joints | • Condyle<br>• Head | • Rounded, articulating knob<br>• Prominent, rounded, articulating end of a bone | • Condyle of the humerus<br>• Head of the femur |
| **Depressions and openings**<br>• Sites for blood vessel, nerve, and duct passage | • Foramen<br><br><br>• Fissure<br>• Meatus<br><br>• Sinus | • Rounded opening through a bone to accommodate blood vessels and nerves<br>• Narrow, slitlike opening<br>• Canal-like passageway into a bone<br><br>• Cavity or hollow space in a bone | • Foramen of the skull through which cranial nerves pass<br><br>• Fissure of the sphenoid bone<br>• External auditory meatus of the temporal bone<br>• Cavity of frontal sinus containing a duct that carries secretions to the upper part of the nasal cavity |

## Divisions of the Skeletal System

The skeletal system of a human adult consists of 206 individual bones. However, only the major bones are discussed. For anatomical purposes, the human skeleton is divided into the axial skeleton and appendicular skeleton. (See Figure 10–4.)

**Axial skeleton.** The axial skeleton is divided into three major regions: skull, rib cage, and vertebral column. It contributes to the formation of body cavities and provides protection for internal organs, such as the brain, spinal cord, and organs enclosed in the thorax. The axial skeleton is distinguished with bone color in Figure 10–4.

*Skull.* The bony structure of the skull consists of **cranial bones** and **facial bones.** (See Figure

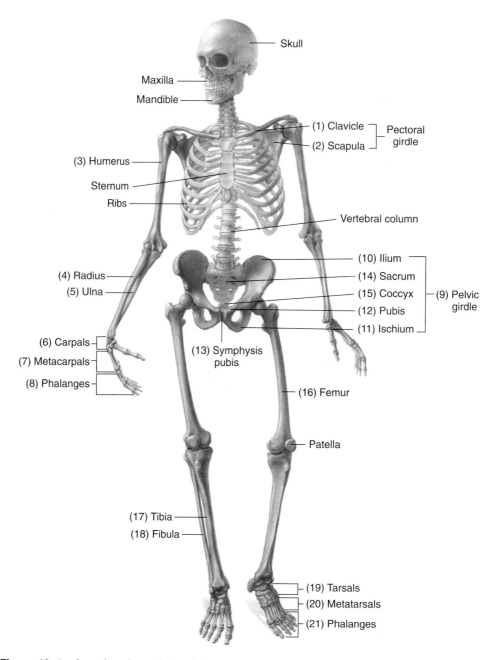

**Figure 10–4**  Anterior view of the skeleton.

10–5.) With the exception of one facial bone, all other bones of the skull are joined together by *sutures*. Sutures are the lines of junction between two bones, especially of the skull, and are usually immovable.

**CRANIAL BONES.** Eight bones, collectively known as the *cranium (skull)*, enclose and protect the brain and the organs of hearing and equilibrium. Cranial bones are connected to muscles to provide head movements, chewing motions, and facial expressions.

An infant's skull contains membranous areas called *fontanels* or "soft spots" where the bone-making process is not yet complete. Their chief function is to allow a small compression of the skull during the delivery process. With age they ossify and become fixed.

The (1) **frontal bone** forms the anterior portion of the skull (forehead) and the roof of the bony cavities that contain the eyeballs. One (2) **parietal bone** is situated on each side of

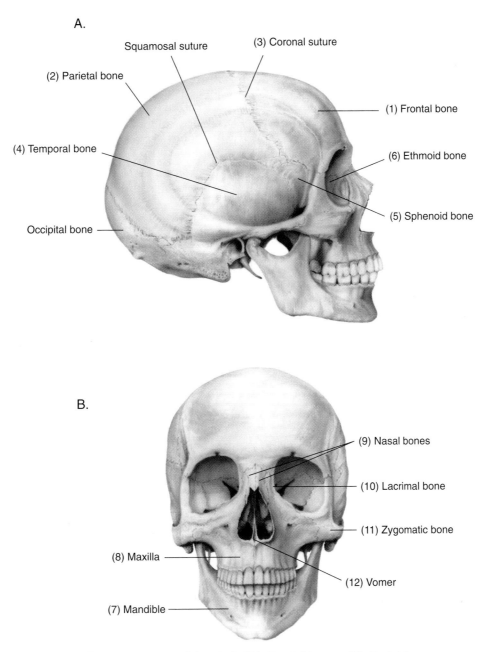

**Figure 10–5** Bony structures of the skull. (A) Cranial bones. (B) Facial bones.

the skull just behind the frontal bone. Together, they form the upper sides and roof of the cranium. Each parietal bone meets the frontal bone along the (3) **coronal suture.** A single *occipital bone* forms the back and base of the skull. It contains an opening in its base through which the spinal cord passes. Two (4) **temporal bones,** one on each side of the skull, form part of the lower cranium. Each temporal bone has a complicated shape that contains various cavities and recesses associated with the internal ear, the essential part of the organ of hearing. The temporal bone projects downward to form the *mastoid process,* which provides a point of attachment for several neck muscles. The (5) **sphenoid bone,** located at the middle part of the base of the skull, forms a central wedge that joins with all other cranial bones, holding them together. A very light and spongy bone, the (6) **ethmoid bone,** forms most of the bony area between the nasal cavity and parts of the orbits of the eyes.

**FACIAL BONES.** All facial bones, with the exception of the (7) **mandible** (lower jaw bone), are joined together by sutures and are immovable. Movement of the mandible is needed for speaking and chewing **(mastication).** The (8) **maxillae,** paired upper jawbones, are fused in the midline by a suture. They form the upper jaw and hard palate (roof of the mouth). If the maxillary bones do not fuse properly before birth, a congenital defect called *cleft palate* results. The maxillae (singular, maxilla) and the mandible contain sockets for the roots of the teeth. Two thin and nearly rectangular bones, the (9) **nasal bones,** lie side by side and are fused medially, forming the shape and the bridge of the nose. Two paired (10) **lacrimal bones** are located at the corner of each eye. These thin, small bones unite to form the groove for the lacrimal sac and canals through which the tear ducts pass into the nasal cavity. The paired (11) **zygomatic bones** are located on the side of the face below the eyes and form the higher portion of the cheeks below and to the sides of the eyes. The zygomatic bone is commonly referred to as the *cheekbone.* The (12) **vomer** is a single, thin bone that forms the lower part of the nasal septum.

**Figure 10–6**  Paranasal sinuses.

Other important structures, the **paranasal sinuses,** are cavities located within the cranial and facial bones. As their name implies, the frontal, ethmoidal, sphenoidal, and maxillary sinuses are named after the bones in which they are located. (See Figure 10–6.) The paranasal sinuses open into the nasal cavities and are lined with *ciliary epithelium* that is continuous with the mucosa of the nasal cavities. When sinuses are unable to drain properly, a feeling of being "stuffed up" ensues. This commonly occurs during upper respiratory infections or with allergies.

***Thorax.*** The internal organs of the chest (thorax), including the heart and lungs, are enclosed and protected by a bony rib cage. The thorax consists of 12 pairs of ribs, all attached to the spine. (See Figure 10–7.) The first seven pairs, the (1) **true ribs,** are attached directly to the (2) **sternum** by a strip of (3) **costal cartilage.** The costal cartilage of the next five pairs of ribs is not fastened directly to the sternum, so these ribs are known as (4) **false ribs.** The last two pairs of false ribs are not joined, even indirectly, to the sternum but attach posteriorly to the thoracic vertebrae. These last two pairs of false ribs are known as (5) **floating ribs.**

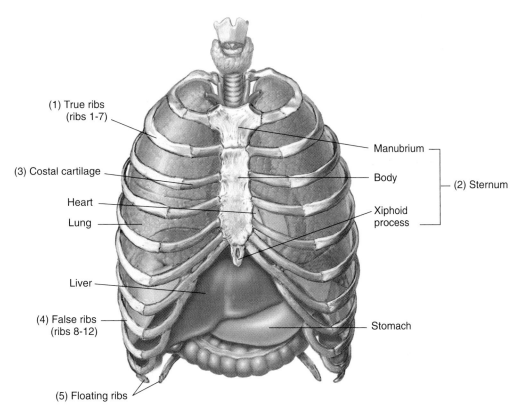

**Figure 10–7**   Thorax.

***Vertebral column.*** The vertebral column of the adult is composed of 26 bones called *vertebrae* (singular, *vertebra*). The vertebral column supports the body and provides a protective bony canal for the spinal cord. A healthy, normal spine has four curves that help make it resilient and maintain balance. The cervical and lumbar regions curve forward, whereas the thoracic and sacral regions curve backward. Abnormal curves may be due to a congenital defect, poor posture, or bone disease. (See Figure 10–8.)

The vertebral column consists of five regions of bones, each deriving its name from its location within the spinal column. The seven (1) **cervical vertebrae** form the skeletal framework of the neck. The first cervical vertebra, the (2) **atlas,** supports the skull. The second cervical vertebra, the (3) **axis,** makes possible the rotation of the skull on the neck. Under the

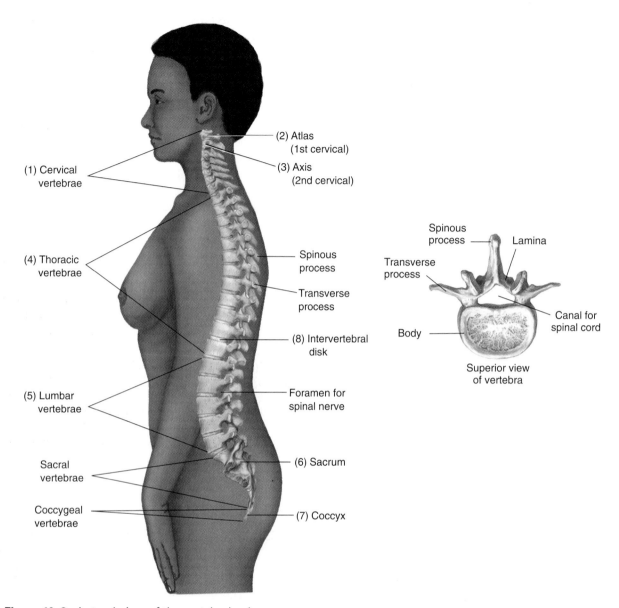

**Figure 10–8**   Lateral view of the vertebral column.

seventh cervical vertebra are twelve (4) **thoracic vertebrae,** which support the chest and serve as a point of articulation for the ribs. The next five vertebrae, the (5) **lumbar vertebrae,** are situated in the lower back area and carry most of the weight of the torso. Below this area are five sacral vertebrae, which are fused into a single bone in the adult and are referred to as the (6) **sacrum.** The tail of the vertebral column consists of four or five fragmented fused vertebrae referred to as the (7) **coccyx.**

Vertebrae are separated by flat, round structures, the (8) **intervertebral disks,** which are composed of a fibrocartilaginous substance with a gelatinous mass in the center (nucleus pulposus). When disk material protrudes into the neural canal, pressure on the adjacent nerve root causes pain. This condition is referred to as *herniation of an intervertebral disk,* **herniated nucleus pulposus (HNP),** *ruptured disk,* or *slipped disk.*

**Appendicular skeleton.**   The appendicular skeleton consists of bones of the upper and lower limbs and their girdles that attach the limbs to the axial skeleton. The appendicular skeleton is distinguished with blue color in Figure 10–4. The difference between the axial and appendicular skeletons is that the axial skeleton protects internal organs, and provides central support for the body; the appendicular skeleton enables the body to move. The ability to walk, run, or catch a ball is possible because of the movable joints of the limbs that make up the appendicular skeleton.

*Pectoral (shoulder) girdle.* The pectoral girdle consists of two bones, the anterior (1) **clavicle** (collarbone) and the posterior (2) **scapula** (triangular shoulder blade). The primary function of the pectoral girdle is to attach the bones of the upper limbs to the axial skeleton and provide attachments for muscles that aid upper limb movements. The paired pectoral structures and their associated muscles form the shoulders of the body.

*Upper limbs.* The skeletal framework of each upper limb includes the arm, forearm, or hand. Anatomically speaking, the arm is only that part of the upper limb between the shoulder and elbow. Each limb or appendage consists of a (3) **humerus** (upper arm bone). The humerus articulates with the (4) **radius** and (5) **ulna** at the elbow. The radius and ulna form the skeleton of the forearm. The bones of the hand include eight (6) **carpals** (wrist); five radiating (7) **metacarpals** (palm); and ten radiating (8) **phalanges** (fingers).

*Pelvic (hip) girdle.* The (9) **pelvic girdle** is a basin-shaped structure that attaches the lower limbs to the axial skeleton. Along with its associated ligaments, it supports the trunk of the body, and provides protection for the visceral organs of the pelvis (lower organs of digestion and urinary and reproductive structures).

Male and female pelves (singular, *pelvis*) differ considerably in size and shape but share the same basic structures. Some of the differences are attributable to the function of the female pelvis during childbearing. The female pelvis is shallower than the male pelvis but wider in all directions. The female pelvis not only supports the enlarged uterus as the fetus matures but also provides a large opening to allow the infant to pass through during birth. Even so, female and male pelves are divided into the (10) **ilium,** (11) **ischium,** and (12) **pubis.** These three bones are fused together in the adult to form a single bone called the *innominate (hip) bone.* The bladder is located behind the (13) **symphysis pubis;** the rectum is in the curve of the (14) **sacrum** and (15) **coccyx.** In the female, the uterus, fallopian tubes, ovaries, and vagina are located between the bladder and the rectum.

*Lower limbs.* The lower limbs support the complete weight of the erect body and are subjected to exceptional stresses, especially in running or jumping. To accommodate for these types of forces, the lower limb bones are stronger and thicker than comparable bones of the upper limbs. The difference between the upper and lower limb bones is that the lighter bones of the upper limbs are adapted for mobility and flexibility; the massive bones of the lower limbs are specialized for stability and weight bearing. There are three parts of each lower limb: the thigh, the leg, and the foot.

The thigh consists of a single bone called the (16) **femur.** It is the largest, longest, and strongest bone in the body. The leg is formed by two parallel bones: the (17) **tibia** and the (18) **fibula.** The seven (19) **tarsals** (ankle bones) resemble metacarpals (wrist bones) in structure. Lastly, the bones of the foot include the (20) **metatarsals,** which consists of five small long bones numbered 1 to 5 beginning with the great toe on the medial side of the foot, and the much smaller (21) **phalanges** (toes).

## Joints or Articulations

To allow for body movements, bones must have points where they meet **(articulate).** These articulating points form joints that have various degrees of mobility. Some are freely movable **(diarthroses),** others are only slightly movable **(amphiarthroses),** and the remaining are totally immovable **(synarthroses).** All three types are necessary for smooth, coordinated body movements.

Joints that allow movement are called synovial joints. The ends of the bones that comprise these joints are encased in a sleevelike extension of the periosteum called the *joint capsule*. This capsule binds the articulating bones to each other. In most synovial joints, the capsule is strengthened by ligaments that lash the bones together, providing additional strength to the joint capsule. A membrane called the *synovial membrane* surrounds the inside of the capsule. It secretes a lubricating fluid **(synovial fluid)** within the entire joint capsule. The ends of each of the bones are covered with a smooth layer of cartilage that serves as a cushion.

 **It is time to review skeletal structures by completing Learning Activity 10–3.**

## Medical Word Elements

This section introduces combining forms, suffixes, and prefixes related to the musculoskeletal system. Word analyses are also provided.

| Element | Meaning | Word Analysis |
|---|---|---|
| **COMBINING FORMS** | | |
| **Skeletal System** | | |
| *General* | | |
| **ankyl/o** | stiffness; bent, crooked | ankyl/osis (ăng-kĭ-LŌ-sĭs): immobility and stiffness of a joint<br>*-osis:* abnormal condition; increase (used primarily with blood cells)<br>*Ankylosis may be the result of trauma, surgery, or disease and most commonly occurs in rheumatoid arthritis.* |
| **arthr/o** | joint | arthr/itis (ăr-THRĪ-tĭs): inflammation of a joint<br>*-itis:* inflammation |
| **kyph/o** | hill, mountain | kyph/osis (kĭ-FŌ-sĭs): humpback posture<br>*-osis:* abnormal condition; increase (used primarily with blood cells) |
| **lamin/o** | lamina (part of vertebral arch) | lamin/ectomy (lăm-ĭ-NĔK-tō-mē): excision of the lamina<br>*-ectomy:* excision, removal<br>*Laminectomy is usually performed to relieve compression of the spinal cord or to remove a lesion or herniated disk.* |
| **lord/o** | curve, swayback | lord/osis (lor-DŌ-sĭs): swayback posture<br>*-osis:* abnormal condition; increase (used primarily with blood cells) |
| **myel/o** | bone marrow; spinal cord | myel/o/pathy (mī-ĕ-LŎP-ă-thē): any pathological condition of the spinal cord<br>*-pathy:* disease |

| Element | Meaning | Word Analysis |
|---------|---------|---------------|
| **orth/o** | straight | orth/o/ped/ist (or-thō-PĒ-dĭst): physician who specializes in the treatment of musculoskeletal disorders<br><br>*ped:* foot; child<br>*–ist:* specialist<br><br>*Initially, an orthopedist corrected deformities and straightened children's bones. In today's medical practice, however, the orthopedist treats musculoskeletal disorders and associated structures in persons of all ages.* |
| **oste/o** | bone | oste/oma (ŏs-tē-Ō-mă): benign bony tumor<br><br>*-oma:* tumor |
| **ped/o**<br>**ped/i** | foot; child | ped/o/graph (PĔD-ō-grăf): imprint of the foot on paper<br>ped/i/cure (PĔD-ĭ-kūr): care of feet |
| **scoli/o** | crooked, bent | scoli/osis (skō-lē-Ō-sĭs): abnormal curvature of the spine<br><br>*-osis:* abnormal condition; increase (used primarily with blood cells) |
| **thorac/o** | chest | thorac/o/dynia (thō-răk-ō-DĬN-ē-ă): chest pain<br><br>*-dynia:* pain |

## Specific Bones

| Element | Meaning | Word Analysis |
|---------|---------|---------------|
| **acromi/o** | acromion (projection of scapula) | acromi/al (ăk-RŌ-mē-ăl): relating to the acromion<br><br>*-al:* pertaining to, relating to |
| **brachi/o** | arm | brachi/algia (brā-kē-ĂL-jē-ă): pain in the arm<br><br>*-algia:* pain |
| **calcane/o** | calcaneum (heel bone) | calcane/o/dynia (kăl-kăn-ō-DĬN-ē-ă): pain in the heel when standing or walking<br><br>*-dynia:* pain |
| **carp/o** | carpus (wrist bone) | carp/o/ptosis (kăr-pŏp-TŌ-sĭs): wrist drop<br><br>*-ptosis:* prolapse, downward displacement |
| **cephal/o** | head | cephal/ad (SĔF-ă-lăd): toward the head<br><br>*-ad:* toward |
| **cervic/o** | neck; cervix uteri (neck of uterus) | cervic/o/dynia (sĕr-vĭ-kō-DĬN-ē-ă): pain or cramp of the neck; also called *cervical neuralgia*<br><br>*-dynia:* pain |
| **clavicul/o** | clavicle (collarbone) | clavicul/ar (klă-VĬK-ū-lăr): pertaining to the clavicle<br><br>*-ar:* pertaining to, relating to |
| **cost/o** | ribs | cost/ectomy (kŏs-TĔK-tō-mē): excision or resection of a rib<br><br>*-ectomy:* excision, removal |
| **crani/o** | cranium (skull) | crani/o/tomy (krā-nē-ŎT-ō-mē): incision of the cranium<br><br>*-tomy:* incision |

*(Continued)*

| Element | Meaning | Word Analysis | (Continued) |
|---------|---------|---------------|-------------|
| **dactyl/o** | fingers; toes | dactyl/o/megaly (dăk-tĭ-lō-MĔG-ă-lē): abnormally large size of fingers and toes<br><br>*-megaly:* enlargement | |
| **femor/o** | femur (thigh bone) | femor/al (FĔM-or-ăl): pertaining to the femur<br><br>*-al:* pertaining to, relating to | |
| **fibul/o** | fibula (smaller bone of lower leg) | fibul/o/calcane/al (fĭb-ū-lō-kăl-KĀ-nē-ăl): pertaining to the fibula and calcaneus<br><br>*calcane:* calcaneum (heel bone)<br>*-al:* pertaining to, relating to | |
| **humer/o** | humerus (upper arm bone) | humer/o/scapul/ar (hū-mĕr-ō-SKĂP-ū-lăr): concerning the humerus and scapula<br><br>*scapul:* scapula (shoulder blade)<br>*-ar:* pertaining to, relating to | |
| **ili/o** | ilium (lateral, flaring portion of hip bone) | ili/o/pelv/ic (ĭl-ē-ō-PĔL-vĭk): concerning the iliac area of the pelvis<br><br>*pelv:* pelvis<br>*-ic:* pertaining to, relating to | |
| **ischi/o** | ischium (lower portion of hip bone) | ischi/o/dynia (ĭs-kē-ō-DĬN-ē-ă): pain in the ischium<br><br>*-dynia:* pain | |
| **lumb/o** | loins (lower back) | lumb/o/dynia (lŭm-bō-DĬN-ē-ă): pain in the lumbar region of the back; also called *lumbago*<br><br>*-dynia:* pain | |
| **metacarp/o** | metacarpus (hand bone) | metacarp/ectomy (mĕt-ă-kăr-PĔK-tō-mē): surgical excision or resection of one or more metacarpal bones<br><br>*-ectomy:* excision, removal | |
| **metatars/o** | metatarsus (foot bone) | metatars/algia (mĕt-ă-tăr-SĂL-jē-ă): pain that emanates from the heads of the metatarsus and worsens with weight bearing or palpation<br><br>*-algia:* pain | |
| **patell/o** | patella (kneecap) | patell/ectomy (păt-ĕ-LĔK-tō-mē): removal of the patella<br><br>*-ectomy:* excision, removal | |
| **pelv/i** | pelvis | pelv/i/metry (pĕl-VĬM-ĕt-rē): act or process of determining the dimension of the bony birth canal<br><br>*-metry:* act of measuring | |
| **pod/o** | foot | pod/iatry (pō-DĪ-ă-trē): treatment and prevention of conditions of the feet<br><br>*-iatry:* medicine, treatment | |
| **phalang/o** | phalanges (bones of fingers and toes) | phalang/ectomy (făl-ăn-JĔK-tō-mē): excision of one or more phalanges<br><br>*-ectomy:* excision, removal | |

| Element | Meaning | Word Analysis |
|---|---|---|
| **pub/o** | pelvis bone (anterior part of pelvic bone) | pub/o/coccyg/eal (pū-bō-kŏk-SĬJ-ē-ăl): pertaining to the pubis and the coccyx<br><br>*coccyg:* coccyx (tailbone)<br>*-eal:* pertaining to, relating to |
| **radi/o** | radiation, x-ray; radius (lower arm bone on thumb side) | radi/al (RĀ-dē-ăl): pertaining to the radius<br><br>*-al:* pertaining to, relating to |
| **spondyl/o** (used to make words about conditions of structure) | vertebrae (backbone) | spondyl/itis (spŏn-dĭl-Ī-tĭs): inflammation of the vertebrae<br>*-itis:* inflammation |
| **vertebr/o** (used to make words that describe structure for anatomy) | | inter/vertebr/al (ĭn-tĕr-VĔRT-ĕ-brĕl): relating to the area between two adjacent vertebrae<br><br>*inter-:* between<br>*-al:* pertaining to, relating to |
| **stern/o** | sternum (breastbone) | stern/ad (STĔR-năd): toward the sternum<br><br>*-ad:* toward |
| **tibi/o** | tibia (larger bone of lower leg) | tibi/o/femor/al (tĭb-ē-ō-FĔM-or-ăl) pertaining to the tibia and femur<br><br>*femor:* femur<br>*-al:* pertaining to, relating to |

## Muscular System

| Element | Meaning | Word Analysis |
|---|---|---|
| **leiomy/o** | smooth muscle (visceral) | leiomy/oma (lī-ō-mi-Ō-mă): tumor consisting principally of smooth muscle tissue<br><br>*-oma:* tumor |
| **muscul/o** | muscle | muscul/ar (MŬS-kū-lăr): pertaining to muscles<br><br>*-ar:* pertaining to, relating to |
| **my/o** | | my/oma (mi-Ō-mă): tumor containing muscle tissue |
| **rhabd/o** | rod-shaped (striated) | rhabd/oid (RĂB-doyd): resembling a rod<br><br>*-oid:* resembling |
| **rhabdomy/o** | rod-shaped (striated) muscle | rhabdomy/oma (răb-dō-mi-Ō-mă): tumor composed of striated muscular tissue<br><br>*-oma:* tumor |

## Related Structures

| Element | Meaning | Word Analysis |
|---|---|---|
| **chondr/o** | cartilage | chondr/itis (kŏn-DRĪ-tĭs): inflammation of cartilage<br><br>*-itis:* inflammation |

*(Continued)*

| Element | Meaning | Word Analysis | (Continued) |
|---|---|---|---|
| **fasci/o** | band, fascia (fibrous membrane supporting and separating muscles) | fasci/o/plasty (FĂSH-ē-ō-plăs-tē): surgical repair of fascia<br>*-plasty:* surgical repair | |
| **fibr/o** | fiber, fibrous tissue | fibr/oma (fī-BRŌ-mă): encapsulated tumor consisting of fibrous connective tissue<br>*-oma:* tumor | |
| **synov/o** | synovial membrane, synovial fluid | synov/ectomy (sĭn-ō-VĔK-tō-mē): removal of a synovial membrane<br>*-ectomy:* excision, removal | |
| **ten/o** | tendon | ten/o/desis (těn-ŎD-ě-sĭs): surgical binding or fixation of a tendon<br>*-desis:* binding, fixation (of a bone or joint) | |
| **tend/o** | | tend/o/plasty (TĔN-dō-plăs-tē): surgical repair of a tendon<br>*-plasty:* surgical repair | |
| **tendin/o** | | tendin/itis (těn-dĭn-Ī-tĭs): inflammation of a tendon<br>*-itis:* inflammation | |

## SUFFIXES

| Element | Meaning | Word Analysis | |
|---|---|---|---|
| **-asthenia** | weakness, debility | my/asthenia (mī-ăs-THĒ-nē-ă): muscle weakness and abnormal fatigue<br>*my:* muscle | |
| **-blast** | embryonic cell | my/o/blast (MĪ-ō-blăst): embryonic cell that develops into a muscle cell<br>*my/o:* muscle | |
| **-clasia** | to break; surgical fracture | oste/o/clasia (ŏs-tē-ō-KLĀ-zē-ă): surgical fracture of a bone to remedy a deformity; bony tissue absorption and destruction; also called *osteoclasis*<br>*oste/o:* bone | |
| **-clast** | | oste/o/clast (ŎS-tē-ō-klăst): device used to fracture a bone to correct a deformity; large multinuclear cell formed in the bone marrow of growing bones | |
| **-desis** | binding, fixation (of a bone or joint) | arthr/o/desis (ăr-thrō-DĒ-sĭs): binding together of a joint<br>*arthr/o:* joint | |
| **-malacia** | softening | chondr/o/malacia (kŏn-drō-măl-Ā-shē-ă): softening of the articular cartilage, usually involving the patella<br>*chondr/o:* cartilage | |
| **-physis** | growth | epi/physis (ě-PĬF-ĭ-sĭs): end of a long bone; upper, growing part of a bone<br>*epi-:* above, upon | |

| Element | Meaning | Word Analysis |
|---------|---------|---------------|
| **-porosis** | porous | oste/o/porosis (ŏs-tē-ō-pŏ-RŌ-sĭs): disorder characterized by loss of bone density<br><br>*oste/o:* bone<br><br>*Osteoporosis may cause pain, especially in the lower back; pathological fractures; loss of stature; and various deformities.* |
| **-scopy** | visual examination | arthr/o/scopy (ăr-THRŎS-kō-pē): endoscopic examination of the interior of a joint<br><br>*arthr/o:* joint<br><br>*Arthroscopy is performed by inserting small surgical instruments to remove and repair damaged tissue, such as cartilage fragments or torn ligaments.* |
| **PREFIXES** | | |
| **a-** | without, not | a/trophy (ĂT-rō-fē): wasting; decrease in size of an organ or tissue<br><br>*-trophy:* development, nourishment |
| **sub-** | under, below | sub/patell/ar (sŭb-pă-TĔL-ăr): beneath the patella<br><br>*patell:* patella (kneecap)<br>*-ar:* pertaining to, relating to |
| **supra-** | above; excessive; superior | supra/cost/al (soo-pră-KŎS-tăl): above the ribs<br><br>*cost:* ribs<br>*-al:* pertaining to, relating to |
| **syn-** | union, together, joined | syn/dactyl/ism (sĭn-DĂK-tĭl-ĭzm): fusion of two or more fingers or toes<br><br>*dactyl:* fingers, toes<br>*-ism:* condition |

 **It is time to review medical word elements by completing Learning Activity 10–4.**

 **Pathology**

Joints are especially vulnerable to constant wear and tear. Repeated motion, disease, trauma, and aging affect joints as well as muscles and tendons. Overall, disorders of the musculoskeletal system are more likely to be caused by injury than disease. Other disorders of structure and bone strength—such as osteoporosis, which occurs primarily in elderly women—affect the health of the musculoskeletal system.

For diagnosis, treatment, and management of musculoskeletal disorders, the medical services of a specialist may be warranted. *Orthopedics* is the branch of medicine concerned with the prevention, diagnosis, care, and treatment of musculoskeletal disorders. The physician who specializes in the diagnoses and treatment of musculoskeletal disorders is known as an *orthopedist*. These professionals employ medical, physical, and surgical methods to restore function that has been lost as a result of musculoskeletal injury or disease. Another physician who specializes in treating joint disease is the *rheumatologist*. Still another physician, the *osteopathic physician (DO)*, maintains that good health requires proper alignment of bones, muscles, ligaments, and nerves. Like the MD, osteopathic physicians combine manipulative procedures with state-of-the-art methods of medical treatment, including prescribing drugs and performing surgeries.

## Bone Disorders

Disorders involving the bones include fractures, infections, osteoporosis, and spinal curvatures.

### Fractures

When a bone is broken, it is called a *fracture*. The different types of fractures are classified by extent of damage. (See Figure 10–9.) A (1) **closed, or simple, fracture** is one in which the bone is broken but no external wound exists. An (2) **open, or compound, fracture** involves a broken bone and an external wound that leads to the site of fracture. Fragments of bone often protrude through the skin. A (3) **complicated fracture** is one in which a broken bone has injured some internal organ, such as when a broken rib pierces a lung. In a (4) **comminuted fracture,** the bone has broken or splintered into pieces. An (5) **impacted fracture** occurs when the bone is broken and one end is wedged into the interior of the other bone. An (6) **incomplete fracture** is when the line of fracture does not include the whole bone. A (7) **greenstick fracture** occurs when one side of a long bone is broken and the other side is bent. It occurs in children because their bones contain more collagen than adult bones and tend to splinter rather than break completely. A (8) **Colles fracture,** a break at the lower end of the radius, occurs just above the wrist. It causes displacement of the hand and usually occurs as a result of flexing a hand to cushion a fall. A **hairline fracture** is a minor fracture in which all portions of the bone are in perfect alignment. The fracture is seen on radiographic examination as a very thin hairline between the two segments but not extending entirely through the bone. **Pathological (spontaneous) fractures** are usually caused by a disease process such as a neoplasm or osteoporosis.

Unlike other repairs of the body, bones sometimes require months to heal. Several factors influence the rate at which fractures heal. Some fractures need to be immobilized to ensure that bones unite soundly in a suitable position. In most cases this is achieved with bandages, casts, traction, or a fixation device. Certain fractures, particularly those with bone fragments, require surgery to reposition and fix bones securely, so that surrounding tissues heal. In addition to promoting healing, immobilization prevents further injury and reduces pain.

Some bones have a natural tendency to heal more rapidly than others. For instance, the long bones of the arms usually mend twice as fast as those of the legs. Age also plays an important role in bone fracture healing rate; older patients require more time for healing. In addition, an adequate blood supply to the injured area and the nutritive state of the individual are crucial to the healing process.

### Infections

Infection of the bone and bone marrow is called *osteomyelitis*. It may be acute or chronic. Bone infections are primarily caused by pus-forming **(pyogenic)** bacteria. The disease usually begins with local trauma to the bone causing a blood clot **(hematoma).** Bacteria from an acute infection in another area of the body find their way to the injured bone and establish the infection.

Most bone infections are more difficult to effectively treat than soft tissue infections. Eventually, some bone infections result in destruction **(necrosis)** of the bone and stiffening, or

**Figure 10–9**  Types of fractures.

freezing, of the joints **(ankylosis).** Osteomyelitis may be acute or chronic. With early treatment, prognosis for acute osteomyelitis is good; prognosis for the chronic form of the disease is poor.

*Paget disease,* also known as *osteitis deformans,* is a chronic inflammation of bones, resulting in thickening and softening of bones. It can occur in any bone but most commonly affects the long bones of the legs, the lower spine, the pelvis, and the skull. This disease is found in the population older than age 40. Although a variety of causes have been proposed, a slow virus (not yet isolated) is currently thought to be the most likely cause.

## Osteoporosis

Osteoporosis is a common metabolic bone disorder in the elderly, particularly in post-menopausal women and especially women older than age 60. It is characterized by decreased bone density that occurs when the rate of bone resorption (loss of substance) exceeds the rate of bone formation. Among the many causes of osteoporosis are disturbances of protein metabolism, protein deficiency, disuse of bones due to prolonged periods of immobilization, estrogen deficiencies associated with menopause, a diet lacking vitamins or calcium, and long-term administration of high doses of corticosteroids.

Patients with osteoporosis commonly complain of bone pain, typically in the back, which may be caused by repeated microscopic fractures. Thin areas of porous bone are also evident. Deformity associated with osteoporosis is usually the result of pathological fractures.

## Spinal Curvatures

Any persistent, abnormal deviation of the vertebral column from its normal position may cause a spinal curvature. Three common deviations are *scoliosis, kyphosis,* and *lordosis.* (See Figure 10–10.)

An abnormal lateral curvature of the spine, either to the right or left, is called *scoliosis.* Some rotation of a portion of the vertebral column may also occur. Scoliosis, or *C-shaped curvature of the spine,* may be congenital, caused by chronic poor posture during childhood while the vertebrae are still growing, or the result of one leg being longer than the other. Treatment depends on the severity of the curvature and may vary from exercises, physical therapy, and back braces to surgical intervention. Untreated scoliosis may result in pulmonary insufficiency (curvature may decrease lung capacity), back pain, sciatica, disk disease, or even degenerative arthritis.

An abnormal curvature of a portion of the spine is called *kyphosis,* more commonly known as *humpback* or *hunchback.* Rheumatoid arthritis, rickets, poor posture, or chronic respiratory diseases may cause kyphosis. Treatment consists of spine-stretching exercises, sleeping with a board under the mattress, and wearing a brace to straighten the kyphotic curve; surgery is rarely required.

An abnormal, inward curvature of a portion of the spine is called *lordosis,* more

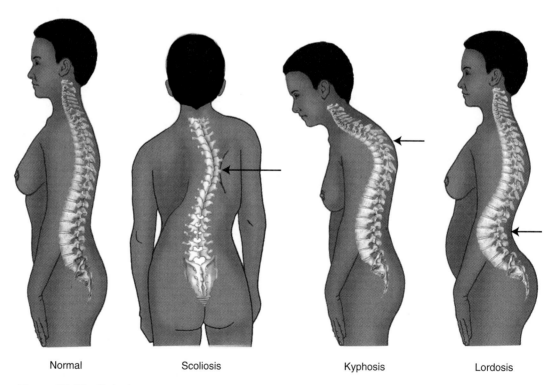

Normal                Scoliosis                Kyphosis                Lordosis

**Figure 10–10**  Spinal curvatures.

commonly known as *swayback*. It may be caused by increased weight of the abdominal contents, resulting from obesity or excessive weight gain during pregnancy. Kyphosis and lordosis also occur in combination with scoliosis. Scoliosis also occurs in combination with kyphosis and lordosis.

## Joint Disorders

**Arthritis**, a general term for many joint diseases, is an inflammation of a joint usually accompanied by pain, swelling and, commonly, changes in structure. Because of their location and constant use, joints are prone to stress injuries and inflammation. The main types of arthritis include rheumatoid arthritis, osteoarthritis, and gouty arthritis, or gout.

Rheumatoid arthritis (RA), a systemic disease characterized by inflammatory changes in joints and their related structures, results in crippling deformities. (See Figure 10–11.) This form of arthritis is believed to be caused by an autoimmune reaction of joint tissue. It occurs most commonly in women between ages 23 and 35 but can affect people of any age group. Intensified aggravations **(exacerbations)** of this disease are commonly associated with periods of increased physical or emotional stress. In addition to joint changes, muscles, bones, and skin adjacent to the affected joint atrophy. There is no specific cure, but **nonsteroidal anti-inflammatory drugs (NSAIDs),** physical therapy, and orthopedic measures are used in treatment of less severe cases.

**Figure 10–11**  Rheumatoid arthritis.

Osteoarthritis, also called *degenerative joint disease (DJD),* is the most common type of connective tissue disease. Cartilage destruction and new bone formation at the edges of joints **(spurs)** are the most common pathologies seen with osteoarthritis. Even though osteoarthritis is less crippling than rheumatoid arthritis, it may result in fusion of two bone surfaces, thereby completely immobilizing the joint. In addition, small, hard nodules may form at the distal interphalangeal joints of the fingers **(Heberden nodes).**

Gouty arthritis, also called *gout,* is a metabolic disease caused by the accumulation of uric acid crystals in blood. These crystals may become deposited in joints and soft tissue near joints, causing painful swelling and inflammation. Although the joint chiefly affected is the big toe, any joint may be involved. Commonly, renal calculi (**nephrolithiasis**) form because of uric acid crystals collecting in the kidney.

## Muscle Disorders

Disorders involving the muscles include muscular dystrophy and myasthenia gravis.

### Muscular Dystrophy

Muscular dystrophy, a genetic disease, is characterized by gradual **atrophy** and weakening of muscle tissue. There are several types of muscular dystrophy. The most common type, *Duchenne dystrophy,* affects children, boys more commonly than girls. It is transmitted as a sex-linked disease passed from mother to son. As muscular dystrophy progresses, the loss of muscle function affects not only skeletal muscle but also cardiac muscle. At present, there is no cure for this disease, and most children with muscular dystrophy die before the age of 20 years.

### Myasthenia Gravis

Myasthenia gravis (MG), a neuromuscular disorder, causes fluctuating weakness of certain skeletal muscle groups (of the eyes, face and, to a lesser degree, the limbs). It is characterized by destruction of the receptors in the synaptic region that respond to acetylcholine, a substance that transmits nerve impulses (**neurotransmitter**). As the disease progresses, the muscle becomes increasingly weak and may eventually cease to function altogether. Women tend to be affected slightly more than men. Initial symptoms include a weakness of the eye muscles and difficulty swallowing (**dysphagia**). Later, the individual has difficulty chewing and talking. Eventually, the muscles of the limbs may become involved.

## Oncology

The two major types of malignancies that affect bone are those that arise directly from bone or bone tissue, called *primary bone cancer,* and those that arise in another region of the body and spread (metastasize) to bone, called *secondary bone cancer.* Primary bone cancers are very rare, but secondary bone cancers are quite prevalent. They are usually caused by malignant cells that have metastasized to the bone from the lungs, breast, or prostate.

Malignancies that originate from bone, fat, muscle, cartilage, bone marrow, and cells of the lymphatic system are called *sarcomas.* Three major types of sarcomas include *fibrosarcoma, osteosarcoma,* and *Ewing sarcoma.* Fibrosarcoma develops in cartilage and generally affects the pelvis, upper legs, and shoulders. The fibrosarcoma patient population is usually between ages 50 and 60. Osteosarcoma develops from bone tissue, and generally affects the knees, upper arms, and upper legs. The osteosarcoma patient population is usually between ages 20 and 25. Ewing sarcoma develops from primitive nerve cells in bone marrow. It usually affects the shaft of long bones but may occur in the pelvis or other bones of the arms or legs. This disease usually affects young boys between ages 10 and 20.

Signs and symptoms of sarcoma include swelling and tenderness, with a tendency toward fractures in the affected area. MRI, bone scan, and CT scan are diagnostic tests that assist in identifying bone malignancies. All malignancies, including Ewing sarcoma, are staged and graded to determine the extent and degree of malignancy. This staging helps the physician determine an appropriate treatment modality. Generally, combination therapy is used, including chemotherapy for management of metastasis and radiation when the tumor is radiosensitive. In some cases, amputation is required.

## Diagnostic, Symptomatic, and Related Terms

This section introduces diagnostic, symptomatic, and related terms and their meanings. Word analyses for selected terms are also provided.

| Term | Definition |
|---|---|
| **ankylosis**<br>ăng-kĭ-LŌ-sĭs<br><br>*ankyl:* stiffness, bent, crooked<br>*-osis:* abnormal condition, increase (used primarily with blood cells) | Stiffening and immobility of a joint as a result of disease, trauma, surgery, or abnormal bone fusion |
| **carpal tunnel syndrome (CTS)**<br>KĂR-păl | Painful condition resulting from compression of the median nerve within the carpal tunnel (wrist canal through which the flexor tendons and the median nerve pass) |
| **claudication**<br>klăw-dĭ-KĀ-shŭn | Lameness, limping |
| **contracture**<br>kŏn-TRĂK-chūr | Fibrosis of connective tissue in skin, fascia, muscle, or joint capsule that prevents normal mobility of the related tissue or joint |
| **crepitation**<br>krĕp-ĭ-TĀ-shŭn | Dry, grating sound or sensation caused by bone ends rubbing together, indicating a fracture or joint destruction |
| **electromyography**<br>ē-lĕk-trō-mi-ŎG-ră-fē<br><br>*electr/o:* electric<br>*my/o:* muscle<br>*-graphy:* process of recording | Use of electrical stimulation to record the strength of muscle contraction |
| **exacerbation**<br>ĕks-ăs-ĕr-BĀ-shŭn | Increase in severity of a disease or of any of its symptoms |
| **ganglion cyst**<br>GĂNG-lē-ŏn  SĬST | Tumor of tendon sheath or joint capsule, commonly found in the wrist<br>*The cyst is aspirated and injected with an anti-inflammatory agent.* |
| **hypotonia**<br>hi-pō-TŌ-nē-ă<br><br>*hypo-:* under, below, deficient<br>*ton:* tension<br>*–ia:* conditon | Loss of muscular tone or a diminished resistance to passive stretching |
| **hemarthrosis**<br>hĕm-ăr-THRŌ-sĭs<br><br>*hem:* blood<br>*arthr:* joint<br>*-osis:* abnormal condition; increase (used primarily with blood cells) | Effusion of blood into a joint cavity |

*(Continued)*

| Term | Definition | (Continued) |
|---|---|---|
| **multiple myeloma**<br>MŬL-tĭ-p'l<br>mī-ĕ-LŌ-mă<br><br>  *myel:* bone marrow; spinal cord<br>  *-oma:* tumor | Primary malignant tumor that infiltrates the bone and red bone marrow<br><br>*Multiple myeloma is a progressive and typically fatal disease that causes multiple tumor masses, which commonly cause bone fractures.* | |
| **osteophyte**<br>ŎS-tē-ō-fīt | Bony outgrowth that occasionally develops on the vertebra and may exert pressure on the spinal cord | |
| **phantom limb**<br>FĂN-tŭm  LĬM | Perceived sensation, following amputation of a limb, that the limb still exists<br><br>*The sensation that pain exists in the removed part is known as phantom limb pain.* | |
| **prosthesis**<br>prŏs-THĒ-sĭs | Replacement of a missing part by an artificial substitute, such as an artificial extremity | |
| **rickets, rachitis**<br>RĬK-ĕts,  ră-KĪ-tĭs | Form of osteomalacia in children caused by vitamin D deficiency | |
| **sequestrum**<br>sē-KWĔS-trŭm<br><br>  *sequestr:* separation<br>  *-um:* structure, thing | Fragment of necrosed bone that has become separated from surrounding tissue | |
| **spondylolisthesis**<br>spŏn-dĭ-lō-lĭs-<br>THĒ-sĭs | Any forward slipping (subluxation) of a vertebra over the one below it | |
| **spondylosis**<br>spŏn-dĭ-LŌ-sĭs<br><br>  *spondyl:* vertebrae (backbone)<br>  *-osis:* abnormal condition; increase (used primarily with blood cells) | Degeneration of the cervical, thoracic, and lumbar vertebrae and related tissues<br><br>*Spondylosis may cause pressure on nerve roots with subsequent pain or paresthesia in the extremities.* | |
| **sprain**<br>SPRĀN | Tearing of ligament tissue that may be slight, moderate, or complete<br><br>*A complete tear of a major ligament is especially painful and disabling. Ligamentous tissue does not heal well because of poor blood supply. Treatment usually consists of surgical reconstruction of the severed ligament.* | |
| **strain**<br>STRĀN | To exert physical force in a manner that may result in injury, usually muscular | |
| **subluxation**<br>sŭb-lŭk-SĀ-shŭn | Partial or incomplete dislocation | |

| Term | Definition |
|---|---|
| **talipes**<br>TĂL-ĭ-pēz | Any number of foot deformities, especially those occurring congenitally; also called *clubfoot* (See Figure 10–12.) |

**Figure 10–12**   Talipes.

 It is time to review pathological, diagnostic, symptomatic, and related terms by completing Learning Activity 10–5.

 ## Diagnostic and Therapeutic Procedures

This section introduces procedures used to diagnose and treat musculoskeletal disorders. Descriptions are provided as well as pronunciations and word analyses for selected terms.

| Procedure | Description |
|---|---|
| **DIAGNOSTIC PROCEDURES** | |
| Radiographic | |
| **arthrography**<br>ăr-THRŎG-ră-fē<br><br>*arthr/o:* joint<br>*-graphy:* process of recording | Series of radiographs taken after injection of a radiopaque substance into a joint cavity, especially the knee or shoulder, to outline the contour of the joint |

*(Continued)*

| Procedure | Description | (Continued) |
|---|---|---|
| **computed tomography (CT) scan** <br> kŏm-PŪ-tĕd <br> tō-MŎG-ră-fē <br><br> *tom/o:* to cut <br> *-graphy:* process of recording | Imaging technique achieved by rotating an x-ray emitter around the area to be scanned and measuring the intensity of transmitted rays from different angles; formerly called *computerized axial tomography* (See Figure 4–4D.) <br><br> *A bone scan is performed to evaluate skeletal involvement related to connective tissue disease; a joint scan is performed to determine joint damage throughout the entire body and is one of the most sensitive studies for early detection of joint disease.* | |
| **dual energy x-ray absorptiometry (DEXA)** | Technique to measure bone density for purposes of diagnosis and management of osteoporosis | |
| **discography** | Radiological examination of the intervertebral disk structures by injecting a contrast medium <br><br> *Discography is used to diagnose suspected cases of herniated disk.* | |
| **lumbosacral spinal radiography (LS spine)** <br> LŬM-bō-sā-krăl <br> SPĪ-năl <br><br> *lumb/o:* loins (lower back) <br> *sacr:* sacrum <br> *-al:* pertaining to, relating to <br> *radi/o:* radiation, x-ray, radius (lower arm bone on thumb side) <br> *-graphy:* process of recording | Radiography of the five lumbar vertebrae and the fused sacral vertebrae, including anteroposterior, lateral, and oblique views of the lower spine <br><br> *The most common indication for lumbosacral spine radiography is lower back pain. It is used to identify or differentiate traumatic fractures, spondylosis, spondylolisthesis, and metastatic tumor.* | |
| **myelography** <br> MĪ-ĕ-lŏg-ră-fē <br><br> *myel/o:* bone marrow, spinal cord <br> *-graphy:* process of recording | Radiography of the spinal cord after injection of a contrast medium to identify and study spinal distortions caused by tumors, cysts, herniated intervertebral disks, or other lesions | |

## THERAPEUTIC PROCEDURES

| | | |
|---|---|---|
| **closed reduction** | Manual correction of fractures without incision <br><br> *Following reduction, the bone is immobilized with an external device to maintain proper alignment during the healing process.* | |
| **casting** | Application of a solid, stiff dressing formed with plaster of Paris or other material to a body part to immobilize it during the healing process | |
| **splinting** | Use of an orthopedic device to an injured body part for immobilization, stabilization, and protection during the healing process <br><br> *A splint is constructed from wood, metal, or plaster of Paris and may be movable or immovable.* | |
| **traction** | Using weights and pulleys to align or immobilize a fracture and facilitate the healing process | |

| Procedure | Description |
|---|---|
| **Surgical** | |
| **amputation**<br>ăm-pŭ-TĀ-shŭn | Partial or complete removal of a limb |
| **arthrocentesis**<br>ăr-thrō-sĕn-TĒ-sĭs<br><br>*arthr/o:* joint<br>*-centesis:* surgical puncture | Puncture of a joint space to remove accumulated fluid |
| **arthroclasia**<br>ăr-thrō-KLĀ-zē-ă<br><br>*arthr/o:* joint<br>*-clasia:* to break;<br>surgical fracture | Surgical breaking of an ankylosed joint to provide movement |
| **arthroscopy**<br>ăr-THRŎS-kŏ-pē<br><br>*arthr/o:* joint<br>*-scopy:* visual examination | Visual examination of a joint, especially the knee; used primarily to detect trauma or lesions and to obtain a biopsy of synovial tissue for microscopic examination |
| **bursectomy**<br>bĕr-SĔK-tō-mē | Excision of bursa (padlike sac or cavity found in connective tissue, usually in the vicinity of joints) |
| **bone grafting**<br>BŌN GRĂFT-ĭng | Implanting or transplanting bone tissue from another part of the body or from another person to serve as replacement for damaged or missing bone tissue |
| **laminectomy**<br>lăm-ĭ-NĔK-tō-mē | Excision of the posterior arch of a vertebra<br><br>*Laminectomy is most commonly performed to relieve the symptoms of a ruptured intervertebral (slipped) disk.* |
| **open reduction** | Treatment of bone fractures using surgery to place the bones in proper position |
| **sequestrectomy**<br>sē-kwĕs-TRĔK-tō-mē | Excision of a sequestrum (segment of necrosed bone) |
| **synovectomy**<br>sĭn-ō-VĔK-tō-mē | Excision of a synovial membrane |

## Pharmacology

Unlike other medications that treat specific disease, most pharmacological agents for musculoskeletal disorders are used to treat symptoms. (See Table 10–3.) Acute musculoskeletal conditions, such as strains, sprains, and "pulled muscles," are treated with analgesics and anti-inflammatory drugs. Nonsteroidal anti-inflammatory drugs (NSAIDs), salicylates, muscle relaxants, opioid analgesics, or narcotics are commonly used to treat pain either by anesthetizing (numbing) the area or by decreasing the inflammation. NSAIDs and salicylates are also used to treat arthritis, in addition to gold salts. Calcium supplements are used to treat hypocalcemia.

| Table 10–3 | DRUGS USED TO TREAT MUSCULOSKELETAL DISORDERS |
| --- | --- |

This table lists common drug classifications used to treat musculoskeletal disorders, their therapeutic actions, and selected generic and trade names.

| Classification | Therapeutic Action | Generic and Trade Names |
| --- | --- | --- |
| **calcium** | Treats and prevents hypocalcemia<br><br>*Over-the-counter calcium supplements are numerous and are contained in many antacids as a secondary therapeutic effect. They are used to prevent osteoporosis when normal diet is lacking adequate amounts of calcium.* | **calcium carbonate**<br>KĂL-sē-ŭm KĂR-bòn-āt<br>   *Alka-Mints Calcarb, Calci-Mix,*<br>   *Oystercal, Tums*<br>**calcium citrate**<br>KĂL-sē-ŭm SĬT-rāt<br>   *Cal-Citrate 250, Citracal, Citracal*<br>   *Liquitab* |
| **gold salts** | Treat rheumatoid arthritis by inhibiting activity within the immune system<br><br>*Gold salts contain actual gold in capsules or in solution for injection. This agent prevents further disease progression but cannot reverse past damage.* | **auranofin**<br>aw-RĂN-ă-fĭn<br>   *Ridaura*<br>**aurothioglucose**<br>aw-rō-thĭ-ō-GLOO-kōs<br>   *Solganal*<br>**gold sodium thiomalate**<br>GŌLD SŌ-dē-ŭm thĭ-ō-MĂ-lāt<br>   *Myochrysine* |
| **nonsteroidal anti-inflammatory drugs (NSAIDs)** | Relieve mild to moderate pain and reduce inflammation<br><br>*NSAIDs have fewer GI adverse effects, such as ulcers, than aspirin. They are used to treat acute musculoskeletal conditions, such as sprains and strains, and inflammatory disorders, including rheumatoid arthritis, osteoarthritis, bursitis, gout, and tendinitis.* | **ibuprofen**<br>ī-bū-PRŌ-fĕn<br>   *Advil, Excedrin IB, Medipren,*<br>   *Motrin, Nuprin*<br>**naproxen**<br>nă-PRŎK-sĕn<br>   *Aleve, Anaprox, Anaprox DS,*<br>   *EC-Naprosyn*<br>**ketoprofen**<br>kē-tō-PRŌ-fĕn<br>   *Actron, Orudis* |

| Table 10-3 | DRUGS USED TO TREAT MUSCULOSKELETAL DISORDERS | |
|---|---|---|
| **Classification** | **Therapeutic Action** | **Generic and Trade Names** |
| **opioid analgesics** | Relieve moderate to severe pain<br><br>*Opioid analgesics are narcotic drugs that may be derived from opium or synthetically produced. They provide preoperative and postoperative pain relief and sedation and are given by mouth, intramuscularly (I.M.), subcutaneously as a patch, or intravenously (I.V.). Because narcotics have a strong addictive quality, they are prescribed for short periods and used especially for severe back pain and postoperative orthopedic surgical procedures.* | **fentanyl**<br>FĔN-tă-nĭl<br>  *Sublimaze, Duragesic, Actiq*<br>**hydromorphone**<br>hĭ-drō-MOR-fōn<br>  *Dilaudid, Hydrostat IR, PMS Hydromorphone*<br>**meperidine**<br>mĕ-PĔR-ĭ-dēn<br>  *Demerol*<br>**morphine**<br>MOR-fēn<br>  *Astramorph, Duramorph, MS Contin, Roxanol*<br>**propoxyphene hydrochloride**<br>prō-PŎK-sē-fēn hĭ-drō-KLŌ-rĭd<br>  *Darvon* |
| **salicylates** | Relieve mild to moderate pain and reduce inflammation<br><br>*Salicylates have anti-inflammatory abilities and alleviate pain. Aspirin is in this drug classification and is known as acetylsalicylic acid (ASA), the oldest drug used to treat arthritis.* | **aspirin**<br>ĂS-pĕr-ĭn<br>  *Acuprin, ASA, Aspergum, Bayer Aspirin*<br>**magnesium salicylate**<br>măg-NĒ-zē-ŭm să-LĬS-ĭ-lāt<br>  *Doan's Regular Strength Tablets, Magan, Mobidin* |
| **skeletal muscle relaxants** | Relieve muscle spasms and stiffness<br><br>*Skeletal muscle relaxants are also prescribed to treat conditions involving muscle spasticity, such as cerebral palsy, multiple sclerosis, stroke, and spinal cord injury.* | **baclofen**<br>BĂK-lō-fēn<br>  *Lioresal*<br>**carisoprodol**<br>kăr-ĭ-sō-PRŌ-dōl<br>  *Soma, Vanadom*<br>**chlorzoxazone**<br>klor-ZŎK-să-zōn<br>  *Paraflex, Parafon Forte DSC, Relaxazone, Remular* |

## Abbreviations

This section introduces musculoskeletal-related abbreviations and their meanings.

| Abbreviation | Meaning |
|---|---|
| ACL | anterior cruciate ligament |
| AE | above the elbow |
| AK | above the knee |
| BE | below the elbow |

*(Continued)*

| Abbreviation | Meaning | (Continued) |
|---|---|---|
| BK | below the knee | |
| C1, C2, and so on | first cervical vertebra, second cervical vertebra, and so on | |
| Ca | calcium; cancer | |
| CDH | congenital dislocation of the hip | |
| CTS | carpal tunnel syndrome | |
| DJD | degenerative joint disease | |
| EMG | electromyography | |
| Fx | fracture | |
| HD | hemodialysis; hip disarticulation; hearing distance | |
| HNP | herniated nucleus pulposus (herniated disk) | |
| HP | hemipelvectomy | |
| IS | intracostal space | |
| I.M., IM | intramuscular; infectious mononucleosis | |
| I.V., IV | intravenous | |
| KD | knee disarticulation | |
| L1, L2, and so on | first lumbar vertebra, second lumbar vertebra, and so on | |
| MG | myasthenia gravis | |
| MS | musculoskeletal; multiple sclerosis; mental status; mitral stenosis | |
| NSAIDs | nonsteroidal anti-inflammatory drugs | |
| ORTH, ortho | orthopedics | |
| P | phosphorous; pulse | |
| PCL | posterior cruciate ligament | |
| RA | rheumatoid arthritis | |
| RF | rheumatoid factor | |
| ROM | range of motion | |
| SD | shoulder disarticulation | |
| THA | total hip arthroplasty | |
| THR | total hip replacement | |
| TKA | total knee arthroplasty | |
| TKR | total knee replacement | |

**It is time to review procedures, pharmacology, and abbreviations by completing Learning Activity 10–6.**

# LEARNING ACTIVITIES

The following activities provide review of the musculoskeletal system terms introduced in this chapter. Complete each activity and review your answers to evaluate your understanding of the chapter.

## Learning Activity 10–1

### Identifying muscle structures

*Label the following illustration using the terms listed below.*

Triceps brachii

Triceps brachii

Brachialis

| | | |
|---|---|---|
| *Achilles tendon* | *gastrocnemius* | *rectus abdominus* |
| *biceps brachii* | *gluteus maximus* | *soleus* |
| *biceps femoris* | *masseter* | *sternocleidomastoid* |
| *brachioradialis* | *orbicularis oculi* | *trapezius* |
| *deltoid* | *pectoralis major* | |

 Check your answers by referring to Figure 10–1 on page 265. Review material that you did not answer correctly.

Learning Activity 10–2

## Identifying sections of a typical long bone (femur)

*Label the following illustration using the terms listed below.*

| | | |
|---|---|---|
| *articular cartilage* | *distal epiphysis* | *proximal epiphysis* |
| *compact bone* | *medullary cavity* | *spongy bone* |
| *diaphysis* | *periosteum* | |

Check your answers by referring to Figure 10–3 on page 268. Review material that you did not answer correctly.

# Learning Activity 10–3

## Identifying skeletal structures

*Label the following illustration using the terms listed below.*

Skull

Maxilla

Mandible

Ribs

Vertebral column

Patella

| | | | |
|---|---|---|---|
| *carpals* | *ilium* | *phalanges* | *sternum* |
| *clavicle* | *ischium* | *pubis* | *symphysis pubis* |
| *coccyx* | *metacarpals* | *radius* | *tarsals* |
| *femur* | *metatarsals* | *sacrum* | *tibia* |
| *fibula* | *pectoral girdle* | *scapula* | *ulna* |
| *humerus* | *pelvic girdle* | | |

✓ Check your answers by referring to Figure 10–4 on page 270. Review material that you did not answer correctly.

Learning Activity 10–4

## Building medical words

*Use* oste/o *(bone) to build words that mean:*

1. bone cells _____

2. pain in bones _____

3. disease of bones and joints _____

4. beginning or formation of bones _____

*Use* cervic/o *(neck) to build words that mean:*

5. pertaining to the neck _____

6. pertaining to the neck and arm _____

7. pertaining to the neck and face _____

*Use* myel/o *(bone marrow; spinal cord) to build words that mean:*

8. herniation of the spinal cord _____

9. sarcoma of bone marrow (cells) _____

10. softening of the spinal cord _____

11. resembling bone marrow _____

*Use* stern/o *(sternum) to build words that mean:*

12. pertaining to above the sternum _____

13. resembling the breastbone _____

*Use* arthr/o *(joint) or* chondr/o *(cartilage) to build words that mean:*

14. embryonic cell that forms cartilage _____

15. inflammation of a joint _____

16. inflammation of bones and joints _____

*Use* pelv/i *(pelvis) to build a word that means:*

17. instrument for measuring the pelvis _____

*Use* my/o *(muscle) to build words that mean:*

18. twitching of a muscle _____

19. any disease of muscle _____

20. rupture of a muscle _____

*Build surgical words that mean:*

21. excision of one or more of the phalanges (bones of a finger or toe) _____
22. incision of the thorax (chest wall) _____
23. excision of a vertebra _____
24. binding of a joint _____
25. repair of muscle (tissue) _____

Check your answers in Appendix A. Review material that you did not answer correctly.

**CORRECT ANSWERS** _____ × 4 = _____ **% SCORE**

## Learning Activity 10–5

## Matching pathological, diagnostic, symptomatic, and related terms

*Match the following terms with the definitions in the numbered list.*

| | | | |
|---|---|---|---|
| ankylosis | greenstick fracture | necrosis | scoliosis |
| chondrosarcoma | hematopoiesis | osteoporosis | sequestrum |
| claudication | hypotonia | phantom limb | spondylitis |
| comminuted fracture | kyphosis | prosthesis | spondylolisthesis |
| Ewing sarcoma | muscular dystrophy | pyogenic | subluxation |
| ganglion cyst | myasthenia gravis | rickets | talipes |
| gout | | | |

1. _____ incomplete or partial dislocation
2. _____ softening of the bones caused by vitamin D deficiency
3. _____ slipped vertebrae
4. _____ limping
5. _____ degeneration of the muscles
6. _____ congenital deformity of the foot, which is twisted out of shape or position
7. _____ part of dead or necrosed bone that has become separated from surrounding tissue
8. _____ chronic neuromuscular disorder characterized by weakness manifested in ocular muscles
9. _____ an artificial part used for replacement of a missing limb
10. _____ tendon sheath or joint capsule tumor, frequently found in the wrist
11. _____ loss of muscular tonicity; diminished resistance of muscles to passive stretching
12. _____ type of sarcoma that attacks the shafts rather than the ends of long bones

13. _____ bone that is partially bent and partially broken; occurs in children

14. _____ exaggeration of the thoracic curve of the vertebral column; hunchback

15. _____ decrease in bone density; occurs in the elderly

16. _____ deviation of the spine to the right or left

17. _____ cartilaginous sarcoma

18. _____ bone that has splintered into pieces

19. _____ inflammation of the vertebrae

20. _____ metabolic disease caused by accumulation of uric acid, usually in the big toe

21. _____ development and production of blood cells, normally in the bone marrow

22. _____ formation of pus

23. _____ death of cells, tissues, or organs

24. _____ stiffening and immobility of a joint

25. _____ perceived sensation, following amputation, that the limb still exists

Check your answers in Appendix A. Review material that you did not answer correctly.

**CORRECT ANSWERS** _____ × **4** = _____ **% SCORE**

# Learning Activity 10–6

## Matching procedures, pharmacology, and abbreviations

*Match the following terms with the definitions in the numbered list.*

| | | |
|---|---|---|
| *ACL* | *closed reduction* | *myelography* |
| *amputation* | *corticosteroids* | *open reduction* |
| *arthrodesis* | *gold salts* | *relaxants* |
| *arthrography* | *HNP* | *salicylates* |
| *arthroscopy* | *laminectomy* | *sequestrectomy* |

1. _____ radiograph of spinal cord after injection of a contrast medium
2. _____ treatment of bone fractures by use of surgery to place bones in proper position
3. _____ used to treat rheumatoid arthritis by inhibiting activity with the immune system
4. _____ major anti-inflammatory drugs used for bone and joint disorders
5. _____ excision of the posterior arch of a vertebra
6. _____ series of joint radiographs preceded by injection of a radiopaque substance or air into the joint cavity
7. _____ surgical immobilization of a joint
8. _____ partial or complete removal of a limb
9. _____ herniated nucleus pulposus
10. _____ relieve mild to moderate pain and reduce inflammation
11. _____ visual examination of a joint's interior, especially the knee
12. _____ excising a segment of necrosed bone
13. _____ anterior cruciate ligament
14. _____ relieve muscle spasms and stiffness
15. _____ manipulative treatment of bone fractures by placing the bones in proper position without incision

Check your answers in Appendix A. Review any material that you did not answer correctly.

**CORRECT ANSWERS** _____ × **6.67** = _____ **% SCORE**

# MEDICAL RECORD ACTIVITIES

The two medical records included in the activities that follow use common clinical scenarios to show how medical terminology is used to document patient care. Complete the terminology and analysis sections for each activity to help you recognize and understand terms related to the musculoskeletal system.

## Medical Record Activity 10–1

### Right knee arthroscopy and medial meniscectomy

#### Terminology

The terms listed in the chart come from the medical record *Right Knee Arthroscopy and Medial Meniscectomy* that follows. Use a medical dictionary such as *Taber's Cyclopedic Medical Dictionary*, the appendices of this book, or other resources to define each term. Then review the pronunciations for each term and practice by reading the medical record aloud.

| Term | Definition |
|---|---|
| ACL | |
| arthroscopy<br>ăr-THRŎS-kō-pē | |
| effusions<br>ĕ-FŪ-zhŭnz | |
| intracondylar<br>ĭn-tră-KŎN-dĭ-lăr | |
| Lachman test<br>LĂK-măn | |
| meniscectomy<br>mĕn-ĭ-SĔK-tō-mē | |
| MRI | |
| PCL | |
| synovitis<br>sĭn-ō-VĪ-tĭs | |

#### RIGHT KNEE ARTHROSCOPY AND MEDIAL MENISCECTOMY

**POSTOPERATIVE DIAGNOSIS:** Torn medial meniscus right knee

**TYPE OF ANESTHESIA:** General

**INDICATIONS FOR PROCEDURE:** This 42-year-old woman has jogged for the past 10 years an average of 25 miles each week. She has persistent posterior medial right knee pain with occasional effusions. The patient has MRI documented medial meniscal tear. She now presents for right knee arthroscopy and medial meniscectomy.

**OPERATIVE FINDINGS:** Examination of the knee under anesthesia showed a full range of motion; no effusion, no instability, and negative Lachman and negative McMurray sign tests. Arthroscopic evaluation showed a normal patellar femoral groove and normal intracondylar notch with normal ACL and PCL, some anterior synovitis, and a normal lateral meniscus and lateral compartment to the knee. The medial compartment of the knee showed an inferior surface, posterior and mid-medial meniscal tear that was flipped up on top of itself. This was resected, and then the remaining meniscus contoured back to a stable rim.

## Analysis

**Review the medical record *Right Knee Arthroscopy and Medial Meniscectomy* to answer the following questions.**

1. Describe the meniscus and identify its location.

   _____

2. What is the probable cause of the tear in the patient's meniscus?

   _____

3. What does normal ACL and PCL refer to in the report?

   _____

4. Explain the McMurray sign test.

   _____

5. Because Lachman and McMurray tests were negative (normal), why was the surgery performed?

   _____

Medical Record Activity 10–2

## Radiographic consultation: Tibial diaphysis nuclear scan

### Terminology

The terms listed in the chart come from the medical record *Radiographic Consultation: Tibial Diaphysis Nuclear Scan*. Use a medical dictionary such as *Taber's Cyclopedic Medical Dictionary*, the appendices of this book, or other resources to define each term. Then review the pronunciations for each term and practice by reading the medical record aloud.

| Term | Definition |
| --- | --- |
| buttressing<br>BŬ-trĕs-ĭng | |
| cortical<br>KOR-tĭ-kăl | |
| diaphysis<br>dī-ĂF-ĭ-sĭs | |
| endosteal<br>ĕn-DŎS-tē-ăl | |
| focal<br>FŌ-kăl | |
| fusiform<br>FŪ-zĭ-form | |
| NSAIDs | |
| nuclear scan<br>NŪ-klē-ăr | |
| periosteal<br>pĕr-ē-ŎS-tē-ăl | |
| resorption<br>rē-SORP-shŭn | |
| tibial<br>TĬB-ē-ăl | |

## RADIOGRAPHIC CONSULTATION: TIBIAL DIAPHYSIS NUCLEAR SCAN

Dear Dr. Hammuda:

We are pleased to provide the following in response to your request for consultation.

This is an 18-year-old male cross-country runner. He complains of pain for more than 1-month duration, with persistent symptoms over middle 1/3 of left tibia with resting. He finds no relief with NSAIDs.

**FINDINGS:** Nuclear scan reveals the following. There is focal, increased blood flow, blood pool, and delayed radiotracer accumulation within the left mid-posterior tibial diaphysis. The delayed spot planar images demonstrate focal fusiform uptake involving 50% to 75% of the tibial diaphysis width.

It is our opinion that with continued excessive, repetitive stress, the rate of resorption will exceed the rate of bone replacement. This will lead to weakened cortical bone with buttressing by periosteal and endosteal new bone deposition. If resorption continues to exceed replacement, a stress fracture will occur.

## Analysis

**Review the medical record *Radiographic Consultation: Tibial Diaphysis Nuclear Scan* to answer the following questions.**

1. Where was the pain located?

   _____

2. What medication was the patient taking for pain and did it provide relief?

   _____

3. How was the blood flow to the affected area described by the radiologist?

   _____

4. How was the radiotracer accumulation described?

   _____

5. What will be the probable outcome with continued excessive repetitive stress?

   _____

6. What will happen if resorption continues to exceed replacement?

   _____

# Chapter

# 11

# Genitourinary System

## OBJECTIVES

*Upon completion of this chapter, you will be able to:*

- Locate and describe the urinary structures as well as the structures of the male reproductive system.
- Recognize, pronounce, spell, and build words related to the genitourinary system.
- Describe pathological conditions, diagnostic and therapeutic procedures, and other terms related to the genitourinary system.
- Explain pharmacology related to the treatment of urinary disorders as well as male reproductive disorders.
- Demonstrate your knowledge of this chapter by completing the learning and medical record activities.

**Key Terms**

This section introduces important genitourinary system terms and their definitions. Word analyses are also provided.

| Term | Definition |
|------|-----------|
| **cortex**<br>KOR-tĕks | Outer layer of an organ or body structure |
| **electrolytes**<br>ē-LĔK-trō-līts | Mineral salts (sodium, potassium, and calcium) that carry an electric charge in solution<br><br>*A proper balance of electrolytes is essential to the normal functioning of the entire body but especially nerves, muscles, and heart.* |
| **erythropoietin (EPO)**<br>ĕ-rĭth-rō-POY-ĕ-tĭn | Glycoprotein hormone produced by certain cells in the kidney<br><br>*Erythropoietin responds to a decrease in oxygen concentration in blood by stimulating stem cells in the bone marrow to produce more erythrocytes (red blood cells).* |
| **libido**<br>lĭ-BĒ-dō | Sexual desire or drive, either conscious or unconscious |
| **meatus**<br>mē-Ā-tŭs<br><br>  *meat:* opening, meatus<br>  *-us:* condition; structure | An opening or passage through any part of the body |
| **medulla**<br>mĕ-DŬL-lă | Inner or central portion of an organ |
| **micturition**<br>mĭk-tū-RĬ-shŭn | The discharge of urine; urination |
| **nitrogenous wastes**<br>nī-TRŎJ-ĕn-ŭs | Products of cellular metabolism that contain nitrogen<br><br>*Nitrogenous wastes include urea, uric acid, creatine, creatinine, and ammonia.* |
| **orifice**<br>OR-ĭ-fĭs | Opening, entrance, or outlet of any body cavity |
| **percutaneous**<br>pĕr-kū-TĀ-nē-ŭs<br><br>  *per:* through<br>  *cutane:* skin<br>  *-ous:* pertaining to, relating to | Procedure performed through the skin, as in a biopsy |
| **reflux**<br>RĒ-flŭks | Backward or return flow of a fluid, such as *vesicoureteral reflux*, where urine backs up into the renal pelvis |
| **urea**<br>ū-RĒ-ă | Principal nitrogenous end product of protein metabolism excreted in urine and perspiration |

## Anatomy and Physiology

The male and female urinary systems have similar structures. In the male, however, some of the urinary structures also have reproductive functions. Thus, the *genitourinary system* includes the urinary system of both the male and female and the reproductive system of the male.

## Urinary System

The purpose of the urinary system is to regulate extracellular fluids (plasma, tissue fluid, and lymph) of the body by removing a variety of harmful substances from plasma while retaining useful products. Harmful substances, including **nitrogenous wastes** and excess **electrolytes** (sodium, potassium, and calcium), are excreted from the body as urine, while useful products are returned to the blood. Nitrogenous wastes are toxic to the body, and must be continuously eliminated or death will occur. Electrolyte concentration must remain fairly constant for proper functioning of nerves, heart, and muscles. The kidneys also secrete **erythropoietin,** a hormone that acts on bone marrow to stimulate production of red blood cells when blood oxygen levels are low.

Four major types of structures make up the urinary system:

- two kidneys
- two ureters
- bladder
- urethra (See Figure 11–1.)

The (1) **kidneys,** each about the size of a fist, are located in the abdominal cavity slightly above the waistline. Because they lie outside of the peritoneum, their location is said to be *retroperitoneal.* A concave medial border gives the kidney its beanlike shape. In a frontal section, two distinct areas are visible, an outer section, the (2) **renal cortex,** and a middle area, the (3) **renal medulla,** which contain portions of the microscopic filtering units of the kidney called *nephrons.* Near the medial border is the (4) **hilum (hilus),** an opening through which the (5) **renal artery** enters and the (6) **renal vein** exits the kidney. The renal artery carries blood that contains waste products to the nephrons for filtering. After waste products are removed, blood leaves the kidney by way of the renal vein.

Waste material, now in the form of urine, passes to a hollow chamber, the (7) **renal pelvis.** This cavity is an enlarged, funnel-shaped extension of the (8) **ureter** where the ureter merges with the kidney. Each ureter is a slender tube about 10 to 12 inches long that carries urine in peristaltic waves to the bladder. They pass behind the bladder and enter its base near the (9) **ureteral orifice.**

The (10) **urinary bladder,** an expandable hollow organ, acts as a temporary reservoir for urine. When empty, the bladder has small folds called *rugae* that allow expansion as the bladder fills. A triangular area at the base of the bladder called the *trigone* is delineated by the openings of the ureters and the urethra.

The base of the trigone forms the (11) **urethra,** the tube that discharges urine from the bladder. The length of the urethra is approximately $1\frac{1}{2}$ inches in women and about 7 to 8 inches in men. In the male, the urethra passes through the prostate gland and the penis. During **micturition,** urine is expelled through the urethral opening, the (12) **urinary meatus.**

### Nephron

Microscopic examination of kidney tissue reveals the presence of approximately 1 million nephrons. (See Figure 11–2.) These microscopic structures are responsible for maintaining homeostasis by continually regulating the amount of water, salts, glucose, urea, and other minerals in blood. Substances removed by nephrons are nitrogenous wastes, including

Renal pyramid

(5) Renal artery

Inferior vena cava

(7) Renal pelvis

(4) Hilum

(2) Renal cortex

(3) Renal medulla

(6) Renal vein

(8) Ureter

Cross section of kidney

Adrenal (suprarenal) glands

(1) Left kidney

(1) Right kidney

Inferior vena cava

Abdominal aorta

(8) Ureters

(10) Urinary bladder

(9) Ureteral orifice

Prostate gland (in males)

(11) Urethra

(12) Urinary meatus

**Figure 11–1**    Urinary structures, including a cross-section of the kidney.

urea, uric acid, and creatinine, the end products of protein metabolism. Nephrons also remove excess electrolytes and many other products that exceed the amount tolerated by the body.

Each nephron includes a *renal corpuscle* and a *renal tubule.* The renal corpuscle is composed of a tuft of capillaries called the (1) **glomerulus** and a modified, funnel-shaped end of the renal tubule known as (2) **Bowman capsule.** This capsule encases the glomerulus. A larger (3) **afferent arteriole** carries blood to the glomerulus, and a smaller (4) **efferent arteriole** carries blood from the glomerulus. The difference in the size of these vessels provides the needed pressure to force small molecules out of the blood and into Bowman capsule. This process is nonselective, which means that all small molecules—including those needed by the body as well as waste molecules—enter the lumen of the tubule. As the efferent arteriole passes behind the renal corpuscle, it forms the (5) **peritubular capillaries.** These capillaries allow needed products filtered from the blood in Bowman capsule to re-enter the vascular system. Each renal tubule consists of four sections: the (6) **proximal convoluted tubule,** followed by the narrow (7) **loop of Henle,** then the larger (8) **distal tubule** and, finally, the (9) **collecting tubule.** The collecting tubule transports newly formed urine to the renal pelvis for excretion by the kidneys.

**Figure 11–2**   Nephron with its associated blood vessels.

The nephron performs three physiological activities as it produces urine:

- *Filtration* occurs in the renal corpuscle, where water, electrolytes, sugar, amino acids, and other small molecules are forced from the blood in the glomerulus into Bowman capsule as a result of increased pressure. The fluid that is formed is called *filtrate.*
- *Reabsorption* begins as filtrate passes through the four sections of the tubule. The tubule reclaims needed substances from the filtrate and returns them to the body for reuse. As filtrate travels the long and twisted pathway of the tubule, most of the water and some of the electrolytes and amino acids are returned to the peritubular capillaries, thus re-entering circulating blood.
- *Secretion* occurs when substances in the capillaries surrounding the distal and collecting tubule secrete ammonia, uric acid, and other substances directly into the tubule, a process that resembles reabsorption, but in the opposite direction. The remaining fluid that enters the collecting tubule is then called urine.

 **It is time to review urinary system anatomy by completing Learning Activity 11–1.**

## Male Reproductive System

The purpose of the male reproductive system is to produce, maintain, and transport sperm, the male sex cell required for the fertilization of the egg. It also produces the male hormone, *testosterone,* which is essential to the development of sperm and male secondary sex characteristics.

The primary male reproductive organ consists of two (1) **testes** (singular, **testis**), located in an external sac called the (2) **scrotum.** (See Figure 11–3.) Within the testes are numerous small tubes that twist and coil to form (3) **seminiferous tubules,** which produce sperm. The testes also secrete testosterone, which develops and maintains secondary sex characteristics. Lying over the superior surface of each testis is a single, tightly coiled tube, the (4) **epididymis.** This structure stores sperm after it leaves the seminiferous tubules. The epididymis is the first duct through which sperm passes after its production in the testes. Tracing the duct upward, the epididymis forms the (5) **vas deferens (seminal duct** or **ductus deferens),** a narrow tube that passes through the inguinal canal into the abdominal cavity. The vas deferens extends over the top and down the posterior surface of the bladder, where it joins the (6) **seminal vesicle.** The union of the vas deferens with the duct from the seminal vesicle forms the (7) **ejaculatory duct.** The seminal vesicle contains nutrients that support sperm viability and secretes approximately 60% of the seminal fluid that is ultimately ejaculated during sexual intercourse (coitus). The ejaculatory duct passes at an angle through the (8) **prostate gland,** a triple-lobed organ fused to the base of the bladder. The prostate gland secretes a thin, alkaline substance that accounts for about 30% of seminal fluid. Its alkalinity helps protect sperm from the acidic environments of both the male urethra and the female vagina. The two pea-shaped (9) **bulbourethral (Cowper) glands** are located below the prostate and are connected by a small duct to the urethra. The bulbourethral glands provide alkaline fluid necessary for sperm viability. The (10) **penis** is the male organ of copulation. It is cylindrical and composed of erectile tissue that encloses the (11) **urethra.** The urethra expels both semen and urine from the body. During ejaculation, the sphincter at the base of the bladder closes, which not only stops the urine from being expelled with the semen, but also prevents semen from entering the bladder. The enlarged tip of the penis, the (12) **glans penis,** contains the (13) **urethral orifice (meatus).** A movable hood of skin, called the (14) **prepuce,** or *foreskin,* covers the glans penis.

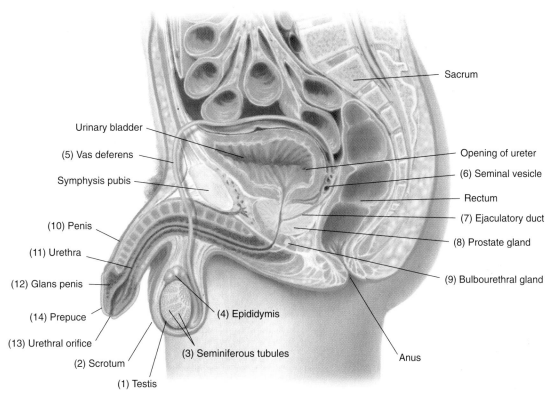

Sacrum

Urinary bladder

(5) Vas deferens

Symphysis pubis

Opening of ureter

(6) Seminal vesicle

Rectum

(10) Penis

(7) Ejaculatory duct

(11) Urethra

(8) Prostate gland

(12) Glans penis

(9) Bulbourethral gland

(14) Prepuce

(4) Epididymis

(13) Urethral orifice

(2) Scrotum

(3) Seminiferous tubules

Anus

(1) Testis

**Figure 11–3**   Midsagittal section of male reproductive structures shown through the pelvic cavity.

  **It is time to review male reproductive anatomy by completing Learning Activity 11–2.**

  ## Medical Word Elements

This section introduces combining forms, suffixes, and prefixes related to the genitourinary system. Word analyses are also provided.

| Element | Meaning | Word Analysis |
|---------|---------|---------------|
| **COMBINING FORMS** | | |
| Urinary System | | |
| **cyst/o** | bladder | cyst/o/scope (SĬST-ō-skōp): instrument used to examine and treat lesions of the bladder and ureters<br>*-scope:* instrument for examining |
| **vesic/o** | | vesic/o/cele (VĔS-ĭ-kō-sēl): herniation of the bladder into the vagina; also called *cystocele*<br>*-cele:* hernia, swelling |

*(Continued)*

| Element | Meaning | Word Analysis | (Continued) |
|---------|---------|---------------|-------------|
| **glomerul/o** | glomerulus | glomerul/o/pathy (glō-měr-ū-LŎP-ă-thē): any disease of the renal glomerulus<br>*-pathy:* disease | |
| **lith/o** | stone, calculus | lith/o/tripsy (LĬTH-ō-trĭp-sē): crushing of a stone<br>*-tripsy:* crushing | |
| **meat/o** | opening, meatus | meat/o/tomy (mē-ă-TŎT-ō-mē): incision of the urinary meatus to enlarge the opening<br>*-tomy:* incision | |
| **nephr/o** | kidney | nephr/o/pexy (NĚF-rō-pěks-ē): fixation of a floating or dropped kidney<br>*-pexy:* fixation (of an organ) | |
| **ren/o** | | ren/al (RĒ-năl): pertaining to the kidney<br>*-al:* pertaining to, relating to | |
| **peritone/o** | peritoneum | peritone/o/clysis (pěr-ĭ-tō-ně-ō-KLĪ-sĭs): introduction of a fluid into the peritoneal cavity<br>*-clysis:* irrigation, washing | |
| **pyel/o** | renal pelvis | pyel/o/plasty (PĪ-ě-lō-plăs-tē): surgical repair of the renal pelvis<br>*-plasty:* surgical repair | |
| **ur/o** | urine | ur/o/lith (Ū-rō-lĭth): concretion or stone in any part of the urinary tract<br>*-lith:* stone, calculus | |
| **ureter/o** | ureter | ureter/ectasis (ū-rē-těr-ĚK-tă-sĭs): dilation of the ureter<br>*-ectasis:* dilation, expansion | |
| **urethr/o** | urethra | urethr/o/stenosis (ū-rē-thrō-stěn-Ō-sĭs): narrowing or stricture of the urethra<br>*-stenosis:* narrowing, stricture | |

## Male Reproductive System

| Element | Meaning | Word Analysis | |
|---------|---------|---------------|---|
| **andr/o** | male | andr/o/gen/ic (ăn-drō-JĚN-ĭk): pertaining to or causing masculinization<br>*gen:* forming, producing, origin<br>*-ic:* pertaining to, relating to | |
| **balan/o** | glans penis | balan/o/plasty (BĂL-ă-nō-plăs-tē): surgical repair of the glans penis<br>*-plasty:* surgical repair | |
| **epididym/o** | epididymis | epididym/o/tomy (ěp-ĭ-dĭd-ĭ-MŎT-ō-mē): incision of the epididymis<br>*-tomy:* incision | |

| Element | Meaning | Word Analysis |
|---|---|---|
| **orch/o** | testis (plural, testes) | orch/itis (or-KĪ-tǐs): inflammation of one or both of the testes<br>*-itis:* inflammation |
| **orchi/o** | | orchi/algia (or-kē-ĂL-jē-ǎ): pain in the testes<br>*-algia:* pain |
| **orchid/o** | | orchid/o/ptosis (or-kǐd-ǒp-TŌ-sǐs): downward displacement of the testes<br>*-ptosis:* prolapse, downward displacement |
| **test/o** | | test/ectomy (tĕs-TĚK-tō-mē): excision of a testis<br>*-ectomy:* excision, removal |
| **prostat/o** | prostate gland | prostat/o/megaly (prŏs-tă-tō-MĚG-ā-lē): enlargement of the prostate gland<br>*-megaly:* enlargement |
| **spermat/o** | spermatozoa, sperm cells | spermat/o/cele (spĕr-MĂT-ō-sēl): cystic tumor of the epididymis containing spermatozoa<br>*-cele:* hernia, swelling |
| **sperm/o** | | sperm/ic (SPĔR-mǐk): pertaining to sperm cells<br>*-ic:* pertaining to, relating to |
| **vas/o** | vessel; vas deferens; duct | vas/ectomy (văs-ĔK-tō-mē): removal of all or part of the vas deferens<br>*-ectomy:* excision, removal |
| **varic/o** | dilated vein | varic/o/cele (VĂR-ǐ-kō-sēl): dilated or enlarged vein of the spermatic cord<br>*-cele:* hernia, swelling |
| **vesicul/o** | seminal vesicle | vesicul/itis (vĕ-sǐk-ū-LĪ-tǐs): inflammation of the seminal vesicle<br>*-itis:* inflammation |

## Other

| Element | Meaning | Word Analysis |
|---|---|---|
| **albumin/o** | albumin, protein | albumin/oid (ăl-BŪ-mǐ-noyd): resembling albumin<br>*-oid:* resembling |
| **azot/o** | nitrogenous compounds | azot/emia (ăz-ō-TĒ-mē-ǎ): presence of nitrogenous products, especially urea in the blood<br>*-emia:* blood condition<br>*Nitrogenous products are toxic, and if not removed from the body death will result.* |
| **bacteri/o** | bacteria | bacteri/uria (băk-tē-rē-Ū-rē-ǎ): presence of bacteria in urine<br>*-uria:* urine |

*(Continued)*

| Element | Meaning | Word Analysis | (Continued) |
|---|---|---|---|
| **crypt/o** | hidden | crypt/orchid/ism (krĭpt-OR-kĭd-ĭzm): failure of the testes to descend into the scrotum<br><br>*orchid:* testis (plural, testes)<br>*-ism:* condition | |
| **gonad/o** | gonads, sex glands | gonad/o/pathy (gŏn-ă-DŎP-ă-thē): any disease of the sex glands<br><br>*-pathy:* disease | |
| **kal/i** | potassium (an electrolyte) | hypo/kal/emia (hī-pō-kă-LĒ-mē-ă): abnormally low concentration of potassium in the blood<br><br>*hypo-:* under, below<br>*-emia:* blood condition<br><br>*Hypokalemia may result from excessive urination, which depletes potassium from the body.* | |
| **keton/o** | ketone bodies (acids and acetone) | keton/uria (kē-tō-NŪ-rē-ă): presence of ketone bodies in the urine<br><br>*-uria:* urine | |
| **noct/o** | night | noct/uria (nŏk-TŪ-rē-ă): excessive and frequent urination after going to bed<br><br>*-uria:* urine<br><br>*Nocturia is associated with prostate disease, urinary tract infection, and uncontrolled diabetes.* | |
| **olig/o** | scanty | olig/o/sperm/ia (ŏl-ĭ-gō-SPĔR-mē-ă): temporary or permanent deficiency of spermatozoa in semen<br><br>*sperm:* spermatozoa, sperm cells<br>*-ia:* condition | |
| **py/o** | pus | py/o/rrhea (pī-ō-RĒ-ă): flow or discharge of pus<br><br>*-rrhea:* discharge, flow | |
| **SUFFIXES** | | | |
| **-cide** | killing | sperm/i/cide (SPĔR-mĭ-sīd): agent that kills or destroys sperm, especially when used as a contraceptive; also called *spermaticide*<br><br>*sperm/i:* spermatozoa, sperm cells | |
| **-genesis** | forming, producing, origin | lith/o/genesis (lĭth-ō-JĔN-ĕ-sĭs): formation or production of stones or calculi<br><br>*lith/o:* stone, calculus | |
| **-iasis** | abnormal condition (produced by something specified) | lith/iasis (lĭth-Ī-ă-sĭs): abnormal condition or presence of stones or calculi<br><br>*lith/o:* stone, calculus | |

| Element | Meaning | Word Analysis |
|---------|---------|---------------|
| -ism | condition | an/orch/ism (ăn-OR-kĭzm): congenital absence of one or both testes<br><br>*an-:* without, not<br>*orch:* testis (plural, testes) |
| -spadias | slit, fissure | hypo/spadias (hī-pō-SPĀ-dē-ăs): congenital defect in which the urethra opens on the underside of the glans penis instead of the tip<br><br>*hypo-:* under, below |
| -uria | urine | poly/uria (pŏl-ē-Ū-rē-ă): excessive formation and excretion of urine<br><br>*poly-:* many, much |
| **PREFIXES** | | |
| dia- | through, across | dia/lysis (dī-ĂL-ĭ-sĭs): procedure that uses a membrane to separate and selectively remove substances from a solution<br><br>*-lysis:* separation; destruction; loosening |
| retro- | backward, behind | retro/peritone/al (rĕt-rō-pĕr-ĭ-tō-NĒ-ăl): pertaining to the area behind or outside of the peritoneum<br><br>*peritone:* peritoneum<br>*-al:* pertaining to, relating to |

**It is time to review medical word elements by completing Learning Activity 11–3.**

## Pathology

Pathology of the urinary system includes a range of disorders from those that are asymptomatic to those that manifest an array of signs and symptoms. Causes for these disorders include congenital anomalies, infectious diseases, trauma, or conditions that secondarily involve the urinary structures. Many times, asymptomatic diseases are initially diagnosed when a routine urinalysis shows abnormalities. Forms of glomerulonephritis and chronic urinary tract infection are two such disorders. Symptoms specific to urinary disorders include changes in urination pattern or output and dysuria. Endoscopic tests, radiological evaluations, and laboratory tests that evaluate renal function are typically required to diagnose disorders of the urinary system.

Signs and symptoms of male reproductive disorders include pain, swelling, erectile dysfunction, and loss of **libido.** Characteristics of infectious diseases, especially those transmitted through sexual activity, commonly include pain, discharge, or lesions as well as a vague feeling of fullness or discomfort in the perineal or rectal area. A complete evaluation of the genitalia, reproductive history, and past and present genitourinary infections and disorders is necessary to identify disorders associated with male reproductive structures.

For diagnosis, treatment, and management of genitourinary disorders, the medical services of a specialist may be warranted. *Urology* is the branch of medicine concerned with male and female urinary disorders and diseases of the male reproductive system. The physician who specializes in the diagnoses and treatment of genitourinary disorders is known as a *urologist*.

## Pyelonephritis

One of the most common forms of kidney disease is *pyelonephritis*, also called *kidney infection* or *complicated urinary tract infection*. In this disorder, bacteria invade the renal pelvis and kidney tissue, often as a consequence of a bladder infection that has ascended to the kidney via the ureters. When the infection is severe, lesions form in the renal pelvis, causing bleeding. The microscopic examination of urine reveals the following: large quantities of bacteria (**bacteriuria**), white blood cells (**pyuria**), and, when lesions are present, red blood cells (**hematuria**). The onset of the disease is usually acute, with symptoms including chills, fever, nausea, and vomiting.

## Glomerulonephritis

Any condition that causes the glomerular walls to become inflamed is referred to as *glomerulonephritis*. One of the most common causes of glomerular inflammation is a reaction to the toxins given off by pathogenic bacteria, especially streptococci, that have recently infected another part of the body, usually the throat. Glomerulonephritis is also associated with autoimmune diseases, such as systemic lupus erythematosus, polyarthritis, scleroderma, and diabetes.

When the glomerular membrane is inflamed, it becomes highly permeable. Red blood cells and protein pass through the glomerulus and enter the tubule as urine is being produced. In some cases, protein solidifies in the nephron tubules and forms solid masses that take the shape of the tubules in which they develop. These masses are called *casts*. They commonly pass out of the kidney by way of the urine and may be visible when urine is examined microscopically. The clinical picture for this disease includes blood and protein in the urine (**hematuria** and **proteinuria**), and red cells casts, along with hypertension, edema, and impaired renal function. Most patients with acute glomerulonephritis associated with a streptococcal infection recover with no residual kidney damage.

## Nephrolithiasis

Stones may form in any part of the urinary tract, but most arise in the kidney; this condition is called *nephrolithiasis*. (See Figure 11–4.) They commonly form when dissolved urine salts begin to solidify. As these stones increase in size, they obstruct urinary structures. As they lodge in the ureters, they cause intense pulsating pain called *colic*. Because urine is hindered from flowing into the bladder, it flows backward (**refluxes**) into the renal pelvis and the tubules, causing them to dilate. This distention is called *hydronephrosis*. Calculi are pulverized using concentrated ultrasound waves or x-rays, called *shockwaves*, directed at the stones from a machine outside the body (**extracorporeal shockwave lithotripsy [ESWL]**). (See Figure 11–5.) For excessively large stones or patients who have contraindications for the procedure, the alternative treatment is stone removal through a small incision in the skin (**percutaneous nephrolithotomy**).

**Figure 11–4**    Kidney stones in the calices and ureter.

**Figure 11–5**    Extracorporeal shockwave lithotripsy.

## Bladder Neck Obstruction

Any blockage of the bladder outlet is referred to as *bladder neck obstruction (BNO)*. Its causes include an enlarged prostate gland and obstructive masses, such as calculi, blood clots, and tumors. The resulting bladder distention may lead to hydronephrosis accompanied by bladder infection **(cystitis).** The patient experiences a need to void but can only void small quantities at a time **(retention with overflow).** Correction of BNO includes surgery that relieves or removes the obstruction.

## Benign Prostatic Hyperplasia

Benign prostatic hyperplasia (BPH), sometimes called *nodular hyperplasia* or *benign prostatic hypertrophy*, is commonly associated with the aging process. (See Figure 11–6.) As the prostate gland enlarges, it decreases the urethral lumen, thus inhibiting complete voiding. Inability to empty the bladder completely may cause cystitis and, ultimately, nephritis. Surgical removal of the prostate may be necessary. Surgical removal may be done through the perineum **(perineal prostatectomy),** urethra **(transurethral resection of the prostate [TURP]),** or an abdominal opening above the pubis and directly over the bladder **(suprapubic prostatectomy).**

Normal prostate

Prostatic hyperplasia

**Figure 11–6**   Prostatic hyperplasia.

## Cryptorchidism

Failure of the testes to descend into the scrotal sac prior to birth is called *cryptorchidism.* In many infants born with this condition, the testes descend spontaneously by the end of the first year. If this does not occur, correction of the disorder involves surgical suspension of the testes (**orchiopexy**) in the scrotum. This procedure is usually done before the child reaches age 2. Because an inguinal hernia commonly accompanies cryptorchidism, the hernia may be sutured (**herniorrhaphy**) at this time.

## Acute Tubular Necrosis

In acute tubular necrosis (ATN), the tubular portion of the nephron is injured through a decrease in blood supply or the presence of toxic substances (usually after ingestion of toxic chemical agents). Two major causes of ATN are ischemia and nephrotoxic injury. Ischemia may be the result of circulatory collapse, severe hypotension, hemorrhage, dehydration, or other disorders that affect blood supply. Signs and symptoms of ATN include scanty urine production (**oliguria**) and increased blood levels of calcium (**hypercalcemia**). When tubular damage is not severe, the disorder is reversible.

## Oncology

The second most common form of cancer in men is carcinoma of the prostate. In the United States, the disease is rarely found in men younger than age 50; however, the incidence dramatically increases with age. Susceptibility to the disease is influenced, to a large extent, by race. Incidence is least in Asians, moderate in whites, and high in blacks. Symptoms include difficulty starting urination (**hesitancy**) and stopping the urinary stream, dysuria, urinary frequency, and hematuria. By the time these symptoms develop and the patient seeks treatment, the disease is quite advanced and long-term survival is not likely. Early presymptomatic tests include a blood test for *prostate-specific antigen (PSA)* and periodic *digital rectal examination (DRE).*

Like other forms of cancer, prostatic carcinomas are staged and graded to determine metastatic potential, response to treatment, survival, and appropriate forms of therapy. Because prostatic cancer is stimulated by testosterone, surgical removal of the testes (**bilateral orchiectomy**) and administration of estrogens temporarily arrest metastatic prostatic cancer.

## Diagnostic, Symptomatic, and Related Terms

This section introduces diagnostic, symptomatic, and related terms and their meanings. Word analyses for selected terms are also provided.

| Term | Definition |
|------|------------|
| **URINARY SYSTEM** | |
| **anuria**<br>ăn-Ū-rē-ă<br><br>  *an-:* without, not<br>  *-uria:* urine | Absence of urine production or urinary output<br>*Anuria may be obstructive, in which there is blockage proximal to the bladder, or unobstructive, which is caused by severe damage to the nephrons of the kidneys.* |
| **azotemia**<br>ăz-ō-TĒ-mē-ă<br><br>  *azot:* nitrogenous<br>  compounds<br>  *-emia:* blood condition | Retention of excessive amounts of nitrogenous compounds (urea, creatinine, and uric acid) in the blood; also called *uremia* |
| **chronic renal failure**<br>KRŎ-nĭk  RĒ-năl | Renal failure that occurs over a period of years, in which the kidneys lose their ability to maintain volume and composition of body fluids with normal dietary intake<br>*Chronic renal failure is the result of decreased numbers of functioning nephrons in the kidneys.* |
| **dysuria**<br>dĭs-Ū-rē-ă<br><br>  *dys-:* bad; painful; difficult<br>  *-uria:* urine | Painful or difficult urination<br>*Dysuria is a symptom of numerous conditions.* |
| **enuresis**<br>ĕn-ū-RĒ-sĭs<br><br>  *en-:* in, within<br>  *ur:* urine<br>  *-esis:* condition | Involuntary discharge of urine; also called *incontinence*<br>*Enuresis that occurs during the night is called* nocturnal enuresis; *during the day,* diurnal enuresis. |
| **fistula**<br>FĬS-tū-lă | Abnormal passage from a hollow organ to the surface or from one organ to another |
| **frequency**<br>FRĒ-kwĕn-sē | Voiding at frequent intervals |
| **hesitancy**<br>HĔZ-ĭ-tĕn-sē | Involuntary delay in initiating urination |

| Term | Definition |
|------|------------|
| **nephrotic syndrome**<br>ně-FRŎT-ĭk<br><br>*nephr/o:* kidney<br>*-tic:* pertaining to, relating to | Loss of large amounts of plasma protein, usually albumin, by way of urine, due to increased permeability of the glomerular membrane<br><br>*Hypoproteinemia, edema, and hyperlipidemia are commonly associated with nephrotic syndrome.* |
| **nocturia**<br>nŏk-TŪ-rē-ă<br><br>*noct:* night<br>*-uria:* urine | Excessive or frequent urination after going to bed<br><br>*Nocturia is typically caused by excessive fluid intake, uncontrolled diabetes mellitus, urinary tract infections, prostate disease, impaired renal function, or the use of diuretics.* |
| **oliguria**<br>ōl-ĭg-Ū-rē-ă<br><br>*olig:* scanty<br>*-uria:* urine | Diminished capacity to form and pass urine so that the end products of metabolism cannot be excreted efficiently<br><br>*Oliguria is usually caused by fluid and electrolyte imbalances, renal lesions, or urinary tract obstruction.* |
| **urgency**<br>ŪR-jĕn-sē | Feeling of the need to void immediately<br><br>*Urinary urgency commonly occurs in urinary tract infections (UTIs).* |
| **urolithiasis**<br>ū-rō-lĭ-THĪ-ă-sĭs<br><br>*ur/o:* urine<br>*lith:* stone, calculus<br>*-iasis:* abnormal condition (produced by something specified) | Presence of stones in any urinary structure<br><br>*Urolithiasis is commonly treated by pulverizing the stones with extracorporeal shockwave lithotripsy.* |
| **Wilms tumor**<br>VĬLMZ TOO-měr | Rapidly developing malignant neoplasm of the kidney that usually occurs in children<br><br>*Diagnosis of Wilms tumor is established by an excretory urogram with tomography. The tumor is well encapsulated in the early stage but may metastasize to other sites, such as lymph nodes and lungs.* |

## Male Reproductive System

| Term | Definition |
|------|------------|
| **anorchidism**<br>ăn-OR-kĭ-dĭzm<br><br>*an-:* without, not<br>*orchid:* testis (plural, testes)<br>*-ism:* condition | Congenital absence of one or both testes; also called *anorchia* or *anorchism*<br><br>*Treatment for anorchidism requires replacement of the male hormone testosterone. Boys affected with anorchidism will need testosterone for puberty to occur.* |
| **aspermia**<br>ă-SPĔR-mē-ă<br><br>*a-:* without, not<br>*sperm:* spermatozoa, sperm cells<br>*-ia:* condition | Failure to form or ejaculate semen |

*(Continued)*

| Term | Definition | (Continued) |
|------|------------|-------------|
| **balanitis**<br>băl-ă-NĪ-tĭs<br><br>*balan:* glans penis<br>*-itis:* inflammation | Inflammation of the skin covering the glans penis<br>*Uncircumcised men with poor personal hygiene are prone to this disorder.* | |
| **epispadias**<br>ĕp-ĭ-SPĀ-dē-ăs<br><br>*epi-:* above, upon<br>*-spadias:* slit, fissure | Malformation in which the urethra opens on the dorsum of the penis | |
| **erectile dysfunction**<br>ĕ-RĔK-tĭl | Repeated inability to get or keep an erection firm enough for sexual intercourse<br>*Any disorder that causes injury to the nerves or impairs blood flow in the penis has the potential to cause erectile dysfunction.* | |
| **hydrocele**<br>HĪ-drō-sēl<br><br>*hydr/o:* water<br>*-cele:* hernia, swelling | Accumulation of serous fluid in a saclike cavity, especially the testes and associated structures<br>*Hydrocele is common in male newborns but usually resolves within the first year.* | |
| **hypospadias**<br>hī-pō-SPĀ-dē-ăs<br><br>*hypo-:* under, below, deficient<br>*-spadias:* slit, fissure | Developmental anomaly in which the urethra opens on the underside of the penis or, in extreme cases, on the perineum | |
| **phimosis**<br>fī-MŌ-sĭs<br><br>*phim:* muzzle<br>*-osis:* abnormal condition; increase (used primarily with blood cells) | Stenosis or narrowing of preputial orifice so that the foreskin cannot be retracted over the glans penis | |
| **sterility**<br>stĕr-ĬL-ĭ-tē | Inability to produce offspring; in the male, inability to fertilize the ovum | |
| **varicocele**<br>VĂR-ĭ-kō-sēl<br><br>*varic/o:* dilated vein<br>*-cele:* hernia, swelling | Swelling and distention of veins of the spermatic cord | |

**It is time to review pathological, diagnostic, symptomatic, and related terms by completing Learning Activity 11–4.**

## Diagnostic and Therapeutic Procedures

This section introduces procedures used to diagnose and treat genitourinary system disorders. Descriptions are provided as well as pronunciations and word analyses for selected terms.

| Procedure | Description |
| --- | --- |
| **DIAGNOSTIC PROCEDURES** | |
| **Clinical** | |
| **digital rectal examination (DRE)** | Screening test that assesses the rectal wall surface for lesions or abnormally firm areas that might indicate cancer<br><br>*In DRE, the physician inserts a gloved, lubricated finger into the rectum. In the male, the physician also evaluates the size and consistency of the prostate.* |
| **electromyography**<br>ē-lĕk-trō-mī-ŎG-ră-fē<br><br>*electr/o:* electricity<br>*my/o:* muscle<br>*-graphy:* process of recording | Measures the contraction of muscles that control urination using electrodes placed in the rectum and urethra<br><br>*Electromyography determines whether incontinence is due to weak muscles or other causes.* |
| **testicular self-examination (TSE)** | Self-examination of the testes for abnormal lumps or swellings in the scrotal sac<br><br>*TSE is increasingly recommended by physicians to detect abnormalities, especially cancer, when the disease is easily treatable. Testicular cancer is the number one cancer killer in men ages 20 to 30.* |
| **Endoscopic** | |
| **endoscopy**<br>ĕn-DŎS-kō-pē<br><br>*endo-:* in, within<br>*-scopy:* examination | Visual examination of a cavity or canal using a specialized lighted instrument called an *endoscope*<br><br>*The organ, cavity, or canal being examined dictates the name of the endoscopic procedure. (See Figure 4–5.) A camera and video recorder are commonly used during the procedure to provide a permanent record.* |
| **cystoscopy**<br>sĭs-TŎS-kō-pē<br><br>*cyst/o:* bladder<br>*-scopy:* examination | Insertion of a cystoscope into the urethra to examine the urinary bladder, obtain biopsies of tumors or other growths, and remove polyps |
| **nephroscopy**<br>nĕ-FRŎS-kō-pē<br><br>*nephr/o:* kidney<br>*-scopy:* examination | Examination of the inside of the kidney(s) using a specialized three-channel endoscope that enables visualization of the kidney and irrigation<br><br>*The nephroscope is passed through a small incision made in the renal pelvis. Kidney pathology and congenital deformities may also be observed.* |
| **urethroscopy**<br>ū-rē-THRŎS-kō-pē<br><br>*urethr/o:* urethra<br>*-scopy:* examination | Visual examination of the urethra, typically for lithotripsy or TURP |

*(Continued)*

| Procedure | Description | (Continued) |
|---|---|---|

### Laboratory

| | |
|---|---|
| **blood urea nitrogen (BUN)**<br>ū-RĒ-ă NĪ-trō-jĕn | Test that determines the amount of urea nitrogen, a waste product of protein metabolism, present in a blood sample<br><br>*Because urea is cleared from the bloodstream by the kidneys, the BUN test can be used as an indicator of kidney function.* |
| **culture and sensitivity (C&S)**<br>KŬL-tūr, sĕn-si-TĬ-vĭ-tē | Test that determines the causative organism of a disease and how the organism responds to various antibiotics<br><br>*C&S tests are performed on urine, blood, and body secretions.* |
| **prostate specific antigen (PSA)**<br>PRŎS-tāt spĕ-SĬF-ĭk<br>ĂN-tĭ-jĕn | Blood test used to detect prostatic disorders, especially prostatic cancer<br><br>*PSA is a substance produced by the prostate and is normally found in a blood sample in small quantities. The level is elevated in prostatitis, benign prostatic hyperplasia, and tumors of the prostate.* |
| **semen analysis**<br>SĒ-mĕn ă-NĂL-ĭ-sĭs | Test that analyzes a semen sample for volume, sperm count, motility, and morphology to evaluate fertility or verify sterilization after a vasectomy |
| **urinalysis (UA)**<br>ū-rĭ-NĂL-ĭ-sĭs | Battery of tests performed on a urine specimen, including physical observation, chemical tests, and microscopic evaluation<br><br>*Urinalysis not only provides information on the urinary structures but may also be the first indicator of such system disorders as diabetes and liver and gallbladder disease.* |

### Radiographic

| | |
|---|---|
| **cystography**<br>sĭs-TŎG-ră-fē<br><br>*cyst/o:* bladder<br>*-graphy:* process of recording | Radiographic examination of the urinary bladder using a contrast medium<br><br>*Cystography is used to diagnose tumors or defects in the bladder wall, vesicoureteral reflux, stones, or other pathological conditions of the bladder.* |
| **cystometrography**<br>sĭs-tō-mĕ-TRŎG-ră-fē<br><br>*cyst/o:* bladder<br>*metr/o:* uterus (womb); measure<br>*-graphy:* process of recording | Procedure that assesses volume and pressure in the bladder at varying stages of filling using saline and a contrast medium introduced into the bladder through a catheter<br><br>*Cystometrography is the primary test used to investigate stress incontinence and urge incontinence.* |

Diagnostic and Ther...

11 • Genito...

328

Procedu...

THER...

Cli...

| Procedure | Description |
|-----------|-------------|
| **cystourethrography**<br>sis-tō-ū-rē-THRŎG-ră-fē<br><br>  *cyst/o:* bladder<br>  *urethr/o:* urethra<br>  *-graphy:* process of recording | Radiographic evaluation of the urina...<br>administration of a contrast mediur... |
|   **voiding (VCUG)** | Cystourethrography with additional rad...<br>the bladder and urethra performed before, durin...<br>voiding<br><br>*Voiding cystourethrography is performed to determine the cause of repeated bladder infections or stress incontinence and to identify congenital or acquired structural abnormalities of the bladder and urethra.* |
| **kidney, ureter, bladder (KUB) radiography** | Radiographic examination to determine the location, size, and shape of the kidneys in relationship to other organs in the abdominopelvic cavity<br><br>*KUB radiography identifies stones and calcified areas and does not require a contrast medium.* |
| **pyelography**<br><br>  *pyel/o:* renal pelvis<br>  *-graphy:* process of recording | Radiographic examination of the ureters and renal pelvis |
|   **intravenous (IVP)**<br>  ĭn-tră-VĒ-nŭs<br><br>    *intra-:* in, within<br>    *ven:* vein<br>    *-ous:* pertaining to, relating to | Radiographic examination of the ureters and renal pelvis after I.V. injection of a contrast medium; also called *excretory urography (EU)* or *intravenous urography (IVU)*<br><br>*IVP detects kidney stones, an enlarged prostate, internal injuries after an accident or trauma, and tumors in the kidneys, ureters, and bladder.* |
| **computed tomography (CT) scan**<br>kŏm-PŪ-těd tō-MŎG-ră-fē | Imaging technique that rotates an x-ray emitter around the area to be scanned and measures the intensity of transmitted rays from different angles<br><br>*In the genitourinary system, CT scans are used to diagnose tumors, cysts, inflammation, abscesses, perforation, bleeding, and obstructions of the kidneys, ureters, and bladder.* |
| **nuclear scan, renal** | Test used to evaluate blood flow, structure, and functions of the kidneys after I.V. injection of a mildly radioactive substance<br><br>*A monitor is used to track the radioactive substance as it passes through the kidney.* |
| **ultrasound**<br>ŬL-tră-sŏwnd | Test that uses high-frequency sound waves (ultrasound) and displays the reflected "echoes" on a monitor; also called *sonography, echography,* or *echo* |
|   **scrotal**<br>  SKRŌ-tăl | Use of ultrasound to assess patency of the vas deferens and other structures |

*(Continued)*

| e | Description | (Continued) |

**APEUTIC PROCEDURES**

nical

**dialysis**
dī-ĂL-ĭ-sĭs

Passage of a solute through a membrane

*dia-:* through, across
*-lysis:* separation;
destruction; loosening

**hemodialysis**
hē-mō-dī-ĂL-ĭ-sĭs

Removal of toxic substances from the blood by shunting blood from the body through a semipermeable membranous tube (See Figure 11–7.)

*hem/o:* blood
*dia-:* through, across
*-lysis:* separation;
destruction; loosening

*At the completion of the process of hemodialysis, the cleansed blood is returned to the body.*

**Figure 11–7**   Hemodialysis.

| Procedure | Description |
|---|---|
| **peritoneal**<br>pĕr-i-tō-NĒ-ăl<br><br>*peritone:* peritoneum<br>*-al:* pertaining to, relating to | Removal of toxic substances from the body by perfusing the peritoneal cavity with a warm, sterile chemical solution (See Figure 11–8.)<br><br>*In peritoneal dialysis, the lining of the peritoneal cavity is used as the dialyzing membrane. Dialyzing fluid remains in the peritoneal cavity for 1 to 2 hours and then is removed. The procedure is repeated as often as necessary.* |
| **lithotripsy**<br>LĬTH-ō-trĭp-sē<br><br>*lith/o:* stone, calculus<br>*-tripsy:* crushing<br><br>**extracorporeal shockwave (ESWL)**<br>ĕks-tră-kor-POR-ē-ăl  SHŎK-wāv | Procedure for eliminating a stone within the urinary system or gallbladder by mechanically crushing the stone through a surgical incision or using a noninvasive method such as ultrasonic shockwaves to shatter it<br><br>Use of shockwaves as a noninvasive method to break up stones in the gallbladder or biliary ducts<br><br>*In ESWL, ultrasound is used to locate the stone or stones and to monitor the destruction of the stones. The patient is usually placed on a course of oral dissolution drugs to ensure complete removal of all stones and stone fragments. (See Figure 11–5.)* |

*(Continued)*

**Figure 11–8**   Peritoneal dialysis. (A) Introducing dialysis fluid into the peritoneal cavity. (B) Draining dialysate with waste products from peritoneal cavity.

| Procedure | Description | (Continued) |
|---|---|---|

### Surgical

| | |
|---|---|
| **circumcision**<br>sĕr-kŭm-SĬ-zhŭn | Removal of all or part of the foreskin, or prepuce, of the penis |
| **nephrolithotomy, percutaneous (PCNL)**<br>nĕf-rō-lĭth-ŎT-ō-mē | Removal of a stone from the kidney through a very small incision in the skin<br>*Percutaneous nephrolithotomy is performed when ESWL is not possible, such as when the stone measures larger than 2 cm. It is less complicated than an open operation, allows a quicker recovery time, and has virtually replaced the open method.* |
| **nephropexy**<br>NĔF-rō-pĕks-ē<br><br>   *nephr/o:* kidney<br>   *-pexy:* fixation (of an organ) | Fixation of a floating or mobile kidney |
| **orchidectomy**<br>or-kĭ-DĔK-tō-mē<br><br>   *orchid:* testis (plural, testes)<br>   *-ectomy:* excision, removal | Removal of one or both testes; also called *orchiectomy*<br>*Orchidectomy may be indicated for serious disease or injury to the testis or to control cancer of the prostate by removing a source of androgenic hormones.* |
| **resection of the prostate**<br>rē-SĔK-shŭn | Partial excision of the prostate gland |
|    **transurethral**<br>   trăns-ū-RĒ-thrăl<br><br>      *trans-:* through, across<br>      *urethr:* urethra<br>      *-al:* pertaining to, relating to | Procedure to remove prostatic tissue by cauterization or cryosurgery<br>*Transurethral resection of the prostate (TURP) is performed using an endoscope passed through the urethra.* |
| **urethrotomy**<br>ū-rē-THRŎT-ō-mē<br><br>   *urethr/o:* urethra<br>   *-tomy:* incision | Incision of a urethral stricture<br>*Urethrotomy corrects constrictions of the urethra that make voiding difficult.* |

| Procedure | Description |
|---|---|
| **vasectomy**<br>văs-ĔK-tō-mē<br><br>*vas:* vessel; vas deferens; duct<br>*-ectomy:* excision, removal | Excision of all or a segment of the vas deferens (See Figure 11–9.)<br><br>*Bilateral vasectomy is the most successful method of male contraception. Although the procedure is considered permanent, with advances in micro-surgery, vasectomy is sometimes reversible.* |

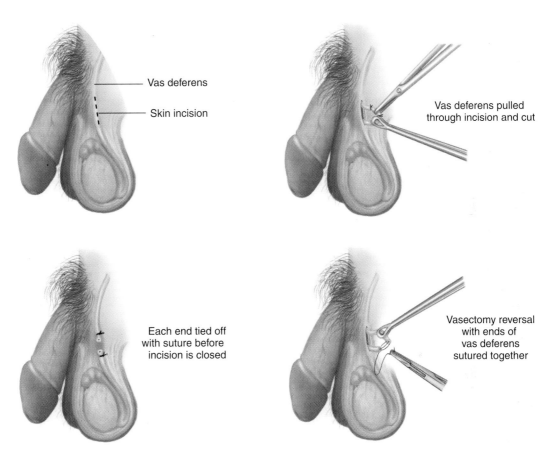

Vas deferens

Skin incision

Vas deferens pulled through incision and cut

Each end tied off with suture before incision is closed

Vasectomy reversal with ends of vas deferens sutured together

**Figure 11–9**   Vasectomy and reversal.

## Pharmacology

This section discusses urinary and male reproductive pharmacologic agents. Urinary tract drugs include antibiotics, diuretics, antidiuretics, urinary antispasmodics, and potassium supplements, commonly taken concurrently with many diuretics to counteract potassium depletion. (See Table 11–1.) Pharmacologic agents are used to treat conditions of the male reproductive system including hypogonadism, erectile disfunction, and reproductive concerns and disorders.

### Table 11–1 DRUGS USED TO TREAT GENITOURINARY DISORDERS

This table lists common drug classifications used to treat urinary and male reproductive disorders, their therapeutic actions, and selected generic and trade names.

| Classification | Therapeutic Action | Generic and Trade Names |
|---|---|---|
| **Urinary System** | | |
| **antibiotics** | Inhibit or kill bacterial microorganisms<br><br>*The most common disorder of the urinary system is urinary tract infection (UTI).* | **ciprofloxacin**<br>sĭp-rō-FLŎCKS-ă-sĭn<br>  *Cipro*<br>**levofloxacin**<br>lē-vō-FLŎKS-ă-sĭn<br>  *Levaquin*<br>**norfloxacin**<br>nor-FLŎKS-ă-sĭn<br>  *Noroxin* |
| **antidiuretics** | Reduce or control excretion of urine | **vasopressin**<br>văs-ō-PRĚS-ĭn<br>  *Pitressin, Pressyn* |
| **antispasmodics** | Decrease spasms in the urethra and bladder by relaxing the smooth muscles lining their walls, thus allowing normal emptying of the bladder<br><br>*Bladder spasms can result from such conditions as UTI and catheterization.* | **neostigmine**<br>nē-ō-STĬG-mĭn<br>  *Prostigmin*<br><br>**oxybutynin**<br>ŏk-sē-BŪ-tĭ-nĭn<br>  *Ditropan* |
| **diuretics** | Promote the excretion of urine<br><br>*Diuretics are grouped by their action and are used to treat edema hypertension, heart failure, and various renal and hepatic diseases.* | **bumetanide**<br>bū-MĚT-ă-nĭd<br>  *Bumex*<br>**furosemide**<br>fū-RŌ-sĕ-mĭd<br>  *Lasix*<br>**spironolactone**<br>spī-rō-nō-LĂK-tōn<br>  *Aldactone* |
| **potassium supplements** | Treat or prevent hypokalemia<br><br>*Potassium supplements are commonly used with diuretics to counteract their potassium-wasting effect. Dietary sources of potassium are usually insufficient to replace potassium lost because of the diuretic.* | **potassium chloride**<br>pō-TĂS-ē-ŭm KLŌ-rĭd<br>  *K-Dur, K-Tab* |

## Table 11-1    DRUGS USED TO TREAT GENITOURINARY DISORDERS

| Classification | Therapeutic Action | Generic and Trade Names |
|---|---|---|
| **Male Reproductive System** | | |
| androgens | Increase testosterone levels<br><br>*Androgens are used to correct hormone deficiency in hypogonadism and treat delayed puberty in males. In females, they are used to suppress tumor growth in some forms of breast cancer.* | **testosterone base**<br>tĕs-TŎS-tĕr-ōn<br>   *Andro, Histerone, Testamone*<br>**testosterone cypionate**<br>tĕs-TŎS-tĕr-ōn SĬP-ē-ō-nāt<br>   *Andronate, depAndro, Depotest* |
| anti-impotence agents | Treat erectile dysfunction by promoting increased blood flow to the corpus cavernosum to maintain an erection sufficient to allow sexual intercourse | **sildenafil citrate**<br>sĭl-DĔN-ă-fĭl SĬT-rāt<br>   *Viagra* |
| spermicides | Chemically destroy sperm before they are able to enter the uterus<br><br>*Spermicides are available in foam, jelly, gel, and suppositories and are used within the female vagina for contraception. If used within an hour of sexual intercourse, spermicide effectiveness is estimated at about 70% to 80%.* | **nonoxynol 9, octoxynol 9**<br>nŏn-ŎK-sĭ-nŏl, ŏk-TŎKS-ĭ-nŏl<br>   *Semicid, Koromex, Ortho-Gynol* |

## Abbreviations

This section introduces genitourinary-related abbreviations and their meanings.

| Abbreviation | Meaning |
|---|---|
| AGN | acute glomerulonephritis |
| ARF | acute renal failure |
| ATN | acute tubular necrosis |
| BNO | bladder neck obstruction |
| BPH | benign prostatic hyperplasia; benign prostatic hypertrophy |
| BUN | blood urea nitrogen |
| C&S | culture and sensitivity |
| cath | catheterization; catheter |
| cysto | cystoscopy |

*(Continued)*

| Abbreviation | Meaning | (Continued) |
|---|---|---|
| DRE | digital rectal examination | |
| ED | erectile dysfunction; emergency department | |
| ESRD | end-stage renal disease | |
| ESWL | extracorporeal shockwave lithotripsy | |
| EU | excretory urography; also called *intravenous pyelography (IVP)* or *intravenous urography (IVU)* | |
| GU | genitourinary | |
| HD | hemodialysis; hip disarticulation; hearing distance | |
| IVP | intravenous pyelography; also called *excretory urography (EU)* or *intravenous urography (IVU)* | |
| IVU | intravenous urography (IVU); also called *excretory urography (EU)* or *intravenous pyelography (IVP)* | |
| K | potassium (an electrolyte) | |
| KUB | kidney, ureter, bladder | |
| Na | sodium (an electrolyte) | |
| PCNL | percutaneous nephrolithotomy | |
| pH | symbol for degree of acidity or alkalinity | |
| PSA | prostate-specific antigen | |
| RP | retrograde pyelography | |
| sp. gr. | specific gravity | |
| TSE | testicular self-examination | |
| TURP | transurethral resection of the prostate (for prostatectomy) | |
| UA | urinalysis | |
| VCUG | voiding cystourethrography | |

 **It is time to review procedures, pharmacology, and abbreviations by completing Learning Activity 11–5**

# LEARNING ACTIVITIES

The activities that follow provide review of the genitourinary system terms introduced in this chapter. Complete each activity and review your answers to evaluate your understanding of the chapter.

Learning Activity 11–1

## Identifying urinary structures

*Label the following illustration using the terms listed below.*

| | | | |
|---|---|---|---|
| *hilum* | *renal medulla* | *right kidney* | *ureteral orifice* |
| *left kidney* | *renal pelvis* | *ureter* | *urinary bladder* |
| *renal artery* | *renal vein* | *urethra* | *urinary meatus* |
| *renal cortex* | | | |

 Check your answers by referring to Figure 11–1 on page 310. Review material that you did not answer correctly.

## Learning Activity 11–2

### Identifying male reproductive structures

*Label the following illustration using the terms listed below.*

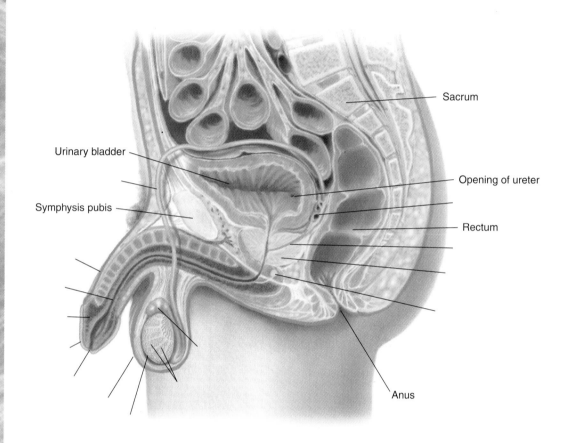

Sacrum

Urinary bladder

Opening of ureter

Symphysis pubis

Rectum

Anus

| | | |
|---|---|---|
| *bulbourethral gland* | *prepuce* | *testis* |
| *ejaculatory duct* | *prostate gland* | *urethra* |
| *epididymis* | *scrotum* | *urethral orifice* |
| *glans penis* | *seminal vesicle* | *vas deferens* |
| *penis* | *seminiferous tubules* | |

 Check your answers by referring to Figure 11–3 on page 313. Review material that you did not answer correctly.

## Building medical words

*Use* **nephr/o** *(kidney) to build words that mean:*

1. stone in the kidney _____
2. abnormal condition of pus in the kidney _____
3. abnormal condition of water in the kidney _____

*Use* **pyel/o** *(renal pelvis) to build words that mean:*

4. dilation of the renal pelvis _____
5. disease of the renal pelvis _____

*Use* **ureter/o** *(ureter) to build words that mean:*

6. dilation of the ureter _____
7. calculus in the ureter _____

*Use* **cyst/o** *(bladder) to build words that mean:*

8. inflammation of the bladder _____
9. instrument to view the bladder _____

*Use* **vesic/o** *(bladder) to build words that mean:*

10. herniation of the bladder _____
11. pertaining to the bladder and prostate _____

*Use* **urethr/o** *(urethra) to build words that mean:*

12. narrowing or stricture of the urethra _____
13. instrument used to incise the urethra _____

*Use* **ur/o** *(urine) to build words that mean:*

14. radiography of urinary (structures) _____
15. disease of the urinary (tract) _____

*Use the suffix* **-uria** *(urine) to build words that mean:*

16. difficult or painful urination _____
17. scanty urination _____

*Use* **orchid/o** *or* **orchi/o** *(testes) to build words that mean:*

18. disease of the testes _____
19. pain in the testes _____

*Use* **balan/o** *(glans penis) to build a word that means:*

20. discharge from the glans penis _____

*Build surgical words that mean:*

21. excision of the testes _____

22. surgical repair of the glans penis _____

23. excision of all or a segment of the vas deferens _____

24. incision of the renal pelvis _____

25. fixation of the bladder _____

Check your answers in Appendix A. Review material that you did not answer correctly.

**CORRECT ANSWERS** _____ × 4 = _____ **% SCORE**

## Learning Activity 11–4

## Matching pathological, diagnostic, symptomatic, and related terms

*Match the following terms with the definitions in the numbered list.*

| | | |
|---|---|---|
| anorchism | epispadias | oliguria |
| anuria | fistula | orchiopexy |
| aspermia | herniorrhaphy | phimosis |
| azotemia | hesitancy | pyuria |
| balanitis | hydrocele | sterility |
| benign prostatic hyperplasia | nephrotic syndrome | urgency |
| enuresis | nocturia | |

1. _____ need to void immediately

2. _____ abnormal passage from a hollow organ to the surface or between organs

3. _____ complete absence of one or both testes

4. _____ absence of urine production

5. _____ metabolic wastes in the blood that contain nitrogen

6. _____ fixation of testes in cryptorchidism

7. _____ nonmalignant enlargement of the prostate

8. _____ difficulty starting urination

9. _____ scanty urine production

10. _____ loss of large amounts of plasma protein resulting in systemic edema

11. _____ stenosis of the preputial orifice

12. _____ inability to produce offspring

13. _____ malformation in which the urethra opens on the dorsum of penis

14. _____ lack of or failure to ejaculate semen

15. _____ pus in the urine

16. _____ suture of hernia
17. _____ excessive urination at night
18. _____ involuntary passage of urine
19. _____ accumulation of fluid in a saclike cavity
20. _____ inflammation of skin covering the penis

✓ Check your answers in Appendix A. Review any material that you did not answer correctly.

**CORRECT ANSWERS** _____ ×5 = _____ **% SCORE**

## Learning Activity 11–5

## Matching procedures, pharmacology, and abbreviations

*Match the following terms with the definitions in the numbered list.*

| | | |
|---|---|---|
| *androgens* | *diuretics* | *potassium supplements* |
| *antibiotics* | *ESWL* | *resection* |
| *C&S* | *KUB* | *semen analysis* |
| *circumcision* | *orchiectomy* | *urethrotomy* |
| *cystoscopy* | *peritoneal dialysis* | *vasectomy* |

1. _____ radiograph that shows the size, shape, and location of the kidneys in relationship to other organs in the abdominopelvic cavity
2. _____ test used to verify sterility after vasectomy
3. _____ visual examination of the urinary bladder
4. _____ inhibit or kill bacterial microorganisms
5. _____ laboratory test that evaluates effect of an antibiotic on an organism
6. _____ drug used to promote the excretion of urine
7. _____ incision of a urethral stricture
8. _____ noninvasive test used to pulverize urinary or bile stones
9. _____ removal of toxic substances by perfusing the peritoneal cavity
10. _____ partial excision of a structure
11. _____ most effective form of male contraception
12. _____ surgical removal of the testes
13. _____ surgical removal of all or part of the foreskin
14. _____ used to increase testosterone levels
15. _____ used to treat or prevent the hypokalemia commonly associated with use of diuretics

✓ Check your answers in Appendix A. Review material that you did not answer correctly.

**CORRECT ANSWERS** _____ × 6.67 = _____ **% SCORE**

# MEDICAL RECORD ACTIVITIES

The two medical records included in the activities that follow use common clinical scenarios to show how medical terminology is used to document patient care. Complete the terminology and analysis sections for each activity to help you recognize and understand terms related to the genitourinary system.

## Medical Record Activity 11–1

### Operative report: Ureterocele

### Terminology

The terms listed in the chart come from the medical record *Operative Report: Ureterocele* that follows. Use a medical dictionary such as *Taber's Cyclopedic Medical Dictionary*, the appendices of this book, or other resources to define each term. Then review the pronunciations for each term and practice by reading the medical record aloud.

| Term | Definition |
|------|------------|
| calculus<br>KĂL-kū-lŭs | |
| cystolithotripsy<br>sĭs-tō-LĬTH-ō-trĭp-sē | |
| cystoscope<br>SĬST-ō-skōp | |
| fulguration<br>fŭl-gŭ-RĀ-shŭn | |
| hematuria<br>hē-mă-TŪ-rē-ă | |
| resectoscope<br>rē-SĔK-tō-skōp | |
| transurethral<br>trăns-ū-RĒ-thrăl | |
| ureterocele<br>ū-RĒ-tĕr-ō-sēl | |
| urethral sound<br>ū-RĒ-thrăl | |

## OPERATIVE REPORT: URETEROCELE

**PREOPERATIVE DIAGNOSIS:** Hematuria with left ureterocele and ureterocele calculus

**POSTOPERATIVE DIAGNOSIS:** Hematuria with left ureterocele and ureterocele calculus

**OPERATION:** Cystoscopy, transurethral incision of ureterocele, extraction of stone, and cystolithotripsy

**ANESTHESIA:** General

**PROCEDURE:** The patient was prepped and draped and placed in the lithotomy position. The urethra was calibrated with ease, using a #26 French Van Buren urethral sound. A #24 resectoscope was inserted with ease. The prostate and bladder appeared normal, except for the presence of a left ureterocele, which was incised longitudinally; a large calculus was extracted from the ureterocele. There was minimal bleeding and no need for fulguration. The stone was crushed with the Storz stone-crushing instrument, and the fragments were evacuated. The bladder was emptied and the procedure terminated.

## Analysis

**Review the medical record *Operative Report: Ureterocele* to answer the following questions.**

1. Why did the doctor perform a cystoscopy?

   _____

2. What was the name and size of the urethral sound used in the procedure?

   _____

3. What is the function of the urethral sound?

   _____

4. In what direction was the ureterocele incised?

   _____

5. Was fulguration required? Why or why not?

   _____

## Medical Record Activity 11–2

## Operative report: Extracorporeal shockwave lithotripsy

### Terminology

The terms listed in the chart come from the medical record *Operative Report: Extracorporeal Shockwave Lithotripsy* that follows. Use a medical dictionary such as *Taber's Cyclopedic Medical Dictionary*, the appendices of this book, or other resources to define each term. Then review the pronunciations for each term and practice by reading the medical record aloud.

| Term | Definition |
|------|------------|
| **calculus** <br> KĂL-kū-lŭs | |
| **calyx** <br> KĀ-lĭx | |
| **cystoscope** <br> SĬST-ō-skōp | |
| **cystoscopy** <br> sĭs-TŎS-kō-pē | |
| **dorsal lithotomy** <br> DOR-săl lĭth-ŎT-ō-mē | |
| **ESWL** | |
| **extracorporeal** <br> ĕks-tră-kor-POR-ē-ăl | |
| **fluoroscopy** <br> floo-or-ŎS-kō-pē | |
| **lithotripsy** <br> LĬTH-ō-trĭp-sē | |
| **Lt** | |
| **shockwave** | |
| **staghorn calculus** <br> STĂG-horn KĂL-kū-lŭs | |
| **stent** <br> STĚNT | |

### OPERATIVE REPORT: EXTRACORPOREAL SHOCKWAVE LITHOTRIPSY

**PREOPERATIVE DIAGNOSIS:** Lt renal calculus

**POSOPERATIVE DIAGNOSIS:** Lt renal calculus

**PROCEDURE:** Extracorporeal shockwave lithotripsy, cystoscopy with double-J stent removal

**INDICATION FOR PROCEDURE:** This 69-year-old male had undergone ESWL on 5/15/xx, with double-J stent placement to allow stone fragments to pass from the calyx to the bladder. At that time, approximately 50% of a partial staghorn calculus was fragmented. He now presents for the fragmenting of the remainder of the calculus and removal of the double-J stent.

**PROCEDURE:** The patient was brought to the lithotripsy unit and placed in the supine position on the lithotripsy table. After induction of anesthesia, fluoroscopy was used to position the patient in the focal point of the shockwaves. Being well positioned, he was given a total of 4,000 shocks with a maximum power setting of 3.0. After confirming complete fragmentation via fluoroscopy, the patient was transferred to the cystoscopy suite.

The patient was placed in the dorsal lithotomy position and draped and prepped in the usual manner. A cystoscope was inserted into the bladder through the urethra. Once the stent was visualized, it was grasped with the grasping forceps and removed as the scope was withdrawn. The patient tolerated the procedure well and was transferred to Recovery.

## Analysis

**Review the medical record *Operative Report: Extracorporeal Shockwave Lithotripsy* to answer the following questions.**

1. What previous procedures were performed on the patient?

   _____

2. Why is this current procedure being performed?

   _____

3. What imaging technique was used for positioning the patient to ensure that the shockwaves would strike the calculus?

   _____

4. In what position was the patient placed in the cystoscopy suite?

   _____

5. How was the double-J stent removed?

   _____

# Chapter

# 12

# Female Reproductive System

## OBJECTIVES

*Upon completion of this chapter, you will be able to:*

- Locate and describe the structures of the female reproductive system.
- Recognize, pronounce, spell, and build words related to the female reproductive system.

- Describe pathological conditions, diagnostic and therapeutic procedures, and other terms related to the female reproductive system.
- Explain pharmacology related to the treatment of female reproductive disorders.
- Demonstrate your knowledge of this chapter by completing the learning and medical record activities.

 **Key Terms**

This section introduces important female reproductive system terms and their definitions. Word analyses are also provided.

| Term | Definition |
|------|------------|
| **fulguration**<br>fŭl-gū-RĀ-shŭn | Destruction of tissue using a high-frequency electrical current<br>*Fulguration of the oviducts via laparoscopy permits gynecologic sterilization.* |
| **genitalia**<br>jĕn-ĭ-TĀL-ē-ă | The sex, or reproductive, organs visible on the outside of the body<br>*Female genitalia include the vulva, mons pubis, labia majora, labia minora, clitoris, and Bartholin glands. The male genitalia include the penis, scrotum, and testicles.* |
| **gestation**<br>jĕs-TĀ-shŭn | The length of time from conception to birth<br>*The human gestational period typically extends approximately 280 days from the last menstrual period. A gestation (pregnancy) of less than 37 weeks is regarded as premature.* |
| **glans**<br>GLĂNZ | Small, rounded mass or glandlike body; erectile tissue at the ends of the clitoris and the penis |
| **lactation**<br>lăk-TĀ-shŭn | Production and release of milk by mammary glands |
| **orifice**<br>OR-ĭ-fĭs | Mouth; entrance or outlet of any anatomic structure |
| **puerperium**<br>pū-ĕr-PĒ-rē-ŭm | Time after childbirth that lasts approximately 6 weeks, during which the anatomic and physiological changes brought about by pregnancy resolve and a woman adjusts to the new or expanded responsibilities of motherhood and nonpregnant life |
| **viable**<br>VĪ-ă-b'l | Capable of sustaining life; denotes a fetus sufficiently developed to live outside of the uterus<br>*A viable infant is one who at birth weighs at least 500 g or is 24 weeks or more of gestational age. Because an infant is determined viable does not mean the baby is born alive.* |

## Anatomy and Physiology

The female reproductive system is composed of internal and external organs of reproduction. The internal organs include the (1) **ovaries,** (2) **fallopian tubes,** (3) **uterus,** (4) **vagina,** and external genitalia. The external genitalia are collectively known as the vulva. Included in these structures are the (5) **labia minora,** (6) **labia majora,** (7) **clitoris,** and (8) **Bartholin glands.** (See Figure 12–1.)

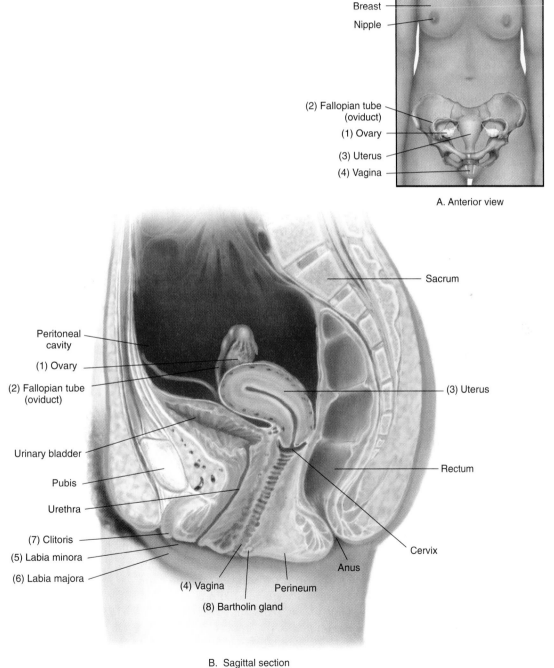

A. Anterior view

B. Sagittal section

**Figure 12–1**  Female reproductive system. (A) Anterior view. (B) Sagittal section showing organs within the pelvic cavity.

The organs of the female reproductive system are designed to produce **ova** (female reproductive cells), transport the cells to the site of fertilization, provide a favorable environment for a developing fetus through pregnancy and childbirth, and produce female sex hormones. Hormones play an important role in the reproductive process, with each providing its influence at critical times during preconception, fertilization, and **gestation.** (See Figure 12–2.)

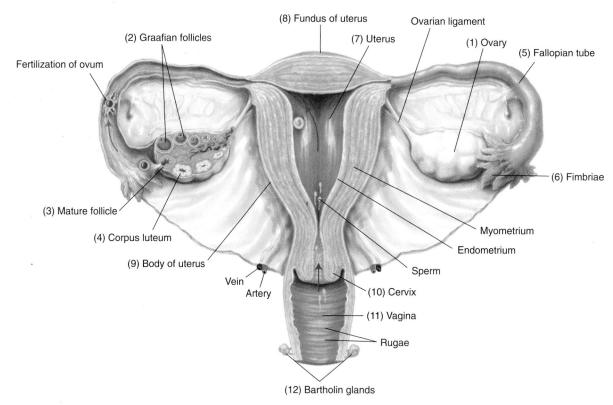

**Figure 12–2**    Anterior view of female reproductive system. The developing follicles are shown in the sectioned left cavity.

## Female Reproductive Organs

Female reproductive organs include the ovaries, fallopian tubes, uterus, and vagina.

### Ovaries

The (1) **ovaries** are almond-shaped glands located in the pelvic cavity, one on each side of the uterus. Each ovary contains thousands of tiny, saclike structures called (2) **graafian follicles.** Each of these structures contains an ovum. When an ovum matures, the (3) **mature follicle** moves to the surface of the ovary, ruptures, and releases the ovum, a process called *ovulation.* After ovulation, the empty follicle is transformed into a very different looking structure called the (4) **corpus luteum,** a small yellow mass that secretes estrogen and progesterone. The corpus luteum ultimately degenerates at the end of a nonfertile cycle. Estrogen and progesterone influence the menstrual cycle and menopause. In addition, both hormones prepare the uterus for implantation of the fertilized egg, help to maintain pregnancy, and promote growth of the placenta. Estrogen and progesterone also play an important role in development of secondary sex characteristics. (See Chapter 13, Endocrine System.)

## Fallopian Tubes

Two (5) **fallopian tubes (oviducts, uterine tubes)** extend laterally from superior angles of the uterus. The (6) **fimbriae** are fingerlike projections that create wavelike currents (peristalsis) in fluid surrounding the ovary to move the ovum into the uterine tube. If the egg unites with a spermatozoon, the male reproductive cell, fertilization or conception takes place. If conception does not occur, the ovum disintegrates within 48 hours and is discharged through the vagina.

## Uterus and Vagina

The (7) **uterus** contains and nourishes the embryo from the time the fertilized egg is implanted until the fetus is born. It is a muscular, hollow, inverted-pear–shaped structure located in the pelvic area between the bladder and rectum. The uterus is normally in a position of anteflexion (bent forward) and consists of three parts: the (8) **fundus,** the upper, rounded part; the (9) **body,** which is the central part; and the (10) **cervix,** also called the *neck of the uterus* or *cervix uteri,* the inferior constricted portion that opens into the vagina.

The (11) **vagina** is a muscular tube that extends from the cervix to the exterior of the body. Its lining consists of folds of mucous membrane that give the organ an elastic quality. During sexual excitement, the vaginal orifice is lubricated by secretions from (12) **Bartholin glands.** In addition to serving as the organ of sexual intercourse and receptor of semen, the vagina discharges menstrual flow. It also acts as a passageway for the delivery of the fetus. The **clitoris** (see Figure 12–1), located anterior to the vaginal orifice, is composed of erectile tissue that is richly innervated with sensory endings. The clitoris is similar in structure to the penis in the male, but is smaller and has no urethra. The area between the vaginal orifice and the anus is known as the **perineum.** (See Figure 12–1.) During childbirth, the obstetrician may decide to surgically incise the area to enlarge the vaginal opening for delivery. If the incision is made, the procedure is called an *episiotomy.*

## Mammary Glands

Although mammary glands (breasts) are present in both sexes, they function only in females. (See Figure 12–3.) The breasts are not directly involved in reproduction but become important after delivery. Their biological role is to secrete milk for the nourishment of the newborn, a process called *lactation.* Breasts begin to develop during puberty as a result of periodic stimulation of the ovarian hormones estrogen and progesterone and are fully developed by age 16. Estrogen is responsible for the development of (1) **adipose tissue,** which enlarges the size of the breasts until they reach full maturity. Breast size is primarily determined by the amount of fat around the glandular tissue but is not indicative of functional ability. Each breast is composed of 15 to 20 lobules of milk-producing glands that are drained by a (2) **lactiferous duct,** which opens on the tip of the raised (3) **nipple.** Circling the nipple is a border of slightly darker skin called the (4) **areola.** During pregnancy, the breasts enlarge and remain so until lactation ceases. At menopause, breast tissue begins to atrophy.

## Menstrual Cycle

The initial menstrual period, *menarche,* occurs at puberty (about age 12) and continues approximately 40 years, except during pregnancy. The duration of the menstrual cycle is approximately 28 days, during which time several phases occur. (See Table 12–1.)

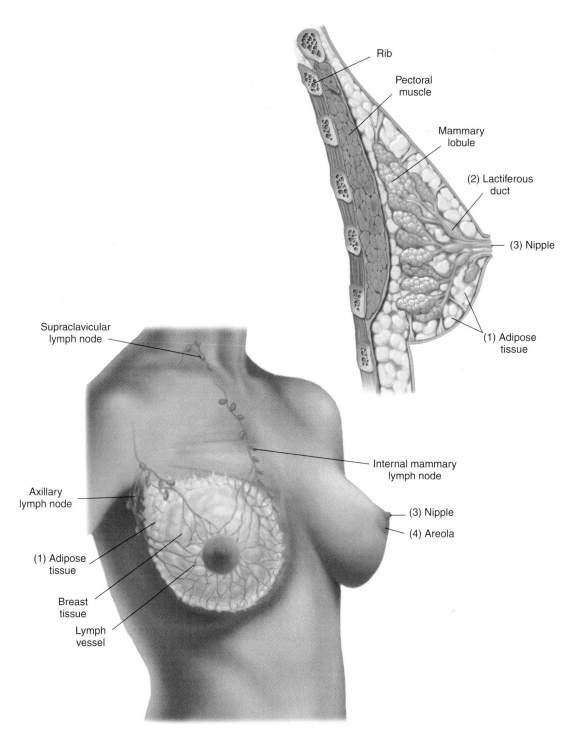

**Figure 12–3**   Structure of mammary glands.

## Table 12-1    CHANGES IN THE MENSTRUAL CYCLE

The menstrual cycle consists of a series of phases, during which the uterine endometrium changes as it responds to changing levels of ovarian hormones. These changes are outlined in the table below. In addition, see Figure 12–4 for an illustration of these changes.

| Phase | Description |
|---|---|
| **Menstrual** Days 1 to 5 | The uterine endometrium sloughs off because of hormonal stimulation, a process that is accompanied by bleeding. The detached tissue and blood are discharged through the vagina as the menstrual flow. |
| **Ovulatory** Days 6 to 14 | When menstruation ceases, the endometrium begins to thicken as new tissue is rebuilt. As the estrogen level rises, several ova begin to mature in the graafian follicles with only one ovum reaching full maturity. About the 14th day of the cycle the graafian follicle ruptures, releasing the egg, a process called *ovulation.* The egg then leaves the ovary and travels down the fallopian tube toward the uterus. |
| **Postovulatory** Days 15 to 28 | The empty graafian follicle fills with a yellow material and is now called the corpus luteum. Secretions of estrogen and progesterone by the corpus luteum stimulate the building of the endometrium in preparation for the implantation of an embryo. If fertilization does not occur, the corpus luteum begins to degenerate as estrogen and progesterone levels decline.* With the decrease of hormone levels, the uterine lining begins to shed, the menstrual cycle starts over again, and the first day of menstruation starts. |

*Some women experience a loose grouping of symptoms called *premenstrual syndrome (PMS).* These symptoms usually occur about 5 days after the decline in hormones and include nervous tension, irritability, headaches, breast tenderness, and a feeling of depression.

## Pregnancy

During pregnancy, the uterus changes its shape, size, and consistency. It increases greatly in size and muscle mass; houses the growing placenta, which nourishes the embryo-fetus; and expels the baby after gestation. To prepare and serve as the birth canal at the end of pregnancy, the vaginal canal elongates as the uterus rises in the pelvis. The mucosa thickens, secretions increase, and the vascularity and elasticity of the cervix and vagina become more pronounced.

The average pregnancy (**gestation**) lasts approximately 9 months and is followed by childbirth (**parturition**). Up to the 3rd month of pregnancy, the product of conception is referred to as the embryo. From the 3rd month to the time of birth, the unborn offspring is referred to as the fetus.

Pregnancy also causes enlargement of the breasts, sometimes to the point of pain. Many other changes occur throughout the body to accommodate the development and birth of the fetus. Toward the end of gestation, the myometrium begins to contract weakly at irregular intervals. At this time, the full-term fetus is usually positioned head down within the uterus.

## Labor and Childbirth

Labor is the physiological process by which the fetus is expelled from the uterus. Labor occurs in three stages. The first is the **stage of dilation,** which begins with uterine contractions and terminates when there is complete dilation of the cervix (10 cm). The second is the **stage of expulsion,** which is the time from complete cervical dilation to birth of the baby. The last stage is the **placental stage,** or *afterbirth.* This stage begins shortly after childbirth, when the uterine contractions discharge the placenta from the uterus. (See Figure 12–5.)

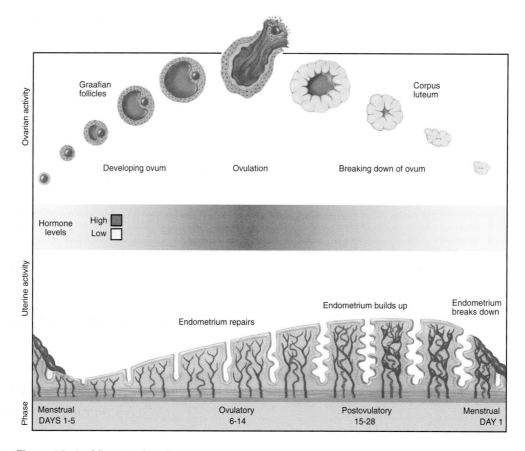

**Figure 12–4**   Menstrual cycle.

## Menopause

Menopause is cessation of ovarian activity and diminished hormone production that occurs at about age 50. Menopause is usually diagnosed if absence of menses (**amenorrhea**) has persisted for 1 year. The period in which symptoms of approaching menopause occur is also known as *change of life* or *climacteric*.

Many women experience hot flashes and vaginal drying and thinning (**vaginal atrophy**) as estrogen levels fall. Although **hormone replacement therapy (HRT)** has become more controversial, it is still used to treat vaginal atrophy and porous bones (**osteoporosis**), and is believed to play a role in heart attack prevention. Restraint in prescribing estrogens for long periods in all menopausal women arises from concern that there is an increased risk that long-term usage will induce neoplastic changes in estrogen-sensitive aging tissue.

 **It is time to review anatomy by completing Learning Activities 12–1 and 12–2.**

(1) Labor begins, membranes intact

(2) Effacement of cervix, which is now partially dilated

(3) When head reaches floor of pelvis, it rotates

(4) Extension of the cervix allows head to pass through

(5) Delivery of head, head rotates to realign itself with body

(6) Delivery of shoulders

(7) Delivery of infant is complete, uterus begins to contract

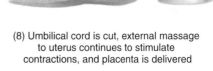

(8) Umbilical cord is cut, external massage to uterus continues to stimulate contractions, and placenta is delivered

**Figure 12–5**    Sequence of labor and childbirth.

## Medical Word Elements

This section introduces combining forms, suffixes, and prefixes related to the female reproductive system. Word analyses are also provided.

| Element | Meaning | Word Analysis |
|---------|---------|---------------|
| **COMBINING FORMS** | | |
| **amni/o** | amnion (amniotic sac) | amni/o/centesis (ăm-nē-ō-sĕn-TĒ-sĭs): transabdominal puncture of the amniotic sac<br>*-centesis:* surgical puncture<br>*Amniocentesis is performed under ultrasound guidance using a needle and syringe to remove amniotic fluid.* |
| **cervic/o** | neck; cervix uteri (neck of uterus) | cervic/itis (sĕr-vĭ-SĪ-tĭs): inflammation of the cervix<br>*-itis:* inflammation |
| **colp/o** | vagina | colp/o/scopy (kŏl-PŎS-kō-pē): visual examination of the vagina<br>*-scopy:* visual examination |
| **vagin/o** | | vagin/o/cele (VĂJ-ĭn-ō-sēl): vaginal hernia; also called *colpocele*<br>*-cele:* hernia, swelling |
| **galact/o** | milk | galact/o/cele (gă-LĂK-tō-sēl): cystic tumor of the female breast caused by occlusion of a milk duct; also called *lactocele*<br>*-cele:* hernia, swelling |
| **lact/o** | | lact/o/gen (LĂK-tō-jĕn): any substance that stimulates milk production<br>*-gen:* forming, producing, origin |
| **gynec/o** | woman, female | gynec/o/logist (gī-nĕ-KŎL-ō-jĭst): physician specializing in treating disorders of the female reproductive system<br>*-logist:* specialist in study of |
| **hyster/o** | uterus (womb) | hyster/ectomy (hĭs-tĕr-ĔK-tō-mē): surgical removal of the uterus<br>*-ectomy:* excision, removal |
| **mamm/o** | breast | mamm/o/gram (MĂM-ō-grăm): radiograph of the breast<br>*-gram:* record, writing |
| **mast/o** | | mast/o/pexy (MĂS-tō-pĕks-ē): surgical fixation of the breast(s)<br>*-pexy:* fixation (of an organ)<br>*Mastopexy is a reconstructive, cosmetic surgical procedure performed to affix sagging breasts in a more elevated position, commonly improving their shape.* |

| Element | Meaning | Word Analysis |
|---------|---------|---------------|
| **men/o** | menses, menstruation | men/o/rrhagia (měn-ō-RĀ-jē-ă): excessive amount of menstrual flow over a longer duration than a normal period<br><br>*-rrhagia:* bursting forth (of) |
| **metri/o** | uterus (womb) | endo/metri/al (ĕn-dō-MĒ-trē-ăl): pertaining to the lining of the uterus<br><br>*endo-:* in, within<br>*-al:* pertaining to, relating to |
| **uter/o** | | uter/o/vagin/al (ū-tĕr-ō-VĂJ-ĭ-năl): relating to the uterus and vagina<br><br>*vagin/o:* vagina<br>*-al:* pertaining to, relating to |
| **metr/o** | uterus (womb); measure | metr/o/ptosis (mē-trō-TŌ-sĭs): prolapse or downward displacement of the uterus<br><br>*-ptosis:* prolapse, downward displacement |
| **nat/o** | birth | pre/nat/al (prē-NĀ-tăl): occurring before birth<br><br>*pre-:* before, in front<br>*-al:* pertaining to, relating to |
| **oophor/o** | ovary | oophor/oma (ō-ŏf-ō-RŌ-mă): ovarian tumor<br><br>*-oma:* tumor |
| **ovari/o** | | ovari/o/rrhexis (ō-vā-rē-ō-RĔK-sĭs): rupture of an ovary<br><br>*-rrhexis:* rupture |
| **perine/o** | perineum | perine/o/rrhaphy (pĕr-ĭ-nē-OR-ă-fē): suture of the perineum<br><br>*-rrhaphy:* suture<br><br>*Perineorrhaphy is used to repair a laceration that occurs or is made surgically during the delivery of the fetus.* |
| **salping/o** | tube (usually fallopian or eustachian [auditory] tubes) | salping/o/plasty (săl-PĬNG-gō-plăs-tē): surgical repair of a fallopian tube<br><br>*-plasty:* surgical repair |

*(Continued)*

| Element | Meaning | Word Analysis | (Continued) |
|---|---|---|---|

### SUFFIXES

| Element | Meaning | Word Analysis |
|---|---|---|
| **-arche** | beginning | men/arche (měn-ĂR-kē): first menstrual period<br>*men:* menses, menstruation |
| **-cyesis** | pregnancy | pseudo/cyesis (soo-dō-si-Ē-sĭs): condition in which a woman believes she is pregnant when she is not; also called *false pregnancy*<br>*pseudo-:* false |
| **-gravida** | pregnant woman | multi/gravida (mŭl-tĭ-GRĂV-ĭ-dă): woman who has been pregnant more than once<br>*multi-:* many, much |
| **-para** | to bear (offspring) | nulli/para (nŭl-ĬP-ă-ră): woman who has never produced a viable offspring<br>*nulli-:* none |
| **-salpinx** | tube (usually fallopian or eustachian [auditory] tubes) | hem/o/salpinx (hē-mō-SĂL-pĭnks): collection of blood in a fallopian tube, commonly associated with a tubal pregnancy; also called *hematosalpinx*<br>*hem/o:* blood |
| **-tocia** | childbirth, labor | dys/tocia (dĭs-TŌ-sē-ă): difficult childbirth<br>*dys-:* bad; painful; difficult |
| **-version** | turning | retro/version (rět-rō-VĔR-shŭn): tipping back of an organ<br>*retro-:* backward, behind<br>*Retroversion of the uterus occurs in one of every four otherwise healthy women.* |

| Element | Meaning | Word Analysis |
|---------|---------|---------------|
| **PREFIXES** | | |
| **ante-** | before, in front of | ante/version (ăn-tē-VĔR-zhŭn): tipping forward of an organ<br>*-version:* turning |
| **dys-** | bad; painful; difficult | dys/men/o/rrhea (dĭs-mĕn-ō-RĒ-ă): pain associated with menstruation<br>*men/o:* menses, menstruation<br>*-rrhea:* discharge, flow |
| **endo-** | in, within | endo/metr/itis (ĕn-dō-mē-TRĪ-tĭs): inflammatory condition of the endometrium<br>*metr:* uterus (womb); measure<br>*-itis:* inflammation |
| **multi-** | many, much | multi/para (mŭl-TĬP-ă-ră): woman who has delivered more than one viable infant<br>*-para:* to bear (offspring) |
| **post-** | after | post/nat/al (pōst-NĀ-tăl): occurring after birth<br>*nat:* birth<br>*-al:* pertaining to, relating to |
| **primi-** | first | primi/gravida (prī-mĭ-GRĂV-ĭ-dă): woman during her first pregnancy<br>*-gravida:* pregnant woman |

 **It is time to review medical word elements by completing Learning Activity 12–3.**

## Pathology

Many female reproductive disorders are caused by infection, injury, or hormonal dysfunction. Although some disorders may be mild and correct themselves over time, others, such as those caused by infection, may require medical attention. Pain, itching, lesions, and discharge are signs and symptoms commonly associated with sexually transmitted diseases and must not be ignored. Other common problems of the female reproductive system are related to hormonal dysfunction that may cause menstrual disorders.

As a preventive measure, a pelvic examination should be performed regularly throughout life. This diagnostic procedure helps identify many pelvic abnormalities and diseases. Cytological and bacteriologic specimens are usually obtained at the time of examination.

**Gynecology** is the branch of medicine concerned with diseases of the female reproductive organs and the breast. **Obstetrics** is the branch of medicine that manages the health of a woman and her fetus during pregnancy, childbirth, and the puerperium. Because of the obvious overlap between gynecology and obstetrics, many practices include both specialties. The physician who simultaneously practices these specialties is called an **obstetrician/gynecologist.**

### Menstrual Disorders

Menstrual disorders are usually caused by hormonal dysfunction or pathological conditions of the uterus and may produce a variety of symptoms. These disorders include:

- Menstrual pain and tension (**dysmenorrhea**) may be the result of uterine contractions, pathological growths, or such chronic disorders as anemia, fatigue, diabetes, and tuberculosis. The female hormone estrogen is used to treat dysmenorrhea and also to regulate menstrual abnormalities.
- Irregular uterine bleeding between menstrual periods (**metrorrhagia**) or after menopause is usually symptomatic of disease, including benign or malignant uterine tumors. Consequently, early diagnosis and treatment are warranted. Metrorrhagia is probably the most significant form of menstrual disorder.
- Profuse or prolonged bleeding during regular menstruation (**menorrhagia** or **hypermenorrhea**) may, during early life, be caused by endocrine disturbances. However, in later life, it is usually due to inflammatory diseases, fibroids, tumors, or emotional disturbances.
- Premenstrual syndrome (PMS) is a disorder with signs and symptoms that range from complaints of headache and fatigue to mood changes, anxiety, depression, uncontrolled crying spells, and water retention. Signs and symptoms involving almost every organ have been attributed to PMS. This syndrome occurs several days before the onset of menstruation and ends when menses begins or a short time after and appears to be related to hormones. The reason most individuals with PMS seek medical assistance is related to mood change. Simple changes in behavior, such as an increase in exercise and a reduction in caffeine, salt, and alcohol use, may be beneficial.

### Endometriosis

Endometriosis is the presence of functional endometrial tissue in areas outside the uterus. (See Figure 12–6.) The endometrial tissue develops into what are called implants, lesions, or growths and can cause pain, infertility, and other problems. The ectopic tissue is usually confined to the pelvic area but may appear anywhere in the abdominopelvic cavity. Like normal endometrial tissue, the ectopic endometrium responds to hormonal fluctuations of the menstrual cycle.

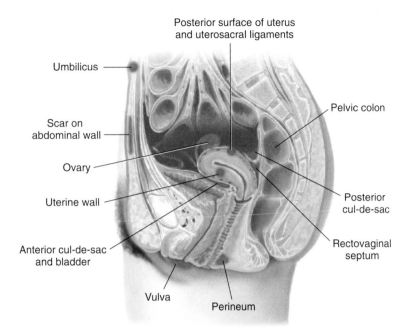

**Figure 12–6**   Endometriosis.

## Pelvic and Vaginal Infections

Pelvic inflammatory disease (PID) is a general term for inflammation of the uterus, fallopian tubes, ovaries, and adjacent pelvic structures and is usually caused by bacterial infection. The infection may be confined to a single organ or it may involve all the internal reproductive organs. The disease-producing organisms (pathogens) generally enter through the vagina during coitus, induced abortion, childbirth, or the postpartum period. As an ascending infection, the pathogens spread from the vagina and cervix to the upper structures of the female reproductive tract. Two of the most common causes of PID are gonorrhea and chlamydia, both of which are sexually transmitted diseases (STDs). Unless treated promptly, PID may result in scarring of the narrow fallopian tubes and of the ovaries, causing sterility. The widespread infection of the reproductive structures can also lead to fatal septicemia. Because regions of the uterine tubes have an internal diameter as small as the width of a human hair, the scarring and closure of the tubes is one of the major causes of female infertility.

### Vaginitis

The vagina is generally resistant to infection because of the acidity of vaginal secretions. Occasionally, however, localized infections and inflammations occur from viruses, bacteria, or yeast. If confined to the vagina, these infections are called vaginitis. Although symptoms may be numerous and varied, including painful intercourse, the most common symptoms are genital itching and a foul-smelling vaginal discharge. It is not uncommon for vaginitis to be accompanied by urethral inflammation (urethritis) because of the proximity of the urethra to the vagina. Two of the most common types of vaginitis are candidiasis and trichomoniasis.

Candidiasis, also called *moniliasis,* is caused by *Candida albicans,* a yeast that is present as part of the normal flora of the vagina. Steroid therapy, diabetes, or pregnancy may cause a change in the vaginal environment that disrupts the normal flora and promotes the overgrowth of this organism, resulting in a yeast **(fungal)** infection. The use of antibiotics may also disrupt the normal balance of microorganisms in the vagina by destroying friendly bacteria, thus allowing the overpopulation of yeast. Antifungal agents (**mycostatics**) that suppress the growth of fungi are used to treat this disease. Trichomoniasis, caused by the protozoan *Trichomonas vaginalis,* is now known to be one of the most common causes of sexually transmitted lower genital tract infections. Trichomoniasis is discussed more fully in the sexually transmitted disease section that follows.

## Sexually Transmitted Disease

Sexually transmitted disease (STD), also called venereal disease, is any of several contagious diseases acquired as a result of sexual activity with an infected partner. As many as 20 different STDs have been identified, of which the newest and most serious is acquired immunodeficiency syndrome (AIDS). (For a full description of AIDS, see Chapter 9, Blood, Lymph, and Immune Systems.) In the United States, the widespread occurrence of STDs is regarded as an epidemic. As a group, STDs are the single most important cause of reproductive disorders. Until recently, gonorrhea and syphilis were the most common STDs but, over the past few decades, chlamydia has become the most widespread STD. Viral diseases such as genital herpes and genital warts are also increasing in prevalence. The current STDs of medical concern are gonorrhea, syphilis, chlamydia, genital herpes, genital warts, and trichomoniasis. Each is described, along with signs and symptoms for males and females.

### Gonorrhea

Gonorrhea is caused by the bacterium *Neisseria gonorrhoeae* and involves the mucosal surface of the genitourinary tract and, possibly, the rectum and pharynx. This disease may be acquired through sexual intercourse and through orogenital and anogenital contact. Some women do not experience pain or manifest overt clinical symptoms (**asymptomatic**) until the disease has spread to the ovaries (**oophoritis**) and uterine tubes (**salpingitis**), causing PID. The most common symptom of gonorrhea in women is a greenish-yellow cervical discharge. The organism may infect the eyes of the newborn during vaginal delivery, which may result in blindness. As a precaution, silver nitrate is instilled in the eyes of newborns immediately after delivery as a preventive measure to ensure that this infection does not occur. The most common sign of gonorrhea in males is a discharge of pus from the penis. Other signs and symptoms include inflammation of the urethra (**urethritis**), which may cause painful urination (**dysuria**). If left untreated, the disease may infect the bladder (**cystitis**) and inflame the joints (**arthritis**). In addition, sterility may result from formation of scars that close the reproductive tubes of both sexes. Both sex partners must be treated because the infection can recur.

### Syphilis

Although less common than gonorrhea, syphilis is the more serious of the two diseases. It is caused by infection with the bacterium *Treponema pallidum.* Syphilis is a chronic, infectious, multisystemic disease acquired through sexual contact or at birth (congenitally). A primary sore (chancre) develops at the point where the bacteria entered the body. The chancre is an ulcerated sore with hard edges that contains contagious organisms for 10 days to 3 months. In pregnancy, the fetus is infected from the mother through the placenta. However, the vast majority of cases are contracted through sexual activity. The danger of transmission is greatest in the early stage of syphilis. If left untreated, the end result is systemic infection that commonly leads to blindness, insanity, and eventual death.

## Chlamydia

Chlamydia, caused by infection with the bacterium *Chlamydia trachomatis*, is the most prevalent and one of the most damaging STDs in the United States. In women, chlamydial infections are associated with mucopurulent discharge and inflammation of the cervix uteri (cervicitis) that may lead to PID. Chlamydia can be transmitted to the newborn baby during the birth process and cause a form of conjunctivitis or pneumonia. In men, chlamydial infections are associated with a whitish discharge from the penis that may lead to urethritis or epididymitis. Chlamydia in men, women, and babies can be successfully treated with antibiotics. However, many cases are asymptomatic, especially in women, and the disease commonly remains untreated until irreversible damage to the reproductive structures has occurred.

## Genital Herpes

Genital herpes causes red, blisterlike, painful lesions that closely resemble the common fever blister or cold sore that appears on the lips and around the mouth. Although both diseases are caused by the herpes simplex virus (HSV), genital herpes is associated with type 2 (HSV-2), and the oral herpes is associated with type 1 (HSV-1). Regardless, both forms can cause oral and genital infection through oral-genital sexual activity. The fluid in the blisters is highly infectious and contains the active virus. However, this disease is associated with a phenomenon called viral shedding. During viral shedding, the virus is present on the skin of the infected patient, and can be transmitted to sexual partners, even when no lesions are present. Individuals with herpes infection may have only one episode or may have repeated attacks that usually lessen in severity over the years. The disease may be transmitted to a baby during the birth process and, although rare, may lead to death of the infant. In females, the lesions appear around the vaginal area, buttocks, and thighs. In men, lesions appear on the glans, foreskin, or penile shaft.

## Genital Warts

Genital warts (condylomas) are caused by the human papilloma virus (HPV). Of the 100 identified types of HPV, only about 30 are spread through sexual contact. The warts may be very small and almost unnoticeable or may be large and appear in clusters. In females, the lesions may be found on the vulva, in the vagina, or on the cervix. In males, the lesions commonly appear on the penis or around the rectum. Many warts disappear without treatment, but there is no way to determine which ones will resolve. When treatment is required, surgical excision or freezing the wart is the usual method. HPV infection has been found to increase the risk of certain cancers, including penile, vaginal, cervical, and anal cancer. The virus is linked to 80% of all cases of invasive cervical cancer. Thus, women who have been diagnosed with HPV infection are urged to have Pap smears every 6 months after diagnosis. There is also a much greater incidence of miscarriages in individuals with HPV disease.

## Trichomoniasis

Trichomoniasis, caused by the protozoan *Trichomonas vaginalis*, affects both males and females but symptoms are more common in females. In women, it causes vaginitis, urethritis, and cystitis. Signs and symptoms include a frothy, yellow-green vaginal discharge with a strong odor. The infection may also cause discomfort during intercourse and urination. Irritation and itching in the female genital area and, in rare cases, lower abdominal pain can also occur. When symptoms are present in males, they include irritation inside the penis, mild discharge, or slight burning after urination or ejaculation. Treatment is generally very effective but reinfection is common if sexual partners are not treated simultaneously.

## Uterine Fibroids

About 30% to 40% of all women develop benign tumors called *fibroids* (also called *leiomyomas* or, more commonly, *myomas*). These benign tumors develop slowly between ages 25 and 40 and commonly enlarge in response to fluctuating endocrine stimulation after this period. Although some individuals are asymptomatic with these types of tumors, when present they include menorrhagia, backache, constipation, and urinary symptoms. In addition, such tumors commonly cause metrorrhagia and even sterility.

Treatment of uterine fibroid tumors depends on their size and location. If the patient plans to have children, treatment is as conservative as possible. As a rule, large tumors that produce pressure symptoms should be removed. Usually, the uterus is removed (**hysterectomy**), but the ovaries are preserved. (See Figure 12–10.) If the tumor is small, a myomectomy may be performed. However, when the tumor is producing excessive bleeding, both the uterus and the tumor are excised.

## Oncology

The two most common forms of cancer involving the female reproductive system are breast cancer and cervical cancer.

### Breast Cancer

Breast cancer, also called *carcinoma of the breast,* is the most common malignancy of women in the United States. This disease appears to be associated with ovarian hormonal function. In addition, a diet high in fats appears to increase the incidence of breast cancer. Other contributing factors include a family history of the disease and possibly the use of hormone replacement therapy (HRT). Women who have not borne children (**nulliparous**) or those who have had an early onset of menstruation (**menarche**) or late onset of menopause are also more likely to develop breast cancer. Because this type of malignancy is highly responsive to treatment when detected early, women are urged to practice breast self-examination monthly and to receive periodic mammography after age 40. Many breast malignancies are detected by the patient.

### Cervical Cancer

Cancer of the cervix most commonly affects women between ages 40 and 49. Statistics indicate that infection associated with sexual activity has some relationship to the incidence of cervical cancer. First coitus at a young age, large number of sex partners, infection with certain sexually transmitted viruses, and frequent intercourse with men whose previous partners had cervical cancer are all associated with increased risk of developing cervical cancer.

A cytological examination known as a *Papanicolaou (Pap) test* can detect cervical cancer before the disease becomes clinically evident. Abnormal cervical cytology routinely calls for colposcopy, which can detect the presence and extent of preclinical lesions requiring biopsy and histological examination. Treatment of cervical cancer consists of surgery, radiation, and chemotherapy. If left untreated, the cancer will eventually metastasize and lead to death.

**Diagnostic, Symptomatic, and Related Terms**

This section introduces diagnostic, symptomatic, and related terms and their meanings. Word analyses for selected terms are also provided.

| Term | Definition |
|---|---|
| **FEMALE REPRODUCTIVE SYSTEM** | |
| **adnexa**<br>ăd-NĔK-să | Accessory parts of a structure<br>*Adnexa uteri are the ovaries and fallopian tubes.* |
| **atresia**<br>ă-TRĒ-zē-ă | Congenital absence or closure of a normal body opening, such as the vagina |
| **choriocarcinoma**<br>kō-rē-ō-kăr-sĭ-NŌ-mă<br><br>  *chori/o:* chorion<br>  *carcin:* cancer<br>  *-oma:* tumor | Malignant neoplasm of the uterus or at the site of an ectopic pregnancy<br>*Although its actual cause is unknown, choriocarcinoma is a rare tumor that may occur after pregnancy or abortion.* |
| **corpus luteum**<br>KOR-pŭs LŪ-tē-ŭm | Ovarian scar tissue that results from rupturing of a follicle during ovulation and becomes a small yellow body that produces progesterone after ovulation |
| **contraceptive diaphragm**<br>kŏn-tră-SĔP-tĭv DI-ă-frăm | Contraceptive device consisting of a hemisphere of thin rubber bonded to a flexible ring; inserted into the vagina together with spermicidal jelly or cream up to 2 hours before coitus so that spermatozoa cannot enter the uterus, thus preventing conception |
| **dyspareunia**<br>dĭs-pă-RŪ-nē-ă | Occurrence of pain during sexual intercourse |
| **endocervicitis**<br>ĕn-dō-sĕr-vĭ-SĪ-tĭs<br><br>  *endo-:* in, within<br>  *cervic:* neck; cervix uteri<br>  (neck of the uterus)<br>  *-itis:* inflammation | Inflammation of the mucous lining of the cervix uteri<br>*Endocervicitis is usually chronic, commonly due to infection, and accompanied by cervical erosion.* |
| **fibroids**<br>FĪ-broyds<br><br>  *fibr:* fiber, fibrous tissue<br>  *-oids:* resembling | Benign uterine tumors composed of muscle and fibrous tissue; also called *leiomyomas (myomas)* and *fibromyoma uteri*<br>*Myomectomy or hysterectomy may be indicated if the fibroids grow too large, causing such symptoms as metrorrhagia, pelvic pain, and menorrhagia.* |
| **infertility**<br>ĭn-fĕr-TĬL-ĭ-tē | Inability or diminished ability to produce offspring |
| **hormonal contraception**<br>hor-MŌ-năl kŏn-tră-SĔP-shŭn | Use of hormones to suppress ovulation and prevent conception |
|   **oral contraceptive pills (OCPs)**<br>  OR-ăl kŏn-tră-SĔP-tĭv | Birth control pills containing estrogen and progesterone in varying proportions<br>*When taken according to schedule, oral contraceptives are about 98% effective.* |

*(Continued)*

| Term | Definition | (Continued) |
|------|------------|-------------|
| **menarche**<br>měn-ĂR-kē<br><br>*men:* menses, menstruation<br>*-arche:* beginning | Beginning of menstrual function | |
| **oligomenorrhea**<br>ŏl-ĭ-gō-měn-ō-RĒ-ă<br><br>*olig/o:* scanty<br>*men/o:* menses, menstruation<br>*-rrhea:* discharge, flow | Scanty or infrequent menstrual flow | |
| **perineum**<br>pĕr-ĭ-NĒ-ŭm | Region between the vulva and anus that constitutes the pelvic floor | |
| **puberty**<br>PŪ-bĕr-tē | Period during which secondary sex characteristics begin to develop and the capability of sexual reproduction is attained | |
| **pyosalpinx**<br>pi-ō-SĂL-pĭnks<br><br>*py/o:* pus<br>*-salpinx:* tube (usually fallopian or eustachian [auditory] tubes) | Pus in the fallopian tube | |
| **retroversion**<br>rĕt-rō-VĔR-shŭn<br><br>*retro-:* backward, behind<br>*-version:* turning | Turning or state of being turned back, especially an entire organ, such as the uterus, being tipped from its normal position | |
| **sterility**<br>stĕr-ĬL-ĭ-tē | Inability of the female to become pregnant or the male to impregnate the female | |
| **vaginismus**<br>văj-ĭn-ĬZ-mŭs | Painful spasm of the vagina from contraction of the muscles surrounding the vagina | |

## OBSTETRICS

| Term | Definition | |
|------|------------|--|
| **abruptio placentae**<br>ă-BRŬP-shē-ō plă-SĔN-tē | Premature separation of a normally situated placenta | |
| **abortion**<br>ă-BOR-shŭn | Termination of pregnancy before the embryo or fetus is capable of surviving outside the uterus | |
| **amnion**<br>ĂM-nē-ŏn | Membrane, continuous with and covering the fetal side of the placenta, that forms the outer surface of the umbilical cord<br>*The fetus is suspended in amniotic fluid.* | |
| **breech presentation** | Common abnormality of delivery in which the fetal buttocks or feet present rather than the head | |
| **Down syndrome, trisomy 21**<br>DOWN SĬN-drōm, TRĪ-sō-mē | Congenital condition characterized by physical malformations and some degree of mental retardation<br>*Trisomy (of chromosome) 21 usually occurs in 1 of 700 live births. The terms Down syndrome and trisomy 21 are preferred to the term mongolism.* | |

| Term | Definition |
|------|-----------|
| **dystocia**<br>dĭs-TŌ-sē-ă<br><br>*dys-:* bad; painful; difficult<br>*-tocia:* childbirth, labor | Difficult labor, which may be produced by the large size of the fetus or the small size of the pelvic outlet |
| **eclampsia**<br>ĕ-KLĂMP-sē-ă | Most serious form of toxemia during pregnancy<br><br>*Signs of eclampsia include high blood pressure, edema, convulsions, renal dysfunction, proteinuria and, in severe cases, coma.* |
| **ectopic pregnancy**<br>ĕk-TŎP-ĭk PRĔG-năn-sē | Pregnancy in which the fertilized ovum does not reach the uterine cavity but becomes implanted on any tissue other than the lining of the uterine cavity, such as a fallopian tube, an ovary, the abdomen, or even the cervix uteri (See Figure 12–7.)<br><br>*Kinds of ectopic pregnancy include abdominal pregnancy, ovarian pregnancy, and tubal pregnancy.* |
| **gravida**<br>GRĂV-ĭ-dă | Pregnant woman<br><br>*The term gravida may be followed by numbers, indicating number of pregnancies, such as gravida 1, 2, 3, 4 or I, II, III, IV, and so forth.* |
| **multigravida**<br>mŭl-tĭ-GRĂV-ĭ-dă<br><br>*multi-:* many, much<br>*-gravida:* pregnant woman | Woman who has been pregnant more than once |
| **multipara**<br>mŭl-TĬP-ă-ră<br><br>*multi-:* many, much<br>*-para:* to bear (offspring) | Woman who has delivered more than one viable infant |
| **para**<br>PĂR-ă | Woman who has given birth to one or more viable infants<br><br>*Para followed by a Roman numeral or preceded by a Latin prefix (primi-, quadri-, and so forth) designates the number of times a pregnancy has culminated in a single or multiple birth. For example, para I and primipara refer to a woman who has given birth for the first time. Para II refers to a woman who has given birth a second time. Whether the births were multiple (twins, triplets) is irrelevant.* |
| **parturition**<br>păr-tū-RĬSH-ŭn | Process of giving birth |
| **pelvimetry**<br>pĕl-VĬM-ĕ-trē *pelv/i:* pelvis<br>*-metry:* act of measuring | Measurement of the pelvic dimensions or proportions, which helps determine whether it will be possible to deliver a fetus through the normal route<br><br>*Pelvimetry is performed by various methods, including manually or radiogically.* |
| **placenta previa**<br>plă-SĔN-tă PRĒ-vē-ă | Condition in which the placenta is attached near the cervix and ruptures prematurely, with spotting as the early symptom<br><br>*Prevention of hemorrhage may necessitate a cesarean delivery.* |

*(Continued)*

| Term | Definition | (Continued) |
|---|---|---|
| **primigravida**<br>prī-mĭ-GRĂV-ĭ-dă<br><br>*primi-:* first<br>*-gravida:* pregnant woman | Woman pregnant for the first time | |
| **primipara**<br>prī-MĬP-ă-ră<br><br>*primi-:* first<br>*-para:* to bear (offspring) | Woman who has given birth to one viable infant, her first child, indicated by the notation *para I* on the patient's chart | |
| **puerperium**<br>pū-ĕr-PĒ-rē-ŭm | Period of 42 days after childbirth and expulsion of the placenta and membranes, during which the reproductive organs usually return to normal | |

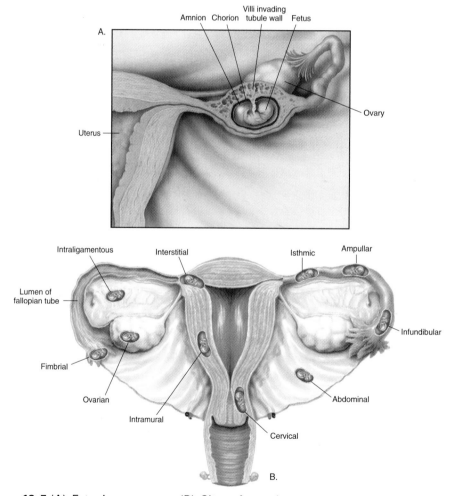

**Figure 12–7** (A) Ectopic pregnancy  (B) Sites of ectopic pregnancy.

 **It is time to review pathological, diagnostic, symptomatic, and related terms by completing Learning Activity 12–4.**

## Diagnostic and Therapeutic Procedures

This section introduces procedures used to diagnose and treat female reproductive disorders. Descriptions are provided as well as pronunciations and word analyses for selected terms.

| Procedure | Description |
|---|---|
| **DIAGNOSTIC PROCEDURES** | |
| **Clinical** | |
| **amniocentesis**<br>ăm-nē-ō-sĕn-TĒ-sĭs<br><br>   *amni/o:* amnion (amniotic sac)<br>   *-centesis:* surgical puncture | Transabdominal puncture of the amniotic sac under ultrasound guidance using a needle and syringe to remove amniotic fluid (See Figure 12–8.)<br><br>*The sample obtained in amniocentesis is chemically and cytologically studied to detect genetic and biochemical disorders and fetal maturity. The procedure also allows for transfusion of platelets or blood to the fetus and instillation of drugs for treating the fetus.* |

*(Continued)*

**Figure 12–8**    Amniocentesis.

| Procedure | Description | (Continued) |
|---|---|---|

| **insufflation**<br>ĭn-sŭ-FLĀ-shŭn | Delivery of pressurized air or gas into a cavity, chamber, or organ to allow visual examination, remove an obstruction, or apply medication<br><br>*Insufflation is performed to increase the distance between structures so the physician can see more clearly and better diagnose possible disorders.* |
|---|---|
| **tubal**<br>TŪ-bǎl | Test for patency of the uterine tubes made by transuterine insufflation with carbon dioxide; also called *Rubin test* |

### Endoscopic

| **colposcopy**<br>kŏl-PŎS-kō-pē<br><br>*colp/o:* vagina<br>*-scopy:* visual examination | Visual examination of the vagina and cervix with an optical magnifying instrument (colposcope)<br><br>*Colposcopy is used chiefly to identify areas of cervical dysplasia in women with abnormal Papanicolaou smears and as an aid in biopsy or excision procedures, including cautery, cryotherapy, and loop electrosurgical excision.* |
|---|---|
| **laparoscopy**<br>lăp-ăr-ŎS-kō-pē<br><br>*lapar/o:* abdomen<br>*-scopy:* visual examination | Visual examination of the abdominal cavity with a laparoscope through one or more small incisions in the abdominal wall, usually at the umbilicus (See Figure 12–9.)<br><br>*Laparoscopy has become a standard technique for many routine surgical procedures, including gynecologic sterilization by fulguration of the oviducts or tubal ligation.* |

**Figure 12–9**   Laparoscopy.

| Procedure | Description |
|---|---|
| **Laboratory** | |
| **chorionic villus sampling (CVS)**<br>kor-ē-ŎN-ĭk VĬL-ŭs SĂM-plĭng | Sampling of placental tissues for prenatal diagnosis of potential genetic defects<br><br>*The sample is obtained through a catheter inserted into the uterus. The advantage of CVS over amniocentesis is that it can be undertaken in the 1st trimester of pregnancy.* |
| **endometrial biopsy**<br>ĕn-dō-MĒ-trē-ăl BĪ-ŏp-sē<br><br>*endo-:* in, within<br>*metri:* uterus(womb); measure<br>*-al:* pertaining to, relating to | Removal of a sample of uterine endometrium for microscopic study<br><br>*Endometrial biopsy is commonly used in fertility assessment to confirm ovulation and as a diagnostic tool to determine the cause of dysfunctional and postmenopausal bleeding.* |
| **Papanicolaou (Pap) test**<br>pă-pă-ni-kō-LĂ-oo | Cytological study used to detect abnormal cells sloughed from the cervix and vagina, usually obtained during routine pelvic examination<br><br>*A Pap test is commonly used to diagnose and prevent cervical cancer. It may also be used to evaluate cells from any organ, such as the pleura and peritoneum, to detect changes that indicate malignancy.* |
| **Radiographic** | |
| **mammography**<br>măm-ŎG-ră-fē<br><br>*mamm/o:* breast<br>*-graphy:* process of recording | Radiographic examination of the soft tissues of the breast<br>*Mammography is used to identify various benign and malignant neoplastic processes and may identify a malignant lesion. The record produced by mammography is called a* mammogram. |
| **hysterosalpingography**<br>hĭs-tĕr-ō-săl-pin-GŎG-ră-fē<br><br>*hyster/o:* uterus (womb)<br>*salping/o:* tube (usually fallopian or eustachian [auditory] tubes)<br>*-graphy:* process of recording<br>*-gram:* record, writing | Radiography of the uterus and uterine tubes (oviducts) following injection of a contrast medium<br>*Hysterosalpingography is used to determine pathology in the uterine cavity, evaluate tubal patency, and determine the cause of infertility. The record produced by hysterosalpingography is called hysterosalpingogram.* |
| **ultrasonography**<br>ŭl-tră-sŏn-ŎG-ră-fē<br><br>*ultra-:* excess, beyond<br>*son/o:* sound<br>*-graphy:* process of recording | Process by which high-frequency sound waves (ultrasound) produce and display an image from reflected "echoes" on a monitor; also called *ultrasound, sonography,* and *echo.* (See Figure 4–4B.)<br>*The record produced by ultrasonography is called* ultrasonogram. |
| **pelvic**<br>PĔL-vĭk | Ultrasound of the pelvic region used to evaluate abnormalities in the female reproductive system as well as the fetus in the obstetric patient |
| **transvaginal**<br>trănz-VĂJ-ĭ-năl<br><br>*trans-:* through, across<br>*vagin:* vagina<br>*-al:* pertaining to, relating to | Ultrasound of the pelvic area performed with a probe inserted into the vagina, which provides sharper images of pathological and normal structures within the pelvis |

*(Continued)*

| Procedure | Description | (Continued) |
|---|---|---|

## THERAPEUTIC PROCEDURES

### Surgical

| Procedure | Description |
|---|---|
| **cerclage**<br>sĕr-KLĂZH | Procedure in which a nonabsorbable ligature is applied around the cervix uteri to treat incompetent uterus, thus decreasing the chance of a spontaneous abortion |
| **cesarean birth**<br>sē-SAR-ē-ăn | Incision of the abdomen and uterus to remove the fetus; also called *C-section*<br><br>*Cesarean birth is most commonly used in the event of cephalopelvic disproportion, presence of sexually transmitted disease organisms in the birth canal, fetal distress, and breech presentation.* |
| **colpocleisis**<br>kŏl-pō-KLĪ-sĭs<br><br>*colp/o:* vagina<br>*-cleisis:* closure | Surgical closure of the vaginal canal |
| **conization**<br>kŏn-ĭ-ZĀ-shŭn | Excision of a cone-shaped piece of tissue, such as mucosa of the cervix, for histological examination |
| **cordocentesis**<br>kor-dō-sĕn-TĒ-sĭs | Sampling of fetal blood drawn from the umbilical vein and performed under ultrasound guidance<br><br>*Cord blood is evaluated in the laboratory to identify hemolytic diseases or genetic abnormalities.* |
| **cryosurgery, cryocautery**<br>krī-ō-SĔR-jĕr-ē, krī-ō-KAW-tĕr-ē | Process of freezing tissue to destroy cells<br><br>*Cryosurgery is used for chronic cervical infections and erosions because offending organisms may be entrenched in cervical cells and glands. The process destroys these infected areas and, in the healing process, normal cells are replenished. This procedure may also be used when a patient shows atypical or possible malignancy, as seen on a Pap smear.* |
| **dilatation and curettage (D&C)**<br>dĭl-ă-TĀ-shŭn, kū-rĕ-TĂZH | Widening of the cervical canal with a dilator and scraping of the uterine endometrium with a curette<br><br>*D&C is used to obtain a sample for cytological examination of tissue, control abnormal uterine bleeding, and treat incomplete abortion.* |
| **episiorrhaphy**<br>ĕ-pĭs-ē-OR-ă-fē<br><br>*episi/o:* vulva<br>*-rrhaphy:* suture | Repair of a lacerated vulva or an episiotomy |
| **episiotomy**<br>ĕ-pĭs-ē-ŎT-ō-mē<br><br>*episi/o:* vulva<br>*-tomy:* incision | Incision of the perineum from the vaginal orifice; usually done to prevent tearing of the tissue and to facilitate childbirth |

| Procedure | Description |
|---|---|
| **hysterectomy**<br>hǐs-tĕr-ĔK-tō-mē<br><br>*hyster:* uterus (womb)<br>*-ectomy:* excision, removal | Excision of the uterus (See Figure 12–10.)<br><br>*Indications for hysterectomy include abnormalities of the uterus and cervix (cancer, severe dysfunctional bleeding, large or bleeding fibroid tumors, prolapse of the uterus, or severe endometriosis). The approach to excision may be abdominal or vaginal.* |
| **subtotal** | Hysterectomy where the cervix, ovaries, and fallopian tubes remain |
| **total (complete)** | Hysterectomy where the cervix is removed but the ovaries and fallopian tubes remain |
| **total (complete) plus bilateral salpingo-oophorectomy**<br>bī-LĂT-ĕr-ăl săl-pǐng-gō-ō-ŏf-ō-RĔK-tō-mē | Total hysterectomy, including uterus, cervix, fallopian tubes, and ovaries |

*(Continued)*

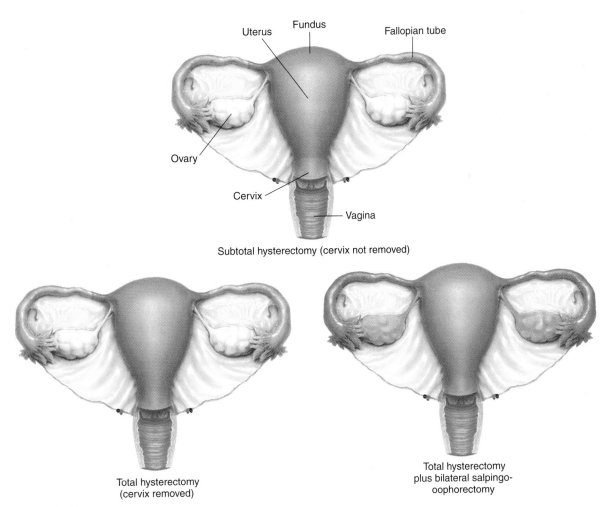

Uterus    Fundus    Fallopian tube

Ovary

Cervix

Vagina

Subtotal hysterectomy (cervix not removed)

Total hysterectomy
(cervix removed)

Total hysterectomy
plus bilateral salpingo-
oophorectomy

**Figure 12–10**   Hysterectomy.

| Procedure | Description | (Continued) |
|-----------|-------------|-------------|
| **intrauterine device (IUD)**<br>ĭn-trā-Ū-tĕr-ĭn dĕ-VĪS | Plastic or metal object placed inside the uterus to prevent implantation of a fertilized egg in the uterine lining | |
| **lumpectomy**<br>lŭm-PĔK-tō-mē | Excision of a small primary breast tumor that leaves the remainder of the breast intact | |
| **mammoplasty, mastoplasty**<br>MĂM-ă-plăs-tē,<br>MĂS-tō-plăs-tē<br><br>*mamm/o:* breast<br>*-plasty:* surgical repair | Surgical reconstruction of the breast(s), sometimes augmented by substances such as fat tissue or silicone to alter size and shape | |
| **mastectomy**<br>măs-TĔK-tō-mē<br><br>*mast:* breast<br>*-ectomy:* excision, removal | Excision of the breast | |
| **radical**<br>RĂD-ĭ-kăl | Removal of the breast and any involved skin, pectoral muscles, axillary lymph nodes, and subcutaneous fat | |
| **myomectomy**<br>mī-ō-MĔK-tō-mē<br><br>*my/o:* muscle<br>*-ectomy:* excision, removal | Excision of a myomatous tumor, generally uterine | |
| **salpingo-oophorectomy**<br>săl-pĭng-gō-ō-ŏf-ō-RĔK-tō-mē<br><br>*salping/o:* tube (usually fallopian or eustachian [auditory] tubes)<br>*oophor:* ovary<br>*-ectomy:* excision, removal | Excision of an ovary and fallopian tube<br><br>*A salpingo-oophorectomy is usually identified as right, left, or bilateral.* | |
| **tubal ligation**<br>TŪ-băl lĭ-GĀ-shŭn | Procedure that ties (ligates) the uterine tubes to prevent pregnancy<br><br>*Tubal ligation is a form of sterilization surgery that is usually performed during laparoscopy.* | |

Hormones perform a vital role in both reproduction and sexual development of the female. Hormone replacement therapy (HRT) is the use of synthetic or natural estrogens or a combination of estrogen and progestin to replace the decline or lack of natural hormones, a condition that accompanies hysterectomy and menopause. (See Table 12–2.) Such symptoms as vaginal dryness, hot flashes, and fatigue are commonly relieved or lessened using HRT. The medical profession is currently rethinking the use of hormone replacement in menopause because of an apparent increased risk of some disorders with extended use of the combination therapy. Use of estrogen alone for HRT is still in clinical trials but has not exhibited the strong contraindications of the combination form of HRT. Estrogen may be administered orally, transdermally, by injection, or as a topical cream (to treat vaginal symptoms only). Other hormones, including oxytocins and prostaglandins, are used for obstetric applications. In addition, pharmacological agents are available for birth control and family planning. These include oral contraceptives, implants, morning-after pills (abortifacients), and spermicides. (See Chapter 11, Genitourinary System.)

**Table 12–2  DRUGS USED TO TREAT OBSTETRIC AND GYNECOLOGIC DISORDERS**

This table lists common drug classifications used to treat obstetric and gynecologic disorders, their therapeutic actions, and selected generic and trade names.

| Classification | Therapeutic Action | Generic and Trade Names |
|---|---|---|
| **antifungals** | Treat vaginal yeast infection<br><br>*Most antifungals used to treat yeast infections are applied topically in the form of ointments, suppositories, or vaginal tablets.* | **miconazole**<br>mĭ-KŎN-ă-zōl<br>  *Monistat*<br>**nystatin**<br>NĬS-tă-tĭn<br>  *Mycostatin, Nilstat* |
| **estrogens** | Treat adverse symptoms of menopause, including hot flashes, vaginal dryness, and fatigue, through hormone replacement therapy (HRT)<br><br>*HRT also reduces the risk of osteoporosis and helps keep cholesterol levels low.* | **conjugated estrogens**<br>KŎN-jū-gā-tĕd ĔS-trō-jĕnz<br>  *Cenestin, Premarin* |
| **oral contraceptives** | Prevent pregnancy<br><br>*Oral contraceptives, or birth control pills, exert a hormonal influence to suppress ovulation and prevent pregnancy. Most contain a combination of estrogen and progestin and are highly effective (95% to 99%) in preventing pregnancy if taken as directed.* | **desogestrel/ethinyl estradiol**<br>dĕz-ō-JĔS-trăl/ĔTH-i-nĭl ĕs-tră-DĪ-ōl<br>  *Desogen, Ortho-Cept*<br>**ethinyl estradiol/ norgestrel**<br>ĔTH-ĭ-nĭl ĕs-tră-DĪ-ōl/nor-JĔS-trĕl<br>  *Lo/Ovral, Ovral* |
| **oxytocics** | Induce labor at term by increasing the strength and frequency of uterine contractions<br><br>*Oxytocics are also used during the postpartum period to control bleeding after the expulsion of the placenta.* | **oxytocin**<br>ŏk-sē-TŌ-sin<br>  *Pitocin, Syntocinon* |

*(Continued)*

| Table 12-2 | DRUGS USED TO TREAT OBSTETRIC AND GYNECOLOGIC DISORDERS *(Continued)* | |
|---|---|---|
| **Classification** | **Therapeutic Action** | **Generic and Trade Names** |
| prostaglandins | Terminate pregnancy<br><br>*Large doses of certain prostaglandins can cause the uterus to contract strongly enough to spontaneously abort a fetus.* | **dinoprostone**<br>di-nō-PRŎS-tōn<br>  *Prostin E2, Cervidil*<br>**mifepristone**<br>mĭ-fē-PRĬS-tōn<br>  *RU 486* |

## Abbreviations

This section introduces female reproductive-related abbreviations and their meanings.

| Abbreviation | Meaning |
|---|---|
| **GYNECOLOGIC** | |
| **AB; ab** | abortion; antibodies |
| **AI** | artificial insemination |
| **BSE** | breast self-examination |
| **D&C** | dilatation (dilation) and curettage |
| **DUB** | dysfunctional uterine bleeding |
| **FSH** | follicle-stimulating hormone |
| **G** | gravida (pregnant) |
| **GC** | gonorrhea |
| **GYN** | gynecology |
| **HRT** | hormone replacement therapy |
| **HSG** | hysterosalpingography |
| **HSV** | herpes simplex virus |
| **IUD** | intrauterine device |
| **LH** | luteinizing hormone |
| **LMP** | last menstrual period |

| Abbreviation | Meaning |
| --- | --- |
| LSO | left salpingo-oophorectomy |
| OCPs | oral contraceptive pills |
| Pap | Papanicolaou smear |
| PID | pelvic inflammatory disease |
| PMP | previous menstrual period |
| PMS | premenstrual syndrome |
| RSO | right salpingo-oophorectomy |
| STD | sexually transmitted disease |
| TAH | total abdominal hysterectomy |
| TVH | total vaginal hysterectomy |
| VD | venereal disease |

## FETAL-OBSTETRIC

| Abbreviation | Meaning |
| --- | --- |
| CPD | cephalopelvic disproportion |
| CS, C-section | cesarean section |
| CVS | chorionic villus sampling |
| CWP | childbirth without pain |
| FECG; FEKG | fetal electrocardiogram |
| FHR | fetal heart rate |
| FHT | fetal heart tone |
| FTND | full-term normal delivery |
| IUGR | intrauterine growth rate; intrauterine growth retardation |
| IVF-ET | in vitro fertilization and embryo transfer |
| LBW | low birth weight |
| NB | newborn |
| OB | obstetrics |
| para 1, 2, 3 | unipara, bipara, tripara (number of viable births) |
| UC | uterine contractions |

 **It is time to review procedures, pharmacology, and abbreviations by completing Learning Activity 12–5.**

# LEARNING ACTIVITIES

The activities that follow provide review of the female reproductive system terms introduced in this chapter. Complete each activity and review your answers to evaluate your understanding of the chapter.

## Learning Activity 12–1

### Identifying female reproductive structures (lateral view)

*Label the following illustration using the terms listed below.*

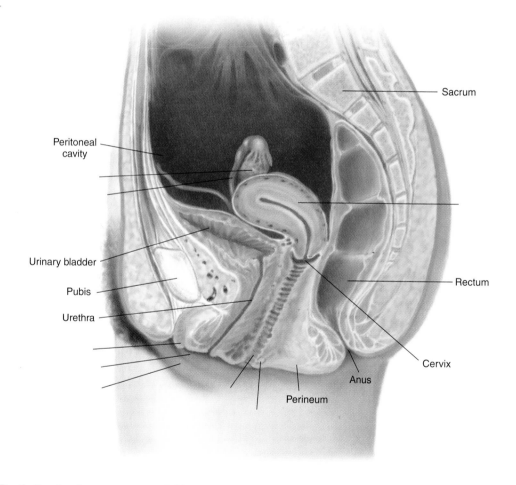

| | | |
|---|---|---|
| *Bartholin gland* | *labia majora* | *uterus* |
| *clitoris* | *labia minora* | *vagina* |
| *fallopian tube* | *ovary* | |

 Check your answers by referring to Figure 12–1 on page 347. Review material that you did not answer correctly.

## Learning Activity 12-2

### Identifying female reproductive structures (anterior view)

*Label the following illustration using the terms listed below.*

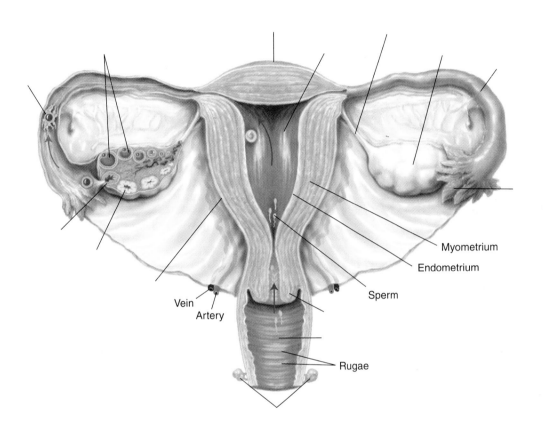

Myometrium

Endometrium

Vein

Artery

Sperm

Rugae

| | | |
|---|---|---|
| *Bartholin glands* | *fertilization of ovum* | *ovarian ligament* |
| *body of the uterus* | *fimbriae* | *ovary* |
| *cervix* | *fundus of uterus* | *uterus* |
| *corpus luteum* | *graafian follicles* | *vagina* |
| *fallopian tube* | *mature follicle* | |

✓ Check your answers by referring to Figure 12–2 on page 348. Review material that you did not answer correctly.

Learning Activity 12–3

## Building medical words

Use **gynec/o** *(woman, female) to build words that mean:*

1. disease (specific to) women _____
2. physician who specializes in diseases of the female _____

Use **cervic/o** *(neck; cervix uteri) to build words that mean:*

3. inflammation of the cervix uteri and vagina _____
4. pertaining to the cervix uteri and bladder _____

Use **colp/o** *(vagina) to build words that mean:*

5. instrument used to examine the vagina _____
6. visual examination of the vagina _____

Use **vagin/o** *(vagina) to build words that mean:*

7. inflammation of the vagina _____
8. herniation of the vagina _____

Use **hyster/o** *(uterus) to build words that mean:*

9. myoma of the uterus _____
10. disease of the uterus _____
11. radiography of the uterus and oviducts _____

Use **metr/o** *(uterus) to build words that mean:*

12. hemorrhage from the uterus _____
13. inflammation around the uterus _____

Use **uter/o** *(uterus) to build words that mean:*

14. herniation of the uterus _____
15. relating to the uterus and cervix _____
16. pertaining to the uterus and bladder _____

Use **oophor/o** *(ovary) to build words that mean:*

17. inflammation of an ovary _____
18. inflammation of an ovary and oviduct _____

Use **salping/o** *(fallopian tube) to build words that mean:*

19. herniation of a fallopian tube _____
20. radiography of the uterine tubes _____

*Build surgical words that mean:*

21. fixation of (a displaced) ovary _____

22. excision of the uterus and ovaries _____

23. suturing the perineum _____

24. excision of the uterus, oviducts, and ovaries _____

25. puncture of the amnion (amniotic sac) _____

✓ Check your answers in Appendix A. Review material that you did not answer correctly.

**CORRECT ANSWERS** _____ × 4 = _____ **% SCORE**

## Learning Activity 12–4

### Matching pathological, diagnostic, symptomatic, and related terms

*Match the following terms with the definitions in the numbered list.*

| | | |
|---|---|---|
| asymptomatic | dystocia | parturition |
| atresia | eclampsia | primigravida |
| candidiasis | gestation | primipara |
| chancre | leiomyoma | pruritus vulvae |
| condylomas | menarche | pyosalpinx |
| congenital | metrorrhagia | retroversion |
| Down syndrome | oligomenorrhea | viable |

1. _____ accumulation of pus in a uterine tube

2. _____ woman who has had one pregnancy that has resulted in a viable offspring

3. _____ pregnancy; 40 weeks in human beings

4. _____ primary syphilitic sore

5. _____ an entire organ, such as the uterus, that is tipped backward from its normal position

6. _____ present at birth

7. _____ difficult labor or childbirth

8. _____ congenital absence of a normal body opening, such as the vagina

9. _____ trisomy 21

10. _____ intense itching of the external female genitalia

11. _____ without symptoms

12. _____ irregular uterine bleeding between menstrual periods

13. _____ beginning of menstrual function

14. _____ benign uterine tumor composed of muscle and fibrous tissue

15. _____ infrequent menstrual flow

16. _____ process of giving birth

17. _____ most serious form of toxemia of pregnancy

18. _____ capable of living outside the uterus

19. _____ genital warts

20. _____ woman during her first pregnancy

✓ Check your answers in Appendix A. Review material that you did not answer correctly.

**CORRECT ANSWERS** _____ × 5 = _____ **% SCORE**

Learning Activity 12–5

## Matching procedures, pharmacology, and abbreviations

*Match the following terms with the definitions in the numbered list.*

| | | |
|---|---|---|
| *amniocentesis* | *episiotomy* | *oxytocins* |
| *antifungals* | *estrogens* | *Pap test* |
| *chorionic villus sampling* | *hysterosalpingography* | *prostaglandins* |
| *colpocleisis* | *IUD* | *total abdominal hysterectomy (TAH)* |
| *cordocentesis* | *laparoscopy* | *tubal ligation* |
| *cryocautery* | *lumpectomy* | *ultrasonography* |
| *D&C* | *OCPs* | |

1. _____ cytological study used to detect cancer in cells that an organ has shed

2. _____ radiography of the uterus and oviducts after a contrast medium is injected into those organs

3. _____ transabdominal puncture of the amniotic sac to remove amniotic fluid for biochemical and cytological study

4. _____ class of drugs used to treat vaginal yeast infections

5. _____ surgical closure of the vaginal canal

6. _____ procedure that widens the cervical canal with a dilator and scrapes the uterine endometrium with a curette

7. _____ excision of the entire uterus, including the cervix, through an abdominal incision

8. _____ tying the uterine tubes to prevent pregnancy

9. _____ birth control pills taken orally

10. _____ examination of the abdominal cavity using an endoscope

11. _____ incision of the perineum to facilitate childbirth

12. _____ noninvasive ultrasound technique used to produce images of internal structures in the body

13. _____ test to detect chromosomal abnormalities that can be done earlier than amniocentesis

14. _____ hormone replacement to reduce adverse symptoms of menopause

15. _____ agents used to induce labor and to rid uterus of unexpelled placenta or fetus that has died

16. _____ freezing tissue to destroy cells

17. _____ birth control method in which object is placed inside the uterus to prevent pregnancy

18. _____ sampling of fetal blood drawn from the umbilical vein

19. _____ excision of a small primary breast tumor

20. _____ agents used to terminate pregnancy

Check your answers in Appendix A. Review any material that you did not answer correctly.

**CORRECT ANSWERS** \_\_\_\_\_ × 5 = \_\_\_\_\_ **% SCORE**

# MEDICAL RECORD ACTIVITIES

The two medical records included in the activities that follow use common clinical scenarios to show how medical terminology is used to document patient care. Complete the terminology and analysis sections for each activity to help you recognize and understand terms related to the female reproductive system.

## Medical Record Activity 12-1

### Primary herpes 1 infection

#### Terminology

The terms listed in the chart come from the medical record *Primary Herpes 1 Infection* that follows. Use a medical dictionary such as *Taber's Cyclopedic Medical Dictionary*, the appendices of this book, or other resources to define each term. Then review the pronunciations for each term and practice by reading the medical record aloud.

| Term | Definition |
|---|---|
| **adenopathy**<br>ăd-ĕ-NŎP-ă-thē | |
| **chlamydia**<br>klă-MĬD-ē-ă | |
| **GC screen** | |
| **herpes lesions**<br>HĔR-pēz | |
| **introitus**<br>ĭn-TRŌ-ĭ-tŭs | |
| **labia**<br>LĀ-bē-ă | |
| **LMP** | |
| **lt** | |
| **monilial**<br>mō-NĬL-ē-ăl | |
| **OCPs** | |

| Term | Definition |
|---|---|
| **pruritus** <br> proo-RĪ-tŭs | |
| **R/O** | |
| **rt** | |
| **vulvar** <br> VŬL-văr | |
| **Wet prep** <br> WĔT PRĔP | |

## PRIMARY HERPES 1 INFECTION

**PRESENT ILLNESS:** A 24-year-old patient started having some sore areas around the labia, both rt and lt side. She stated that the last few days she started having a brownish discharge. She has pruritus and pain of her vulvar area with adenopathy and pm fever, and blisters. Apparently her partner had a cold sore and they had oral-genital sex.

The patient has been using condoms since last seen in April. She has not missed any OCPs. LMP 5/15/xx. Patient has what looks like herpes lesions and ulcers all over vulva and introitus area. Rt labia appears as an ulcerlike lesion; it appears to be almost like an infected follicle. Speculum inserted, a brown discharge noted. GC screen, chlamydia screen, and general culture obtained from that. Wet prep revealed monilial forms. Viral culture obtained from the ulcerlike lesion on the right.

**DIAGNOSIS:** Primary herpes 1 infection; will R/O other infectious etiologies.

## Analysis

**Review the medical record *Primary Herpes 1 Infection* to answer the following questions.**

1. Did the patient have any discharge? If so, describe it.

   _____

2. What type of discomfort was the patient experiencing around the vulvar area?

   _____

3. Has the patient been taking her oral contraceptive pills regularly?

   _____

4. Where was the viral culture obtained?

   _____

5. Even though the patient's partner used a condom, how do you think the patient became infected with herpes?

   _____

Medical Record Activity 12–2

## Menometrorrhagia

### Terminology

The terms listed in the chart come from the medical record *Menometrorrhagia* that follows. Use a medical dictionary such as *Taber's Cyclopedic Medical Dictionary*, the appendices of this book, or other resources to define each term. Then review the pronunciations for each term and practice by reading the medical record aloud.

| Term | Definition |
|------|------------|
| **ablation**<br>ăb-LĀ-shŭn | |
| **benign**<br>bē-NĪN | |
| **Cesarean section**<br>sē-SĀR-ē-ăn | |
| **cholecystectomy**<br>kō-lē-sĭs-TĔK-tō-mē | |
| **dysmenorrhea**<br>dĭs-mĕn-ō-RĒ-ă | |
| **endometrial biopsy**<br>ĕn-dō-MĒ-trē-ăl  BĪ-ŏp-sē | |
| **fibroids**<br>FĪ-broyds | |
| **gravida 2**<br>GRĂV-ĭ-dă | |
| **hysterectomy**<br>hĭs-tĕr-ĔK-tō-mē | |
| **laparoscopic**<br>lăp-ă-rō-SKŎP-ĭk | |
| **mammogram**<br>MĂM-ō-grăm | |
| **menometrorrhagia**<br>mĕn-ō-mĕt-rō-RĀ-jē-ă | |
| **palliative**<br>PĂL-ē-ā-tĭv | |
| **para I**<br>PĂR-ă | |
| **postoperative**<br>pōst-ŎP-ĕr-ă-tĭv | |

| Term | Definition |
|------|------------|
| **Premarin** <br> PRĔM-ă-rĭn | |
| **salpingo-oophorectomy** <br> săl-pĭng-gō-ō-ŏf-ō-RĔK-tō-mē | |
| **therapeutic abortion** <br> thĕr-ă-PŪ-tĭk ă-BOR-shŭn | |
| **thyroid function test** <br> THĪ-royd FŬNG-shŭn | |

## Menometrorrhagia

**CHIEF COMPLAINT:** Dysmenorrhea and night sweats

**HISTORY OF PRESENT ILLNESS:** The patient is a 43-year-old gravida 2, para 1 with multiple small uterine fibroids, irregular menses twice a month, family history of ovarian cancer, benign endometrial biopsy, normal Pap, normal mammogram, and normal thyroid function tests. Negative cervical cultures. She has completed childbearing and desires definitive treatment on endometrial ablation, hormonal regulation.

**SURGICAL HISTORY:** Cesarean section, therapeutic abortion, and cholecystectomy

**ASSESSMENT:** This is a patient with menometrorrhagia who declines palliative treatment and desires definitive treatment in the form of a hysterectomy.

**PLAN:** The plan is to perform a laparoscopic assisted vaginal hysterectomy as the patient has essentially no uterine prolapse and desires her ovaries taken out. She desires to be started on Premarin in the postoperative period. She has been counseled concerning the risks of surgery, including injury to bowel or bladder, infection, and bleeding.

She voices understanding and agrees to the plan to perform a laparoscopic assisted vaginal hysterectomy bilateral salpingo-oophorectomy.

### Analysis

**Review the medical record *Menometrorrhagia* to answer the following questions.**

1. How many pregnancies did this patient have? How many viable infants did she deliver?

2. What is a therapeutic abortion?

3. Why did the physician propose to perform a hysterectomy?

4. What is a vaginal hysterectomy?

5. Does the surgeon plan to remove one or both ovaries and fallopian tubes?

6. Why do you think the physician will use the laparoscope to perform the hysterectomy?

# Chapter

# 13

# Endocrine System

## CHAPTER OUTLINE

## OBJECTIVES

*Upon completion of this chapter, you will be able to:*

- Locate and describe the structures of the endocrine system.
- Recognize, pronounce, spell, and build words related to the endocrine system.
- Describe pathological conditions, diagnostic and therapeutic procedures, and other terms related to the endocrine system.
- Explain pharmacology related to the treatment of endocrine disorders.
- Demonstrate your knowledge of this chapter by completing the learning and medical record activities.

**Key Terms**

This section introduces important endocrine system terms and their definitions. Word analyses are also provided.

| Term | Definition |
|------|------------|
| **diabetes insipidus**<br>dī-ă-BĒ-tēz ĭn-SĬ-pĭ-dŭs | Disorder of insufficient secretion of antidiuretic hormone (ADH) by the posterior portion of the pituitary gland<br>*Diabetes insipidus is characterized by polyuria and polydipsia.* |
| **diabetes mellitus**<br>dī-ă-BĒ-tēz MĔ-lĭ-tŭs | Chronic metabolic disorder of impaired carbohydrate, protein, and fat metabolism due to insufficient secretion of insulin or insulin resistance of target tissues<br>*When body cells are deprived of glucose, their principal energy fuel, they begin to metabolize fats and proteins, depositing unusually high levels of wastes in the blood, causing a condition called ketosis. Hyperglycemia and ketosis are responsible for the host of troubling and commonly life-threatening symptoms of diabetes mellitus.* |
| **electrolytes**<br>ē-LĔK-trō-līts | Mineral salts (sodium, potassium, and calcium) that carry an electrical charge in solution<br>*A proper balance of electrolytes is essential to the normal functioning of the entire body.* |
| **glucagon**<br>GLOO-kă-gŏn | Hormone produced by pancreatic alpha cells that increases the blood glucose level by stimulating the liver to change stored glycogen (a starch form of sugar) to glucose<br>*Glucagon opposes the action of insulin and is used to reverse hypoglycemic reactions in insulin shock.* |
| **glucose**<br>GLOO-kōs | Simple sugar that is the end product of carbohydrate digestion<br>*Glucose is the primary source of energy for living organisms.* |
| **homeostasis**<br>hō-mē-ō-STĀ-sĭs<br><br>*homeo-:* same, alike<br>*-stasis:* standing still | The body's internal state of equilibrium that is maintained by the every-changing processes of feedback and regulation in response to external or internal changes |
| **hormone**<br>HOR-mōn | Chemical substances produced by specialized cells of the body that are released slowly in minute amounts directly into the bloodstream<br>*Hormones are produced primarily by endocrine glands and are carried through the bloodstream to the target organ.* |
| **hyperglycemia**<br>hī-pĕr-glī-SĒ-mē-ă<br><br>*hyper-:* excessive, above normal<br>*glyc:* sugar, sweetness<br>*-emia:* blood condition | Greater than normal amount of glucose in the blood; commonly associated with diabetes mellitus |

| Term | Definition |
|---|---|
| **idiopathic**<br>ĭd-ē-ō-PĂTH-ĭk<br><br>   *idi/o:* unknown, peculiar<br>   *path:* disease<br>   *-ic:* pertaining to, relating to | Pertaining to conditions without clear pathogenesis or disease without recognizable cause |
| **insulin**<br>ĬN-sŭ-lĭn | Hormone produced by pancreatic beta cells that acts to clear sugar (glucose) from the blood by promoting its storage in tissues as carbohydrates (glycogen) |
| **mimetic**<br>mĭm-ĔT-ĭk | Imitation or simulation of a certain effect |
| **sympathomimetic**<br>sĭm-pă-thō-mĭm-ĔT-ĭk | Agent that mimics the effects of the sympathetic nervous system<br><br>*Epinephrine and norepinephrine are sympathomimetic hormones because they produce effects that mimic those brought about by the sympathetic nervous system.* |
| **target** | A structure, organ, or tissue to which something is directed<br><br>*In the endocrine system, a target is the structure, organ, or tissue on which a hormone exerts its specific effect.* |

## Anatomy and Physiology

The endocrine system comprises a network of ductless glands that produce specific effects on body functions by slowly discharging **hormones** directly into the bloodstream. The ductless glands of the endocrine system are not to be confused with exocrine glands such as the sweat and oil glands of the skin, which release their secretions externally through ducts. Although the general effects of most hormones are well known, the manner in which specific hormones affect different organs or tissues of the body is just now becoming clear. The organs or tissues that respond to the effects of a hormone are called **target organs** or **target tissues.** The release of a hormone by an endocrine gland to a target organ is determined by the body's need for the hormone at any given time and is regulated to avoid overproduction **(hypersecretion)** or underproduction **(hyposecretion).** Unfortunately, there are times when the body's regulating mechanism does not operate properly and hormonal levels become excessive or deficient, causing various disorders.

This chapter discusses the structure, hormones, and functions of the *pituitary, thyroid, parathyroid, adrenal, pancreatic,* and *pineal glands.* The function of the *thymus* is covered in Chapter 9, the *testes* in Chapter 11, and the *ovaries* in Chapter 12. (See Figure 13–1.)

## Pituitary Gland

The (1) **pituitary gland,** or **hypophysis,** is no larger than a pea and is located at the base of the brain. It is known as the "master gland" because it regulates many body activities and stimu-

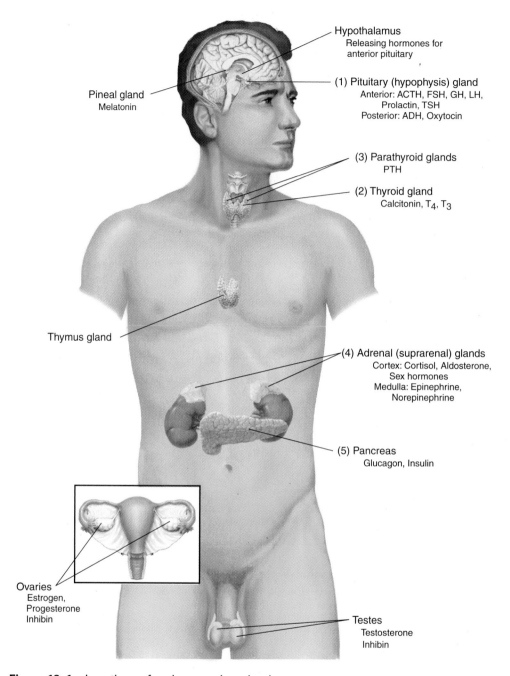

**Figure 13–1** Locations of major exocrine glands.

lates other glands to secrete their own specific hormones. (See Figure 13–2.) The pituitary gland consists of two distinct portions, an anterior lobe (adenohypophysis) and a posterior lobe (neurohypophysis). The anterior lobe, triggered by the action of the hypothalamus, produces at least six hormones. The hypothalamus also produces and secretes two hormones directly to the posterior lobe, where they are stored and released into the bloodstream as needed. (See Table 13–1.)

**Figure 13–2**   Hormones secreted by anterior and posterior pituitary gland along with target organs.

| Table 13–1 | PITUITARY HORMONES |
|---|---|

This table outlines pituitary hormones, along with their target organs and functions and selected associated disorders.

| Hormone | Target Organ and Functions | Disorders |
|---|---|---|
| **Posterior Pituitary Hormones (Neurohypophysis)** | | |
| Antidiuretic hormone (ADH) | • Kidney—increases water reabsorption (water returns to the blood) | • Hyposecretion causes diabetes insipidus. <br>• Hypersecretion causes syndrome of inappropriate antidiuretic hormone (SIADH). |
| Oxytocin | • Uterus—stimulates uterine contractions; initiates labor <br>• Breast—promotes milk secretion from the mammary glands | • Unknown |

*(Continued)*

**Table 13-1    PITUITARY HORMONES** *(Continued)*

| Hormone | Target Organ and Functions | Disorders |
|---|---|---|
| **Anterior Pituitary Hormones (Adenohypophysis)** | | |
| Adrenocorticotropic hormone (ACTH) | • Adrenal cortex—promotes secretions of some hormones by adrenal cortex, especially cortisol | • Hyposecretion is rare.<br>• Hypersecretion causes Cushing disease. |
| Follicle-stimulating hormone (FSH) | • Ovaries—in females, stimulates egg production; increases secretion of estrogen<br>• Testes—in males, stimulates sperm production | • Hyposecretion causes failure of sexual maturation.<br>• Hypersecretion has no known significant effects. |
| Growth hormone (GH) or somatotropin | • Bone, cartilage, liver, muscle, and other tissues—stimulates somatic growth; increases use of fats for energy | • Hyposecretion in children causes pituitary dwarfism.<br>• Hypersecretion in children causes gigantism; hypersecretion in adults causes acromegaly. |
| Luteinizing hormone (LH) | • Ovaries—in females, promotes ovulation; stimulates production of estrogen and progesterone<br>• Testes—in males, promotes secretion of testosterone | • Hyposecretion causes failure of sexual maturation.<br>• Hypersecretion has no known significant effects. |
| Prolactin | • Breast—in conjunction with other hormones, promotes lactation | • Hyposecretion in nursing mothers causes poor lactation.<br>• Hypersecretion in nursing mothers causes galactorrhea. |
| Thyroid-stimulating hormone (TSH) | • Thyroid gland—stimulates secretion of thyroid hormone | • Hyposecretion in infants causes cretinism; hyposecretion in adults causes myxedema.<br>• Hypersecretion causes Graves disease, exophthalmos. (See Figure 13–3.) |

**Figure 13–3** Exophthalmos caused by Graves disease.

## Thyroid Gland

The (2) **thyroid gland** is the largest gland of the endocrine system. An H-shaped organ located in the neck just below the larynx, this gland is composed of two large lobes that are separated by a strip of tissue called an **isthmus.** Thyroid hormone (TH) is the body's major metabolic hormone, which increases the rate of oxygen consumption and thus the rate at which carbohydrates, proteins, and fats are metabolized. TH is actually two active iodine-containing hormones, **thyroxine ($T_4$)** and **triiodothyronine ($T_3$).** Thyroxine is the major hormone secreted by the thyroid; most triiodothyronine is formed at the target tissues by conversion of $T_4$ to $T_3$. Except for the adult brain, spleen, testes, uterus, and the thyroid gland itself, thyroid hormone affects virtually every cell in the body. TH also influences growth hormone and plays an important role in maintaining blood pressure. (See Table 13–2.)

| Table 13–2 | THYROID HORMONES | |
|---|---|---|

This table outlines thyroid hormones, along with their functions and selected associated disorders.

| Hormone | Functions | Disorders |
|---|---|---|
| Calcitonin | • Regulates calcium levels in the blood in conjunction with parathyroid hormone<br>• Secreted when calcium levels in the blood are high in order to maintain homeostasis | • Exerts its most significant effects in childhood when bones are growing and changing dramatically in mass, size, and shape<br>• At best, a weak hypocalcemic agent in adults |
| Thyroxine ($T_4$) and triiodothyronine ($T_3$) | • Increases energy production from all food types<br>• Increases rate of protein synthesis | • Hyposecretion in infants causes cretinism; hyposecretion in adults causes myxedema.<br>• Hypersecretion causes Graves disease, exophthalmos. (See Figure 13–3.) |

## Parathyroid Glands

The (3) **parathyroid glands** consist of at least four separate glands located on the posterior surface of the lobes of the thyroid gland. The only hormone known to be secreted by the parathyroid glands is parathyroid hormone (PTH). PTH helps to regulate calcium balance by stimulating three target organs: bones, kidneys, and intestines. (See Table 13–3.) Because of PTH stimulation, calcium and phosphates are released from bones, increasing concentration of these substances in blood. Thus, calcium that is necessary for the proper functioning of body tissues is available in the bloodstream. At the same time, PTH enhances the absorption of calcium and phosphates from foods in the intestine, causing a rise in the blood levels of calcium and phosphates. PTH causes the kidneys to conserve blood calcium and to increase the excretion of phosphates in the urine.

## Adrenal Glands

The (4) **adrenal glands** are paired organs covering the superior surface of the kidneys. Because of their location, the adrenal glands are also known as *suprarenal glands.* Each adrenal gland is divided into two sections, each of which has its own structure and function. The outer adrenal cortex makes up the bulk of the gland and the adrenal medulla makes up the inner portion. Although these regions are not sharply divided, they represent distinct glands that secrete different hormones.

| Table 13-3 | PARATHYROID HORMONES | |
| --- | --- | --- |

This table outlines parathyroid hormones, along with their target organs and functions and selected associated disorders.

| Hormone | Target Organ and Functions | Disorders |
| --- | --- | --- |
| Parathyroid hormone (PTH) | • Bones—increases the reabsorption of calcium and phosphate from bone to blood<br>• Kidneys—increases calcium absorption and phosphate excretion<br>• Small intestine—increases absorption of calcium and phosphate | • Hyposecretion causes tetany.<br>• Hypersecretion causes osteitis fibrosa cystica. |

## Adrenal Cortex

The adrenal cortex secretes three types of steroid hormones:

1. **Mineralocorticoids,** mainly aldosterone, are essential to life. These hormones act mainly through the kidneys to maintain the balance of sodium and potassium **(electrolytes)** in the body. More specifically, aldosterone causes the kidneys to conserve sodium and excrete potassium. At the same time, it promotes water conservation and reduces urine output.
2. **Glucocorticoids,** mainly cortisol, influence the metabolism of carbohydrates, fats, and proteins. The glucocorticoid with the greatest activity is *cortisol.* It helps to regulate the concentration of glucose in the blood, protecting against low blood sugar levels between meals. Cortisol also stimulates the breakdown of fats in adipose tissue and releases fatty acids into the blood. The increase in fatty acids causes many cells to use relatively less glucose.
3. **Sex hormones,** including androgens, estrogens, progestins, help maintain secondary sex characteristics, such as development of the breasts and adult distribution of hair. (See Table 13–4.)

## Adrenal Medulla

The adrenal medulla cells secrete two closely related hormones, **epinephrine** (adrenaline) and **norepinephrine** (noradrenaline). Both of these hormones are activated when the body responds to crisis situations, and are considered sympathomimetic agents because they produce effects that mimic those brought about by the sympathetic nervous system. Because hormones of the adrenal medulla merely intensify activities set into motion by the sympathetic nervous system, their deficiency is not a problem.

Of the two hormones, epinephrine is secreted in larger amounts. In the physiological response to stress, epinephrine is responsible for maintaining blood pressure and cardiac output, keeping airways open wide, and raising blood glucose levels. All these functions are useful for frightened, traumatized, injured, or sick persons. Norepinephrine reduces the diameter of blood vessels in the periphery (vasoconstriction), thereby raising blood pressure. (See Table 13–4.)

## Pancreas (Islets of Langerhans)

The (5) **pancreas** lies inferior to the stomach in a bend of the duodenum. It functions both as an exocrine and endocrine gland. A large pancreatic duct runs through the gland, carrying enzymes and other exocrine digestive secretions from the pancreas to the small intestine. The endocrine portion of the pancreas consists of groups of cells called islets of Langerhans that produce two distinct types of hormones: alpha cells that produce glucagon and beta cells that produce insulin. Both hormones play important roles in the proper metabolism of sugars and starches in the body.

When blood glucose levels are low **(hypoglycemia),** glucagon stimulates the release of glucose from storage sites in the liver. Because the liver converts stored glycogen to glucose **(glycogenolysis),** the blood glucose level rises. The overall effect, therefore, is a rise in the

## Table 13–4    ADRENAL HORMONES

This table outlines adrenal hormones, along with their target organs and functions and selected associated disorders.

| Hormone | Target Organ and Functions | Disorders |
|---|---|---|
| **Adrenal Cortex Hormones** | | |
| Glucocorticoids (mainly cortisol) | • Body cells—promote gluconeogenesis; regulate metabolism of carbohydrates, proteins, and fats; help depress inflammatory and immune responses | • Hyposecretion causes Addison disease.<br>• Hypersecretion causes Cushing syndrome. (See Figure 13–4.) |
| Mineralocorticoids (mainly aldosterone) | • Kidneys—increase blood levels of sodium and decrease blood levels of potassium in the kidneys | • Hyposecretion causes Addison disease.<br>• Hypersecretion causes aldosteronism. |
| Sex hormones (any of the androgens, estrogens, or related steroid hormones) produced by the ovaries, testes, and adrenal cortices | • In females, possibly responsible for female libido and source of estrogen after menopause; otherwise, effects in adults are insignificant. | • Hypersecretion of adrenal androgen in females leads to virilism (development of male characteristics).<br>• Hypersecretion of adrenal estrogen and progestin secretion in males leads to feminization (development of feminine characteristics).<br>• Hyposecretion has no known significant effects. |
| **Adrenal Medullary Hormones** | | |
| Epinephrine and norepinephrine | • Sympathetic nervous system target organs—hormone effects mimic sympathetic nervous system activation (sympathomimetic); increase metabolic rate and heart rate; raise blood pressure by promoting vasoconstriction | • Hyposecretion has no known significant effects.<br>• Hypersecretion causes prolonged "fight-or-flight" reaction and hypertension. |

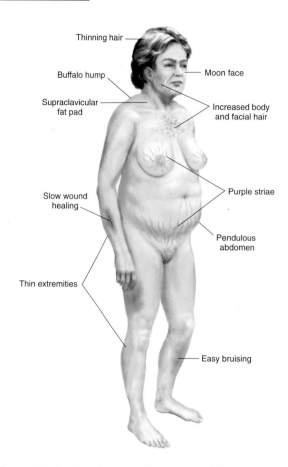

Labels:
- Thinning hair
- Buffalo hump
- Supraclavicular fat pad
- Moon face
- Increased body and facial hair
- Slow wound healing
- Purple striae
- Thin extremities
- Pendulous abdomen
- Easy bruising

**Figure 13–4**  Physical manifestations of Cushing syndrome.

blood glucose level. When blood glucose levels are high **(hyperglycemia),** the pancreatic beta cells are stimulated to produce insulin, which causes glucose to enter body cells to be used for energy and acts to clear glucose from the blood by promoting its storage as glycogen. Insulin and glucagon function as opposites—normal secretion of both hormones ensures a blood glucose level that fluctuates within normal limits. (See Table 13–5.)

## Table 13–5     PANCREATIC HORMONES

This table outlines pancreatic hormones, along with their target organs and functions and selected associated disorders.

| Hormone | Target Organ and Functions | Disorders |
|---------|---------------------------|-----------|
| Glucagon | • Liver and blood—raises blood glucose level by accelerating conversion of glycogen into glucose in the liver (glycogenolysis) and other nutrients into glucose in the liver (gluconeogenesis) and releasing glucose into blood (glycogen to glucose) | • Persistently low blood glucose levels (hypoglycemia) may be caused by deficiency in glucagon. |
| Insulin | • Tissue cells—lowers blood glucose level by accelerating glucose transport into cells and the use of that glucose for energy production (glucose to glycogen) | • Hyposecretion of insulin causes diabetes mellitus.<br>• Hypersecretion of insulin causes hyperinsulinism. |

## Pineal Gland

The (6) **pineal gland,** which is shaped like a pinecone, is attached to the posterior part of the third ventricle of the brain. Although the exact functions of this gland have not been established, there is evidence that it secretes the hormone melatonin. It is believed that melatonin may inhibit the activities of the ovaries. When melatonin production is high, ovulation is blocked, and there may be a delay in puberty development.

 **It is time to review anatomy by completing Learning Activity 13–1.**

## Medical Word Elements

This section introduces combining forms, suffixes, and prefixes related to the endocrine system. Word analyses are also provided.

| Element | Meaning | Word Analysis |
|---|---|---|
| **COMBINING FORMS** | | |
| **adren/o** | adrenal glands | adren/o/megaly (ăd-rēn-ō-MĔG-ă-lē): enlargement of the adrenal glands<br><br>*-megaly:* enlargement |
| **adrenal/o** | | adrenal/ectomy (ăd-rē-năl-ĔK-tō-mē): excision of one or both adrenal glands<br><br>*-ectomy:* excision, removal |
| **calc/o** | calcium | hyper/calc/emia (hī-pěr-kăl-SĒ-mē-ă): abnormally high level of calcium in the blood<br><br>*hyper-:* excessive, above normal<br>*-emia:* blood condition |
| **crin/o** | secrete | endo/crin/o/logy (ěn-dō-krǐn-ŎL-ō-jē): study of the endocrine glands and their functions<br><br>*endo-:* in, within<br>*-logy:* study of |
| **gluc/o** | sugar, sweetness | gluc/o/genesis (gloo-kō-JĔN-ě-sĭs): forming or producing glucose<br><br>*-genesis:* forming, producing, origin |
| **glycos/o** | | glycos/uria (glī-kō-SŪ-rē-ă): abnormal amount of sugar, especially glucose, in the urine<br><br>*-uria:* urine |
| **glyc/o** | | hypo/glyc/emia (hī-pō-glī-SĒ-mē-ă): abnormally low level of glucose in the blood<br><br>*hypo-:* under, below<br>*-emia:* blood condition<br><br>*Hypoglycemia is usually caused by administration of too much insulin, excessive secretion of insulin by the islet cells of the pancreas, or dietary deficiency.* |

*(Continued)*

| Element | Meaning | Word Analysis | (Continued) |
|---|---|---|---|
| **home/o** | same, alike | home/o/stasis (hō-mē-ō-STĀ-sĭs): state of equilibrium in the internal environment of the body<br>*-stasis:* standing still | |
| **kal/i\*** | potassium (an electrolyte) | kal/emia (kă-LĒ-mē-ă): presence of potassium in the blood<br>*-emia:* blood condition | |
| **pancreat/o** | pancreas | pancreat/o/tomy (păn-krē-ă-TŎT-ō-mē): incision in the pancreas<br>*-tomy:* incision | |
| **parathyroid/o** | parathyroid glands | parathyroid/ectomy (păr-ă-thī-royd-ĔK-tō-mē): excision of one or more of the parathyroid glands<br>*-ectomy:* excision, removal | |
| **thym/o** | thymus gland | thym/oma (thī-MŌ-mă): rare neoplasm of the thymus gland<br>*-oma:* tumor<br>*Treatment for thymoma may include surgical removal, radiation therapy, or chemotherapy.* | |
| **thyr/o**<br><br>**thyroid/o** | thyroid gland | thyr/o/megaly (thī-rō-MĔG-ă-lē): enlargement of the thyroid gland<br>*-megaly:* enlargement<br>hyper/thyroid/ism (hī-pĕr-THĪ-royd-ĭzm): condition characterized by hyperactivity of the thyroid gland<br>*hyper-:* excessive, above normal<br>*-ism:* condition | |
| **toxic/o** | poison | toxic/o/logist (tŏks-ĭ-KŎL-ō-jĭst): specialist in poisons, their effects, and antidotes<br>*-logist:* specialist in study of | |

**SUFFIXES**

| Element | Meaning | Word Analysis | |
|---|---|---|---|
| **-crine** | secrete | endo/crine (ĔN-dō-krĭn): secrete internally or within<br>*endo-:* in, within | |
| **-dipsia** | thirst | poly/dipsia (pŏl-ē-DĬP-sē-ă): excessive thirst<br>*-poly-:* many, much | |
| **-gen** | forming, producing, origin | andr/o/gen (ĂN-drō-jĕn): any steroid hormone that increases masculinization<br>*andr/o:* male | |
| **-toxic** | poison | thyr/o/toxic (thī-rō-TŎKS-ĭk): pertaining to, affected by, or marked by toxic activity of the thyroid gland<br>*thyr/o:* thyroid gland | |
| **-uria** | urine | glycos/uria (glī-kō-SŪ-rē-ă): abnormal amount of glucose in the urine<br>*glycos:* sugar, sweetness | |

| Element | Meaning | Word Analysis |
|---------|---------|---------------|
| **PREFIXES** | | |
| **eu-** | good, normal | eu/thyr/oid (ū-THĪ-royd): pertains to a normal thyroid gland<br><br>*thyr/o:* thyroid gland<br>*-oid:* resembling |
| **exo-** | outside, outward | exo/crine (ĔKS-ō-krĭn): secrete outwardly<br><br>*-crine:* secrete<br><br>*Exocrine denotes a gland that secretes outwardly through excretory ducts* |
| **hyper-** | excessive, above normal | hyper/glyc/emia (hī-pĕr-glī-SĒ-mē-ă): increased blood glucose, as occurs in diabetes<br><br>*glyc:* sugar, sweetness<br>*-emia:* blood condition |
| **hypo-** | under, below | hypo/insulin/ism (hī-pō-ĬN-sŭ-lĭn-izm): deficiency of insulin secretion by cells of the pancreas<br><br>*-ism:* condition |
| **poly-** | many, much | poly/uria (pŏl-ē-Ū-rē-ă): excessive secretion and discharge of urine<br><br>*-uria:* urine<br><br>*Some causes of polyuria are diabetes, use of diuretics, excessive fluid intake, and hypercalcemia.* |

*The combining vowel *i* is used instead of *o*. This is an exception to the rule.

 **It is time to review medical word elements by completing Learning Activity 13–2.**

# Pathology

Disorders of the endocrine system are caused by underproduction (**hyposecretion**) or overproduction (**hypersecretion**) of hormones. In general, hyposecretion is treated with drug therapy in the form of hormone replacement. Hypersecretion is generally treated by surgery. Most hormone deficiencies result from genetic defects in the glands, surgical removal of the glands, or production of poor-quality hormones.

## Pituitary Disorders

Hypersecretion or hyposecretion of growth hormone leads to body-size abnormalities. Abnormal variations of ADH secretion lead to disorders in the composition of blood and marked electrolyte imbalance. (See Table 13–1.)

## Thyroid Disorders

Thyroid gland disorders are common and may develop at any time during life. They may be the result of a developmental problem, injury, disease, or dietary deficiency. One form of hypothyroidism that develops in infants is called *cretinism*. If not treated, this disorder leads to mental retardation, impaired growth, low body temperatures, and abnormal bone formation. Usually these symptoms do not appear at birth because the infant has received thyroid hormones from the mother's blood during fetal development. When hypothyroidism develops during adulthood, it is known as **myxedema.** The characteristics of this disease are edema, low blood levels of $T_3$ and $T_4$, mental retardation, weight gain, and sluggishness.

Hyperthyroidism results from excessive secretions of $T_3$, $T_4$, or both. Two of the most common disorders of hyperthyroidism are **Graves disease** and **toxic goiter.** Graves disease is considerably more prevalent and is characterized by an elevated metabolic rate, abnormal weight loss, excessive perspiration, muscular weakness, and emotional instability. Also, the eyes are likely to protrude **(exophthalmos)** because of edematous swelling in the tissues behind them. (See Figure 13–3.) At the same time, the thyroid gland is likely to enlarge, producing *goiter.* (See Figure 13–5.)

**Figure 13–5**   Enlargement of the thyroid gland in goiter.

It is believed that toxic goiter may occur because of excessive release of thyroid-stimulating hormone (TSH) from the anterior lobe of the pituitary gland. Overstimulation by TSH causes thyroid cells to enlarge and secrete extra amounts of hormones. Treatment for this condition may involve drug therapy to block the production of thyroid hormones or surgical removal of all or part of the thyroid gland. Another method for treating this disorder is to administer a sufficient amount of radioactive iodine to destroy the thyroid secretory cells. (See Table 13–2.)

## Parathyroid Disorders

As with the thyroid gland, dysfunction of the parathyroids is usually characterized by inadequate hormone secretion **(hypoparathyroidism),** or excessive hormone secretion **(hyperparathyroidism).**

Insufficient production of parathyroid hormone (PTH), called *hypoparathyroidism,* can be caused by primary parathyroid dysfunction or by elevated blood calcium levels. This condition can result from an injury or from surgical removal of the glands, sometimes in conjunction with thyroid surgery. The primary effect of hypoparathyroidism is a decreased blood calcium level (**hypocalcemia**). Decreased calcium lowers the electrical threshold, causing neurons to depolarize more easily, and increases the number of nerve impulses, resulting in muscle twitches and spasms (**tetany**).

Excessive production of PTH, called *hyperparathyroidism,* is commonly caused by a benign tumor. The increase in PTH secretion leads to demineralization of bones (**osteitis fibrosa cystica**), making them porous (**osteoporosis**) and highly susceptible to fracture and deformity. When this condition is the result of a benign glandular tumor (**adenoma**) of the parathyroid, the tumor is removed. Treatment may also include orthopedic surgery to correct severe bone deformities. Excess PTH also causes calcium to be deposited in the kidneys. When the disease is generalized and all bones are affected, this disorder is known as *von Recklinghausen disease.* Renal symptoms and kidney stones (**nephrolithiasis**) may also develop. (See Table 13–3.)

## Disorders of the Adrenal Glands

As outlined before, the adrenal glands consist of the adrenal cortex and adrenal medulla. Each has its own structure and function as well as its own set of associated disorders.

### Adrenal Cortex

The adrenal cortex is mainly associated with Addison disease and Cushing syndrome.

**Addison disease.** Addison disease, a relatively uncommon chronic disorder caused by a deficiency of cortical hormones, results when the adrenal cortex is damaged or atrophied. Atrophy of the adrenal glands is probably the result of an autoimmune process in which circulating adrenal antibodies slowly destroy the gland. The gland usually suffers 90% destruction before clinical signs of adrenal insufficiency appear. Hypofunction of the adrenal cortex interferes with the body's ability to handle internal and external stress. In severe cases, the disturbance of sodium and potassium metabolism may be marked by depletion of sodium and water through urination, resulting in severe chronic dehydration. Other clinical manifestations include muscular weakness, anorexia, gastrointestinal symptoms, fatigue, hypoglycemia, hypotension, low blood sodium (**hyponatremia**), and high serum potassium (**hyperkalemia**). If treatment for this condition begins early, usually with adrenocortical hormone therapy, the prognosis is excellent. If untreated, the disease will continue a chronic course with progressive but relatively slow deterioration. In some patients, the deterioration may be rapid.

**Cushing syndrome.** Cushing syndrome is a cluster of symptoms caused by excessive amounts of cortisol, adrenocorticotropin hormone (ACTH), or both circulating in the blood. (See Figure 13–4.) Causes of this excess secretion include:

- long-term administration of steroid drugs (glucocorticoids) in treating such diseases as rheumatoid arthritis, lupus erythematosus, and asthma
- adrenal tumor resulting in excessive production of cortisol
- Cushing disease, a pituitary disorder that results in increased secretion of ACTH.

Regardless of the cause, Cushing syndrome alters carbohydrate and protein metabolism and electrolyte balance. The overproduction of mineralocorticoids and glucocorticoids causes blood glucose concentration to remain high, depleting tissue protein. In addition, sodium retention causes increased fluid in tissue that leads to edema. These metabolic changes produce weight gain and may cause structural changes, such as a moon-shaped face, grossly exaggerated head and trunk, and pencil-thin arms and legs. Other symptoms include fatigue, high blood pressure, and excessive hair growth in unusual places (**hirsutism**), especially in women. The treatment goal for this disease is to restore serum cortisol to normal levels. Nevertheless, treatment varies with the cause and may necessitate radiation, drug therapy, surgery, or a combination of these methods.

## Adrenal Medulla

No specific diseases can be traced directly to a deficiency of hormones from the adrenal medulla. However, medullary tumors sometimes cause excess secretions. The most common disorder is a neoplasm known as *pheochromocytoma,* which produces excessive amounts of epinephrine and norepinephrine. Most of these tumors are encapsulated and benign. These hypersecretions produce stress, fear, palpitations, headaches, visual blurring, muscle spasms, and sweating. Typical treatment consists of antihypertensive drugs and surgery.

## Pancreatic Disorders

Diabetes is a general term that when used alone refers to diabetes mellitus (DM). It is by far the most common pancreatic disorder. DM is a disease in which the body does not produce sufficient insulin or does not utilize it properly. Insulin is an essential hormone for conversion of sugar, starches, and other food into energy required for daily life.

Although genetics and environmental factors, such as obesity and lack of exercise, seem significant in the development of this disease, the cause of diabetes is not always clear. It is characterized by an upset in carbohydrate metabolism and disturbance in protein and fat metabolism with a subsequent rise in the concentration of blood glucose **(hyperglycemia).** Glucose is excreted in the urine **(glycosuria)** along with electrolytes, particularly sodium. Sodium and potassium losses result in muscle weakness and fatigue. Because glucose cannot enter the cells, cellular starvation results and leads to hunger and an increased appetite **(polyphagia).** (See Table 13–5.) Diabetes mellitus occurs in two primary forms:

- *Type 1 diabetes,* also known as *insulin-dependent diabetes mellitus (IDDM),* is usually diagnosed in children and young adults and was previously called *juvenile diabetes.* In type 1 diabetes, the body does not produce insulin. Treatment includes injection of insulin to maintain a normal level of glucose in the blood. (See Table 13–6.)
- *Type 2 diabetes,* also known as *non-insulin-dependent diabetes mellitus (NIDDM),* is the most common form and is distinctively different from type 1. Its onset is usually later in life (maturity onset), and risk factors include a family history of diabetes and obesity. In type 2 diabetes, the body is deficient in producing enough insulin or the body's cells are resistant to insulin action in target tissues. The hyperglycemia that results may cause cell starvation and, over time, may damage the kidneys, eyes, nerves, or heart. Treatment for type 2 diabetes includes exercise, diet, weight loss and, if needed, insulin or oral antidiabetic agents. Oral antidiabetic agents activate the release of pancreatic insulin and improve the body's sensitivity to insulin. (See Table 13–6.)

## Complications

Diabetes is associated with a number of primary and secondary complications. Patients with type 1 diabetes usually report rapidly developing symptoms. With type 2 diabetes, the patient's symptoms are usually vague, long-standing, and develop gradually.

Primary complications of type 1 include diabetic ketoacidosis (DKA). DKA, also referred to as *diabetic acidosis* or *diabetic coma,* may develop over several days or weeks. It can be caused by too little insulin, failure to follow a prescribed diet, physical or emotional stress, or undiagnosed diabetes.

Secondary complications due to long-standing diabetes emerge years after the initial

## Table 13-6    CLINICAL MANIFESTATIONS OF DIABETES

According to the American Diabetes Association, the following signs and symptoms are manifestations of type 1 and type 2 diabetes.

### Type 1 Diabetes

Type 1 diabetes may be suspected if any one of the associated signs and symptoms appears. Children usually exhibit dramatic, sudden symptoms and must receive prompt treatment. Signs and symptoms that signal type 1 diabetes can be remembered using the acronym *CAUTION*. Type 1 diabetes is characterized by the sudden appearance of:
- **C**onstant urination (polyuria) and glycosuria
- **A**bnormal thirst (polydipsia)
- **U**nusual hunger (polyphagia)
- **T**he rapid loss of weight
- **I**rritability
- **O**bvious weakness and fatigue
- **N**ausea and vomiting.

### Type 2 Diabetes

Many adults may have type 2 diabetes with none of the associated signs or symptoms. The disease is commonly discovered during a routine physical examination. In addition to any of the signs and symptoms associated with type 1 diabetes, those for type 2 diabetes can be remembered using the acronym *DIABETES*:
- **D**rowsiness
- **I**tching
- **A** family history of diabetes
- **B**lurred vision
- **E**xcessive weight
- **T**ingling, numbness, and pain in the extremities
- **E**asily fatigued
- **S**kin infections and slow healing of cuts and scratches, especially of the feet.

diagnosis. Common chronic complications include diabetic retinopathy and diabetic nephropathy. In diabetic retinopathy, the retina's blood vessels are destroyed, causing visual loss and, eventually, blindness. In diabetic nephropathy, destruction of the kidneys causes renal insufficiency and commonly requires hemodialysis or renal transplantation. Another secondary complication known as *gestational diabetes* may occur in pregnant women because of the body's hormonal changes during pregnancy. Gestational diabetes usually subsides after the child is born **(parturition).** However, mothers with type 1 or type 2 diabetes mellitus have a two to three times greater risk of giving birth to infants who suffer fetal distress and congenital malformations.

## Oncology

### Pancreatic Cancer

Most carcinomas of the pancreas arise as epithelial tumors **(adenocarcinomas)** and make their presence known by obstruction and local invasion. Because the pancreas is richly supplied with nerves, pain is a prominent feature of pancreatic cancer, whether it arises in the head, body, or tail of the organ.

The prognosis in pancreatic cancer is poor, with only a 2% survival rate in 5 years. Pancreatic cancer is the fourth leading cause of cancer death in the United States. The highest incidence is among people ages 60 to 70. The etiology is unknown, but cigarette smoking, exposure to occupational chemicals, a diet high in fats, and heavy coffee intake are associated with an increased incidence of pancreatic cancer.

## Pituitary Tumors

Pituitary tumors are generally not malignant, however because their growth is invasive, they are considered neoplastic and are usually treated as such. Initial signs and symptoms include headache, blurred vision, and, commonly, personality changes, dementia, and seizures. Tomography, skull radiographs, pneumoencephalography, angiography, and computed tomography scans assist in diagnosis. Depending on the size of the tumor and its location, different treatment modalities are employed. Treatments include surgical removal, radiation, or both.

## Thyroid Carcinoma

Cancer of the thyroid gland, or *thyroid carcinoma,* is classified according to the specific tissue that is affected. In general, however, all types share many predisposing factors, including radiation, prolonged TSH stimulation, familial disposition, and chronic goiter. The malignancy usually begins with a painless, commonly hard nodule or a nodule in the adjacent lymph nodes accompanied with an enlarged thyroid. When the tumor is large, it typically destroys thyroid tissue, which results in symptoms of hypothyroidism. Sometimes the tumor stimulates the production of thyroid hormone, resulting in symptoms of hyperthyroidism. Treatment includes surgical removal, radiation, or both.

# Diagnostic, Symptomatic, and Related Terms

This section introduces diagnostic, symptomatic, and related terms and their meanings. Word analyses for selected terms are also provided.

| Term | Definition |
|------|------------|
| **acromegaly**<br>ăk-rō-MĔG-ă-lē<br><br>*acr/o:* extremity<br>*-megaly:* enlargement | Chronic metabolic disorder characterized by a gradual, marked enlargement and thickening of the bones of the face and jaw<br><br>*Acromegaly afflicts middle-aged and older persons and is caused by over-production of growth hormone (GH). Treatment includes radiation, pharmacological agents, or surgery, which commonly involves partial resection of the pituitary gland.* |
| **diuresis**<br>dī-ū-RĒ-sĭs<br><br>*di-:* double<br>*ur:* urine<br>*-esis:* condition | Abnormal secretion of large amounts of urine<br><br>*Diuresis occurs in such conditions as diabetes mellitus, diabetes insipidus, and acute renal failure.* |
| **glucagon**<br>GLOO-kă-gŏn | Hormone secreted by the pancreatic alpha cells<br><br>*Glucagon increases the blood glucose level by stimulating the liver to change stored glycogen to glucose. Glucagon opposes the action of insulin and is used as an injection in diabetes to reverse hypoglycemic reactions and insulin shock.* |

| Term | Definition |
|---|---|
| **glucose**<br>GLOO-kōs | Simple sugar that is the end product of carbohydrate digestion<br>*Glucose is found in many foods, especially fruits, and is a major source of energy. The determination of blood glucose levels is an important diagnostic test in diabetes and other disorders.* |
| **glycosuria**<br>glī-kō-SŪ-rē-ă<br><br>   *glycos:* sugar, sweetness<br>   *-uria:* urine | Presence of glucose in the urine, abnormal amount of sugar in the urine |
| **Graves disease** | Multisystem autoimmune disorder characterized by pronounced hyperthyroidism usually associated with enlarged thyroid gland and exophthalmos (abnormal protrusion of the eyeball) (See Figure 13–3.) |
| **hirsutism**<br>HŬR-sūt-ĭzm | Excessive distribution of body hair, especially in women<br>*Hirsutism in women is usually caused by abnormalities of androgen production or metabolism.* |
| **hypercalcemia**<br>hī-pĕr-kăl-SĒ-mē-ă<br><br>   *hyper-:* excessive, above normal<br>   *calc:* calcium<br>   *-emia:* blood | Excessive amount of calcium in the blood |
| **hyperkalemia**<br>hī-pĕr-kă-LĒ-mē-ă<br><br>   *hyper-:* excessive, above normal<br>   *kal:* potassium (an electrolyte)<br>   *-emia:* blood | Excessive amount of potassium in the blood<br>*Hyperkalemia is most commonly a result of defective renal excretion of potassium.* |
| **hypervolemia**<br>hī-pĕr-vŏl-Ē-mē-ă<br><br>   *hyper-:* excessive, above normal<br>   *vol:* volume<br>   *-emia:* blood | Abnormal increase in the volume of circulating fluid (plasma) in the body<br>*Hypervolemia commonly results from retention of large amounts of sodium and water by the kidneys. Signs and symptoms of hypervolemia include weight gain, edema, dyspnea, tachycardia, and pulmonary congestion.* |
| **hyponatremia**<br>hī-pō-nă-TRĒ-mē-ă<br><br>   *hypo-:* under, below, deficient<br>   *natr:* sodium (an electrolyte)<br>   *-emia:* blood | Abnormal condition of low sodium in the blood |
| **insulinoma**<br>ĭn-sū-lĭn-Ō-mă<br><br>   *insulin:* insulin<br>   *-oma:* tumor | Tumor of the islets of Langerhans of the pancreas |

*(Continued)*

| Term | Definition | *(Continued)* |
|------|------------|---------------|
| **obesity**<br>ō-BĒ-sĭ-tē | Abnormal increase in the proportion of fat cells, mainly in the viscera and subcutaneous tissues of the body<br><br>*Obesity may be due to an excessive intake of food (exogenous) or metabolic or endocrine abnormalities (endogenous).* | |
| **panhypopituitarism**<br>păn-hī-pō-pĭ-TŪ-ĭ-tăr-ĭzm<br><br>*pan-:* all<br>*hypo:* under, below, deficient<br>*pituitar:* pituitary gland<br>*-ism:* condition | Total pituitary impairment that brings about a progressive and general loss of hormonal activity | |
| **pheochromocytoma**<br>fē-ō-krō-mō-sĭ-TŌ-mă | Small chromaffin cell tumor, usually located in the adrenal medulla | |
| **thyroid storm**<br>THĪ-royd<br><br>*thyr:* thyroid gland<br>*-oid:* resembling | Crisis of uncontrolled hyperthyroidism caused by the release into the bloodstream of increased amount of thyroid hormone; also called *thyroid crisis* or *thyrotoxic crisis*<br><br>*Thyroid storm may occur spontaneously or be precipitated by infection, stress, or thyroidectomy performed on a patient who is inadequately prepared with antithyroid drugs. If left untreated, it may be fatal.* | |
| **virile**<br>VĬR-ĭl | Masculine or having characteristics of a man, especially copulative powers | |
| **virilism**<br>VĬR-ĭl-ĭzm | Masculinization in a woman or development of male secondary sex characteristics in the woman | |

 **It is time to review pathological, diagnostic, symptomatic, and related terms by completing Learning Activity 13–3.**

## Diagnostic and Therapeutic Procedures

This section introduces procedures used to diagnose and treat endocrine disorders. Descriptions are provided as well as pronunciations and word analyses for selected terms.

| Procedure | Description |
|---|---|
| **DIAGNOSTIC PROCEDURES** | |
| *Clinical* | |
| **exophthalmometry**<br>ĕk-sŏf-thăl-MŎM-ĕ-trē<br>   *ex-*: out, out from<br>   *ophthalm/o*: eye<br>   *-metry*: act of measuring | Test that measures the degree of forward displacement of the eyeball (exophthalmos) as seen in Graves disease (See Figure 13–3.)<br>*The test is administered with an instrument called an exophthalmometer, which allows measurement of the distance from the center of the cornea to the lateral orbital rim.* |
| *Laboratory* | |
| **fasting blood glucose (FBG)** | Test that measures blood glucose level after a 12-hour fast |
| **glucose tolerance test (GTT)**<br>GLOO-kōs | Test that measures the body's ability to metabolize carbohydrates by administering a standard dose of glucose and measuring glucose level in blood and urine at regular intervals<br>*GTT is commonly used to help diagnose diabetes or other disorders that affect carbohydrate metabolism.* |
| **insulin tolerance test** | Test that determines insulin levels in serum (blood) by administering insulin and measuring blood glucose level in blood at regular intervals<br>*In hypoglycemia, glucose levels may be lower and return to normal more slowly.* |
| **protein-bound iodine (PBI)** | Test that measures the concentration of thyroxine in a blood sample<br>*Result of the PBI test provides an index of thyroid activity.* |
| **thyroid function test (TFT)** | Test that determines increase or decrease in thyroid function<br>*The thyroid function test measures levels of thyroid-stimulating hormone (TSH), triiodothyronine ($T_3$), and thyroxine ($T_4$).* |
| **total calcium** | Test that measures calcium to detect bone and parathyroid disorders<br>*Hypercalcemia can indicate primary hyperparathyroidism; hypocalcemia can indicate hypoparathyroidism.* |

| Procedure | Description | (Continued) |
|---|---|---|

### Radiographic

| | |
|---|---|
| **computed tomography (CT) scan**<br>kŏm-PŪ-tĕd tō-MŎG-ră-fē<br><br>*tom/o:* to cut<br>*-graphy:* process of recording | Imaging technique achieved by rotating an x-ray emitter around the area to be scanned and measuring the intensity of transmitted rays from different angles<br><br>*In a CT scan, the computer generates a detailed cross-sectional image that appears as a slice. (See Figure 4–4D.) CT scan is used to detect disease and tumors in soft body tissues, such as the pancreas, thyroid, and adrenal glands, and may be used with or without a contrast medium.* |
| **magnetic resonance imaging (MRI)**<br>măg-NĔT-ĭc RĔZ-ĕn-ăns<br>ĬM-ĭj-ĭng | Noninvasive imaging technique that uses radio waves and a strong magnetic field rather than an x-ray beam to produce multiplanar cross-sectional images<br><br>*MRI is the method of choice for diagnosing a growing number of diseases because it provides superior soft-tissue contrast, allows multiple plane views, and avoids the hazards of ionizing radiation. MRI is used to identify abnormalities of pituitary, pancreatic, adrenal, and thyroid glands.* |
| **radioactive iodine uptake (RAIU)** | Administration of radioactive iodine (RAI) orally as a tracer to test how quickly the thyroid gland takes up (uptake) iodine from the blood<br><br>*Results of RAIU test are used to determine thyroid function.* |
| **thyroid scan**<br><br>*thyr:* thyroid gland<br>*-oid:* resembling | Test that involves administration of a radioactive substance that is localized in the thyroid gland and use of a scanner to visualize the gland<br><br>*Thyroid scanning is used to detect pathological formations such as tumors. It is useful in evaluating neck or substernal masses, thyroid nodules, hyperthyroidism, and metastatic tumors.* |

## THERAPEUTIC PROCEDURES

### Surgical

| | |
|---|---|
| **microneurosurgery of pituitary gland**<br>mī-krō-nū-rō-SĔR-jĕr-ē,<br>pĭ-TŪ-ĭ-tār-ē | Microdissection of a tumor using a binocular surgical microscope for magnification |
| **parathyroidectomy**<br>păr-ă-thī-royd-ĔK-tō-mē<br><br>*para-:* near, beside; beyond<br>*thyroid:* thyroid gland<br>*-ectomy:* excision, removal | Excision of one or more of the parathyroid glands, usually to control hyperparathyroidism |
| **pinealectomy**<br>pĭn-ē-ăl-ĔK-tō-mē | Removal of the pineal body |
| **thymectomy**<br>thī-MĔK-tō-mē<br><br>*thym:* thymus gland<br>*-ectomy:* excision, removal | Excision of the thymus gland |

| Procedure | Description |
|---|---|
| **thyroidectomy**<br>thi-royd-ĔK-tō-mē<br><br>  *thyroid:* thyroid gland<br>  *-ectomy:* excision, removal | Excision of the thyroid gland<br><br>*Thyroidectomy is performed for goiter, tumors, or hyperthyroidism that does not respond to iodine therapy and antithyroid drugs.* |
| **partial** | Method of choice for removing a fibrous, nodular thyroid |
| **subtotal** | Removal of most of the thyroid to relieve hyperthyroidism |

## Pharmacology

Common disorders associated with endocrine glands include hyposecretion and hypersecretion of hormones. When deficiencies of this type occur, natural and synthetic hormones, such as insulin and thyroid agents, are prescribed. These agents normalize hormone levels to maintain proper functioning and homeostasis. Therapeutic agents are also available to regulate various substances in the body, such as glucose levels in diabetic patients. Hormone replacement therapy (HRT), such as synthetic thyroid and estrogen, treat these hormonal deficiencies. Although specific drugs are not covered in this section, hormonal chemotherapy drugs are used to treat certain cancers, such as testicular, ovarian, breast, and endometrial cancer. (See Table 13–7.)

## Table 13–7   DRUGS USED TO TREAT ENDOCRINE DISORDERS

This table lists common drug classifications used to treat endocrine disorders, their therapeutic actions, and selected generic and trade names.

| Classification | Therapeutic Action | Generic and Trade Names |
|---|---|---|
| insulins | Treat type 1 diabetes<br><br>*Insulins are classified according to how quickly they act and the duration of their therapeutic action. They are administered by intermittent subcutaneous injection, implanted infusion pump, or directly into the blood-stream by I.V. injection or continuous I.V. infusion through a controlled infusion device. Currently, nasal sprays and oral capsules are being tested as a method of administration. Although type 2 diabetes may be treated with insulin, it is more commonly treated with oral antidiabetics.* | **regular insulin**<br>ĬN-sŭ-lĭn<br>  *Humulin R\*, Novolin R*<br>**NPH insulin**<br>ĬN-sŭ-lĭn<br>  *Humulin N, Novolin N*<br>**NPH/regular insulin mixtures**<br>ĬN-sŭ-lĭn<br>  *Humulin 50/50, Humulin 70/30, Novolin 70/30* |

*(Continued)*

## Table 13-7    DRUGS USED TO TREAT ENDOCRINE DISORDERS
*(Continued)*

| Classification | Therapeutic Action | Generic and Trade Names |
|---|---|---|
| **oral antidiabetics** | Stimulate the pancreas to produce more insulin and increase the number of insulin receptors<br><br>*Contrary to popular opinion, oral antidiabetic drugs are not insulin and are not effective in treating type I diabetes mellitus.* | **glimepiride**<br>GLĪ-mĕ-pi-rĭd<br>*Amaryl*<br>**glipizide**<br>GLĬP-ĭ-zĭd<br>*Glucotrol, Glucotrol XL*<br>**glyburide**<br>GLĪ-bū-rĭd<br>*DiaBeta, Glynase, Micronase*<br>**metformin**<br>mĕt-FOR-mĭn<br>*Glucophage* |
| **antithyroids** | Treat hyperthyroidism by impeding the formation of $T_3$ and $T_4$ hormone<br><br>*Antithyroids are administered in preparation for a thyroidectomy and in thyrotoxic crisis.* | **methimazole**<br>mĕth-ĬM-ă-zōl<br>*Tapazole*<br>**strong iodine solution**<br>Ī-ō-dĭn<br>*Lugol's solution* |
| **corticosteroids** | Replace hormones lost in adrenal insufficiency (Addison disease)<br><br>*Corticosteroids are also widely used to suppress inflammation, control allergic reactions, reduce rejection in transplantation, and treat some cancer.* | **cortisone**<br>KOR-tĭ-sōn<br>*Cortone, Acetate*<br>**hydrocortisone**<br>hi-drō-KOR-tĭ-sōn<br>*A-Hydrocort, Cortef, Hydrocortone, Solu-Cortef* |
| **growth hormone replacements** | Increase skeletal growth in children and growth hormone deficiencies in adults<br><br>*Growth hormones increase spinal bone density and help manage growth failure in children.* | **somatropin (recombinant)**<br>sō-mă-TRO-pĭn<br>*Humatrope, Norditropin, Nutropin, Serostim*<br>**somatrem (recombinant)**<br>SŌ-mă-trĕm<br>*Protropin* |
| **thyroid supplements** | Replace or supplement thyroid hormones<br><br>*Each thyroid supplement contains $T_3$, $T_4$, or a combination of both. Thyroid supplements are also used to treat some types of thyroid cancer.* | **levothyroxine**<br>lē-vō-thi-RŌK-sēn<br>*Levo-T, Levoxyl, Synthroid, $T_4$ Unithroid*<br>**liothyronine**<br>li-ō-THĪ-rō-nēn<br>*Cytomel, l-triiodothyronine, $T_3$, Triostat*<br>**thyroid**<br>THĪ-royd<br>*$T_3/T_4$, Thyrolar* |

*The trade name for all human genetically produced insulins is *Humulin*. Traditionally, insulin has been derived from beef or pork pancreas. Human insulin is genetically produced using recombinant DNA techniques to avoid the potential for allergic reaction.

## Abbreviations

This section introduces endocrine-related abbreviations and their meanings.

| Abbreviation | Meaning |
| --- | --- |
| ACTH | adrenocorticotropic hormone |
| ADH | antidiuretic hormone (vasopressin) |
| BMR | basal metabolic rate |
| DI | diabetes insipidus; diagnostic imaging |
| DKA | diabetic ketoacidosis |
| DM | diabetes mellitus |
| FSH | follicle-stimulating hormone |
| GH | growth hormone |
| IDDM | insulin-dependent diabetes mellitus |
| K | potassium (an electrolyte) |
| LH | luteinizing hormone |
| MSH | melanocyte-stimulating hormone |
| NIDDM | non-insulin-dependent diabetes mellitus |
| NPH | neutral protamine Hagedorn (insulin) |
| PRL | prolactin |
| PGH | pituitary growth hormone |
| PTH | parathyroid hormone; also called *parathormone* |
| RAI | radioactive iodine |
| RAIU | radioactive iodine uptake |
| $T_3$ | triiodothyronine (thyroid hormone) |
| $T_4$ | thyroxine (thyroid hormone) |
| TFT | thyroid function test |
| TSH | thyroid-stimulating hormone |

**It is time to review procedures, pharmacology, and abbreviations by completing Learning Activity13–4.**

# LEARNING ACTIVITIES

The activities that follow provide review of the endocrine system terms introduced in this chapter. Complete each activity and review your answers to evaluate your understanding of the chapter.

## Learning Activity 13–1

### Identifying endocrine structures

*Label the following illustration using the terms listed below.*

| adrenal (suprarenal) glands | parathyroid glands | testes |
| --- | --- | --- |
| *ovaries* | *pineal gland* | *thymus gland* |
| *pancreas* | *pituitary (hypophysis) gland* | *thyroid gland* |

 Check your answers by referring to Figure 13–1 on page 390. Review material that you did not answer correctly.

## Learning Activity 13-2

### Building medical words

*Use* **glyc/o** *(sugar) to build words that mean:*

1. blood condition of excessive glucose _____
2. blood condition of deficiency of glucose _____
3. formation of glycogen _____

*Use* **pancreat/o** *(pancreas) to build words that mean:*

4. inflammation of the pancreas _____
5. destruction of the pancreas _____
6. disease of the pancreas _____

*Use* **thyr/o** *or* **thyroid/o** *(thyroid gland) to build words that mean:*

7. inflammation of the thyroid gland _____
8. enlargement of the thyroid _____

*Build surgical words that mean:*

9. excision of a parathyroid gland _____
10. removal of the adrenal gland _____

Check your answers in Appendix A. Review material that you did not answer correctly.

**CORRECT ANSWERS** _____ × **10** = _____ **% SCORE**

## Learning Activity 13–3

# Matching pathological, diagnostic, symptomatic, and related terms

*Match the following terms with the definitions in the numbered list.*

| | | |
|---|---|---|
| *Addison disease* | *glycosuria* | *myxedema* |
| *cretinism* | *hirsutism* | *pheochromocytoma* |
| *Cushing syndrome* | *hyperkalemia* | *type 1 diabetes* |
| *diuresis* | *hyponatremia* | *type 2 diabetes* |
| *exophthalmic goiter* | *insulin* | *virile* |

1. _____ having characteristics of a man; masculine

2. _____ hypothyroidism acquired in adulthood

3. _____ increased excretion of urine

4. _____ excessive growth of hair or the presence of hair in unusual places, especially in women

5. _____ hypothyroidism that appears as a congenital condition and is commonly associated with other endocrine abnormalities

6. _____ hormone produced by beta cells of the pancreas

7. _____ caused by deficiency in the secretion of adrenocortical hormones

8. _____ characterized by protrusion of the eyeballs, increased heart action, enlargement of the thyroid gland, weight loss, and nervousness

9. _____ excessive amount of potassium in the blood

10. _____ small chromaffin cell tumor, usually located in the adrenal medulla

11. _____ insulin-dependent diabetes mellitus that occurs most commonly in children and adolescents (juvenile onset)

12. _____ decreased concentration of sodium in the blood

13. _____ abnormal presence of glucose in the urine

14. _____ metabolic disorder caused by hypersecretion of the adrenal cortex resulting in excessive production of glucocorticoids, mainly cortisol

15. _____ non-insulin-dependent diabetes mellitus that usually occurs later in life (maturity onset)

✓ Check your answers in Appendix A. Review material that you did not answer correctly.

**CORRECT ANSWERS** _____ × **6.67** = _____ **% SCORE**

# Learning Activity 13–4

## Matching procedures, pharmacology, and abbreviations

*Match the following terms with the definitions in the numbered list.*

| | | |
|---|---|---|
| antithyroids | growth hormone | protein-bound iodine |
| computed tomography (CT) scan | GTT | RAIU |
| corticosteroids | Humulin | $T_3$ |
| exophthalmometry | magnetic resonance imaging (MRI) | $T_4$ |
| FBS | oral antidiabetics | thyroid scan |

1. _____ measures circulating glucose level after a 12-hour fast

2. _____ measures thyroid function and monitors how quickly ingested iodine is taken into the thyroid gland

3. _____ replacement hormones for adrenal insufficiency (Addison disease)

4. _____ increases skeletal growth in children

5. _____ radioactive compound is administered and localizes in the thyroid gland; used to detect thyroid abnormalities

6. _____ thyroxine

7. _____ used to treat type 1 diabetes

8. _____ diagnostic test used to determine hypoglycemia, hyperglycemia, and adjustments in insulin dosage

9. _____ used to treat hyperthyroidism by impeding the formation of $T_3$ and $T_4$ hormone

10. _____ test to measure the concentration of thyroxine in a blood sample

11. _____ triiodothyronine

12. _____ noninvasive imaging technique that uses radio waves and a strong magnetic field to produce multiplanar cross-sectional images

13. _____ test that measures the degree of forward displacement of the eyeball as seen in Graves disease

14. _____ imaging technique achieved by rotating an x-ray emitter around the area to be scanned and measuring the intensity of transmitted rays from different angles; used to detect disease in soft body tissues, such as the pancreas, thyroid, and adrenal glands

15. _____ trade name for all human genetically produced insulins

✓ Check your answers in Appendix A. Review any material that you did not answer correctly.

**CORRECT ANSWERS** _____ × 6.67 = _____ **% SCORE**

# MEDICAL RECORD ACTIVITIES

The two medical records included in the activities that follow use common clinical scenarios to show how medical terminology is used to document patient care. Complete the terminology and analysis sections for each activity to help you recognize and understand terms related to the endocrine system.

## Medical Record Activity 13–1

### Hyperparathyroidism

#### Terminology

The terms listed in the chart come from the medical record *Hyperparathyroidism* that follows. Use a medical dictionary such as *Taber's Cyclopedic Medical Dictionary*, the appendices of this book, or other resources to define each term. Then review the pronunciations for each term and practice by reading the medical record aloud.

| Term | Definition |
|------|------------|
| **adenoma**<br>ăd-ĕ-NŌ-mă | |
| **claudication**<br>klaw-dĭ-KĀ-shŭn | |
| **diabetes mellitus**<br>dĭ-ă-BĒ-tēz  MĔ-lĭ-tŭs | |
| **endocrinologist**<br>ĕn-dō-krĭn-ŎL-ō-jĭst | |
| **hypercalciuria**<br>hi-pĕr-kăl-sē-Ū-rē-ă | |
| **hyperparathyroidism**<br>hi-pĕr-păr-ă-THĪ-roy-dĭzm | |
| **impression**<br>ĭm-PRĔSH-ŭn | |
| **osteoarthritis**<br>ŏs-tē-ō-ăr-THRĪ-tĭs | |
| **parathyroid**<br>păr-ă-THĪ-royd | |
| **peripheral vascular disease**<br>pĕr-ĬF-ĕr-ăl  VĂS-kū-lăr  dĭ-ZĒZ | |

## HYPERPARATHYROIDISM

**HISTORY OF PRESENT ILLNESS:** This 66-year-old former blackjack dealer is under evaluation for hyperparathyroidism. Surgery evidently has been recommended, but there is confusion as to how urgent this is. She has a 13-year history of type 1 diabetes mellitus, a history of shoulder pain, osteoarthritis of the spine, and peripheral vascular disease with claudication. She states her 548-pack-per-year smoking history ended 3.5 years ago. Her first knowledge of parathyroid disease was about 3 years ago when laboratory findings revealed an elevated calcium level. This subsequently led to the diagnosis of hyperparathyroidism. She was further evaluated by an endocrinologist in the Lake Tahoe area, who determined that she also had hypercalciuria, although there is nothing to suggest a history of kidney stones.

**IMPRESSION:** Hyperparathyroidism and hypercalciuria, probably a parathyroid adenoma

## Analysis

**Review the medical record *Hyperparathyroidism* to answer the following questions.**

1. What is an adenoma?

   _____

2. What does the physician suspect caused the patient's hyperparathyroidism?

   _____

3. What type of laboratory findings revealed parathyroid disease?

   _____

4. What is hypercalciuria?

   _____

5. If the patient smoked 548 packs of cigarettes per year, how many packs did she smoke in an average day?

   _____

## Medical Record Activity 13–2

## Diabetes mellitus

### Terminology

The terms listed in the chart come from the medical record *Diabetes Mellitus* that follows. Use a medical dictionary such as *Taber's Cyclopedic Medical Dictionary*, the appendices of this book, or other resources to define each term. Then review the pronunciations for each term and practice by reading the medical record aloud.

| Term | Definition |
|------|------------|
| **Accu-chek** ĂK-ū-chĕk | |
| **morbid obesity** MOR-bĭd ō-BĒ-sĭ-tē | |

*(Continued)*

| Term | Definition | (Continued) |
|------|------------|-------------|
| **obesity, exogenous**<br>ō-BĒ-sĭ-tē,  ĕks-ŎJ-ĕ-nŭs | | |
| **polydipsia**<br>pŏl-ē-DĬP-sē-ă | | |
| **polyphagia**<br>pŏl-ē-FĀ-jē-ă | | |
| **polyuria**<br>pŏl-ē-Ū-rē-ă | | |

## DIABETES MELLITUS

Chart Notes

This 200-pound patient was admitted to the hospital because of a 10-day history of polyuria, polydipsia, and polyphagia. She has been very nervous, irritable, and very sensitive emotionally and cries easily. During this period, she has had headaches and has become very sleepy and tired after eating. On admission, her Accu-Chek was 540.

Family history is significant in that both parents and two sisters have type 1 diabetes.

Physical examination was essentially negative. The abdomen was difficult to evaluate because of morbid obesity.

**DIAGNOSIS:** Diabetes mellitus; obesity, exogenous

## Analysis

**Review the medical record *Diabetes Mellitus* to answer the following questions.**

1.  How long has this patient been experiencing voracious eating?

   _____

2.  Was the patient's obesity due to overeating or metabolic imbalance?

   _____

3.  Why did the doctor experience difficulty in examining the patient's abdomen?

   _____

4.  Was the patient's blood glucose above or below normal on admission?

   _____

5.  What is the reference range for fasting blood glucose?

   _____

# Chapter

# 14

# Nervous System

## CHAPTER OUTLINE

## OBJECTIVES

*Upon completion of this chapter, you will be able to:*

- Locate and describe the structures of the nervous system.
- Recognize, pronounce, spell, and build words related to the nervous system.
- Describe pathological conditions, diagnostic and therapeutic procedures, and other terms related to the nervous system.
- Explain pharmacology related to the treatment of nervous disorders.
- Demonstrate your knowledge of this chapter by completing the learning and medical record activities.

## Key Terms

This section introduces important nervous system terms and their definitions. Word analyses are also provided.

| Term | Definition |
|---|---|
| **blood-brain barrier** | Mechanism that blocks specific substances found in the bloodstream from entering the brain |
| **cell body** | Division of a neuron that includes the nucleus, cell organelles, and surrounding cytoplasm, but does not include the axon or dendrites |
| **motor neuron** | Neuron that transmits impulses from the central nervous system (brain or spinal cord) to a muscle or gland; also called *efferent neuron* |
| **nervous impulse** | Physiological change transmitted through certain tissues, especially nerve fibers and muscles, resulting in activity or inhibition |
| **neurology**<br>nū-RŎL-ō-jē<br><br>*neur/o:* nerve<br>*-logy:* study of | Branch of medicine concerned with diagnosis and treatment of disorders of the nervous system |
| **neurotransmitter**<br>nū-rō-TRĂNS-<br>mĭt-ĕr | Chemical substance that transmits or inhibits nerve impulses at a synapse<br>*Chemical substances that are neurotransmitters include acetylcholine, adrenaline, and dopamine.* |
| **organelle**<br>or-găn-ĔL | Cytoplasm structure that provides specialized function for the cell |
| **psychiatry**<br>si-KĪ-ă-trē<br><br>*psych:* mind<br>*-iatry:* medicine; treatment | Branch of medicine concerned with the diagnosis and treatment of mental disorders |
| **sensory neuron**<br>SĔN-sō-rē | Neuron that transmits impulses from receptors in the skin, sense organs, and internal organs to the central nervous system (brain or spinal cord); also called *afferent neuron* |
| **synapse**<br>SĬN-ăps | Junction where a nerve impulse passes from an axon terminal to a neuron, muscle cell, or gland cell |

## Anatomy and Physiology

The nervous system is one of the most complicated systems of the body in both structure and function. It senses physical and chemical changes in the internal and external environments, processes them, and then responds to maintain homeostasis. Voluntary activities, such as walking and talking, and involuntary activities, such as digestion and circulation, are coordinated, regulated, and integrated by the nervous system. The entire neural network of the body relies on the transmission of electrochemical impulses. Impulses travel from cell to cell as they convey information from one area of the body to another. The speed at which this occurs is almost instantaneous, thus providing an immediate response to change.

## Cellular Structure of the Nervous System

Despite its complexity, the nervous system is composed of only two principal types of cells: **neurons** and **neuroglia.** Neurons are cells that transmit impulses. They are commonly identified by the direction the impulse travels. **Sensory neurons,** also called *afferent nerves,* transmit stimuli to the brain and spinal cord; **motor neurons,** also called *efferent nerves,* transmit impulses from the brain or spinal cord to muscles and glands. Most nerves are composed of both afferent and efferent fibers and, thus, are called *mixed nerves.* Neuroglia are cells that support neurons and bind them to other tissues. They also play an important role when the nervous system suffers an injury or infection.

### Neurons

The three major structures of the neuron are the *cell body,* the *axon,* and the *dendrites.* (See Figure 14–1.) The (1) **cell body** is the enlarged structure of the neuron that contains the (2) **nucleus** of the cell and various **organelles.** Its branching cytoplasmic projections are (3) **dendrites** that carry impulses to the cell body and (4) **axons** that carry impulses from the cell body. Dendrites resemble tiny branches on a tree, providing additional surface area for receiving impulses from other neurons. Axons are long, single projections ranging from a few millimeters to more than a meter in length. Axons transmit impulses to muscles, glands, and other dendrites.

Many axons in both the peripheral nervous system and the autonomic nervous system possess a white, lipoid covering called a (5) **myelin sheath.** This covering acts as an electrical insulator that reduces the possibility of an impulse stimulating adjacent nerves. It also accelerates impulse transmission through the axon. The myelin that covers axons in the brain and spinal cord gives these structures a white appearance and constitutes the white matter of the central nervous system. Unmyelinated fibers, dendrites, and nerve cell bodies make up the gray matter of the brain and spinal cord.

On peripheral nerves, the myelin sheath is formed by a neuroglial cell called a (6) **Schwann cell** that wraps tightly around the axon. It forms a thin cellular membrane called (7) **neurilemma,** or *neurolemma.* The space between adjacent Schwann cells is called the (8) **node of Ranvier.** This space helps maintain the electrical potentials needed for impulse conduction.

Neurons are not continuous with one another. Instead, a small space, known as a (9) **synapse,** is found between the (10) **axon terminal** of one neuron and the dendrite of another. For an impulse to travel from neuron to neuron, it must cross the synapse. The impulse within the neuron causes a chemical substance called a (11) **neurotransmitter** to be released at the end of the axon. The neurotransmitter diffuses across the synapse to receptor sites on the dendrite of the next neuron. Here it generates the next electrical stimulus. The receiving neuron immediately inactivates the neurotransmitter, thereby preventing an unwanted continued stimulation, and prepares the site for another stimulus by a neurotransmitter. Thus, impulses travel through neural pathways.

### Neuroglia

The term **neuroglia** literally means "nerve glue." Scientists once believed that neuroglia served only a supporting role for neurons; however, we now know that neuroglia cells perform many functions. There are four types of neuroglia and each serves a distinct function:

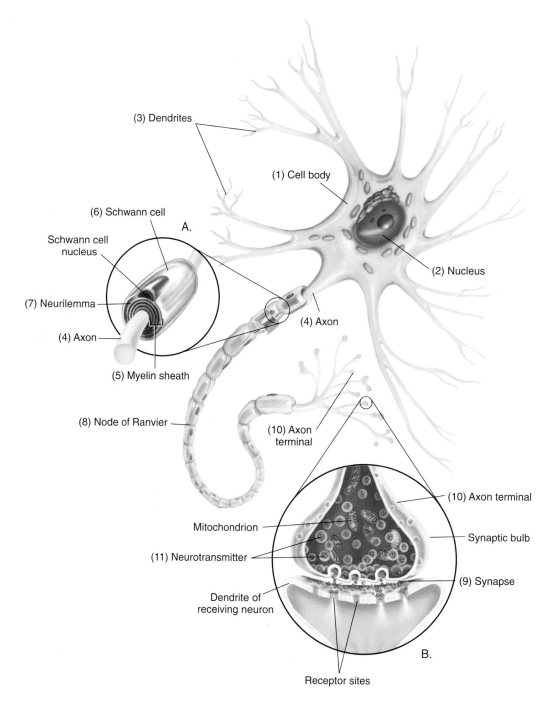

(3) Dendrites

(1) Cell body

(6) Schwann cell

A.

Schwann cell
nucleus

(2) Nucleus

(7) Neurilemma

(4) Axon

(4) Axon

(5) Myelin sheath

(8) Node of Ranvier

(10) Axon
terminal

(10) Axon terminal

Synaptic bulb

Mitochondrion

(11) Neurotransmitter

(9) Synapse

Dendrite of
receiving neuron

B.

Receptor sites

**Figure 14–1**   Neuron. (A) Schwann cell. (B) Axon terminal synapse.

- *Astrocytes,* as their name suggests, are star-shaped neuroglia. They provide three-dimensional mechanical support for neurons and form tight sheaths around the capillaries of the brain. These sheaths provide an obstruction, called the *blood-brain barrier,* that keeps large molecular substances from entering the delicate tissue of the brain. Even so, small molecules, such as water, carbon dioxide, oxygen, and alcohol, readily pass from blood vessels through the barrier and enter the interstitial spaces of the brain. Researchers must take the blood-brain barrier into consideration when developing drugs for treatment of brain disorders.

- *Oligodendrocytes,* also called *oligodendroglia,* help in the development of myelin on neurons of the central nervous system.
- *Microglia,* the smallest of the neuroglia, possess phagocytic properties and may become very active during times of infection.
- *Ependyma* are ciliated cells that line fluid-filled cavities of the central nervous system, especially the ventricles of the brain. They assist in cerebrospinal fluid (CSF) circulation.

## Nervous System Divisions

The nervous system consists of two main divisions, the central nervous system (CNS) and the peripheral nervous system (PNS). The CNS consists of the brain and spinal cord. The PNS consists of 12 pairs of cranial nerves, which emerge from the base of the skull, and 31 pairs of spinal nerves, which emerge from the spinal cord. (See Table 14–1.)

### Central Nervous System

The CNS consists of the brain and spinal cord, which are enclosed within three protective membranes called the *meninges.*

**Brain.** In addition to being one of the largest organs of the body, the brain is highly complex in structure and function. (See Figure 14–2.) It integrates almost every physical and mental activity of the body and is the center for memory, emotion, thought, judgment, reasoning, and consciousness. The brain is composed of four major structures:

## Table 14–1    NERVOUS SYSTEM DIVISIONS AND FUNCTIONS

This table lists the divisions of the nervous system along with their functions.

| Division | Function |
| --- | --- |
| **Central** | |
| Brain | Center for thought and emotion, interpretation of sensory stimuli, and coordination of body functions |
| Spinal cord | Main pathway for transmission of information between the brain and body |
| **Peripheral** | |
| Cranial nerves | Includes 12 pairs of nerves that emerge from the base of the skull and may act in a motor or sensory capacity |
| Spinal nerves | Includes 31 pairs of nerves that emerge from the spine and act in motor and sensory capacities |
| Somatic | Transmits sensory impulses to the central nervous system and motor impulses to voluntary (skeletal) muscles |
| Autonomic<br>• Sympathetic<br><br>• Parasympathetic | Regulates involuntary (visceral) muscles and glands<br>• Division of the autonomic nervous system that prepares the body for "fight or flight"<br>• Division of the autonomic nervous system that moderates or reverses the action of the sympathetic nervous system |

**Figure 14–2**  Brain structures.

- cerebrum
- cerebellum
- diencephalon
- brainstem

*Cerebrum.*  The (1) **cerebrum** is the largest and uppermost portion of the brain. It consists of two hemispheres divided by a deep longitudinal fissure, or groove. The fissure does not completely separate the hemispheres. A structure called the (2) **corpus callosum** joins these hemispheres, permitting communication between the right and left sides of the brain. Each hemisphere is divided into five lobes. Four of these lobes are named for the bones that lie directly above them: (3) **frontal,** (4) **parietal,** (5) **temporal,** and (6) **occipital.** The fifth lobe, the **insula** (not shown in the figure), is hidden from view and can be seen only upon dissection.

The cerebral surface consists of numerous folds, or convolutions, called *gyri.* The gyri are separated by furrows or fissures called *sulci.* A thin gray layer called the *cerebral cortex* covers the entire cerebrum and is composed of millions of cell bodies, which give it its gray color.

The remainder of the cerebrum is primarily composed of white matter (myelinated axons). Major functions of the cerebrum include sensory perception and interpretation, language, voluntary movement, and the emotional aspects of behavior and memory.

*Cerebellum.* The second largest part of the brain, the (7) **cerebellum,** occupies the posterior portion of the brain. All functions of the cerebellum involve movement. When the cerebrum initiates muscular movement, the cerebellum coordinates and refines it. The cerebellum also aids in maintaining equilibrium and balance.

*Diencephalon.* The (8) **diencephalon (interbrain)** is composed of many smaller structures, two of which are the (9) **thalamus** and the (10) **hypothalamus.** The thalamus receives all sensory stimuli except olfactory stimuli and processes and transmits them to the cerebral cortex. In addition, the thalamus receives impulses from the cerebrum and relays them to efferent nerves. The hypothalamus integrates autonomic nerve impulses, regulates body temperature, and controls endocrine functions.

*Brainstem.* The brainstem completes the last major section of the brain. It is composed of three structures: the (11) **midbrain (mesencephalon),** separating the cerebrum from the brainstem; the (12) **medulla,** which attaches to the spinal cord; and (13) the **pons,** or "bridge," connecting the midbrain to the medulla. In general, the brainstem is a pathway for impulse conduction between the brain and spinal cord. The brainstem is the origin of 10 of the 12 pairs of cranial nerves and controls respiration, blood pressure, and heart rate. Because the brainstem is the site that controls the beginning of life (the initiation of the beating heart in a fetus) and the end of life (the cessation of respiration and heart activity) it is sometimes called the *primary brain.*

**Spinal cord.** The spinal cord transmits sensory impulses from the body to the brain and motor impulses from the brain to muscles and organs of the body. The sensory nerve tracts are called *ascending tracts* because the direction of the impulse is upward. Conversely, motor nerve tracts are called *descending tracts* because they carry impulses in a downward direction to muscles and organs. A cross-section of the spinal cord reveals an inner gray area composed of cell bodies and dendrites and a white outer area composed of myelinated tissue of the ascending and descending tracts.

The entire spinal cord is located within the spinal cavity of the vertebral column, with spinal nerves exiting between the intervertebral spaces throughout almost the entire length of the spinal column. Unlike the cranial nerves, which have specific names, the spinal nerves are identified by the region of the vertebral column from which they exit.

**Meninges.** The brain and the spinal cord receive limited protection from three coverings called *meninges* (singular, *meninx*). These coverings include:

- The *dura mater,* the outermost covering, is tough, fibrous, and composed primarily of connective tissue. Beneath the dura mater is a cavity called the **subdural space** filled with serous fluid.
- The *arachnoid,* the middle covering, has (as its name suggests) a spider-web appearance. A **subarachnoid space** contains cerebrospinal fluid (CSF) that provides additional protection for the brain and spinal cord by acting as a shock absorber.

- The *pia mater,* the innermost covering of the meninges, contains numerous blood vessels and lymphatics that nourish the underlying tissues.

Cerebrospinal fluid (CSF) is a colorless fluid that contains proteins, glucose, urea, salts, and some white blood cells. It circulates around the spinal cord and brain and through spaces called *ventricles* located within the inner portion of the brain, and provides nutritive substances to the CNS. Normally, CSF is absorbed as rapidly as it is formed, maintaining a constant fluid volume. Any interference with absorption results in a collection of fluid in the brain, a condition called **hydrocephalus.**

## Peripheral Nervous System

The peripheral nervous system is composed of all nervous tissue located outside of the spinal column and skull. It includes 12 pairs of cranial nerves that carry impulses to and from the brain and 31 pairs of spinal nerves that carry impulses to and from the spinal cord.

Functionally, the PNS is subdivided into two specialized systems: the somatic nervous system (SNS) and the autonomic nervous system (ANS).

**Cranial nerves.** The cranial nerves are designated by name or number. (See Figure 14–3.) Cranial nerves consist of fibers that may serve a sensory or motor function, or a mixture of both. Sensory nerves receive impulses from the sense organs, including the eyes, ears, nose, tongue, and skin, and transmit them to the CNS. Because sensory nerves conduct impulses toward the CNS, they are also known as afferent nerves. Motor nerves, in contrast, conduct impulses away from the CNS, so they are called efferent nerves. They conduct impulses to muscles, causing them to contract, or to glands, causing them to secrete. Nerves composed of both sensory and motor fibers are called mixed nerves. An example of a mixed nerve is the facial nerve. It acts in a motor capacity by transmitting impulses for smiling or frowning. However, it also acts in a sensory capacity by transmitting taste impulses from the tongue to the brain.

**Spinal nerves.** All spinal nerves are mixed nerves. (See Figure 14–4.) They have two points of attachment to the spinal cord: an *anterior root* and a *posterior root.* The anterior root contains motor fibers and the posterior root contains sensory fibers. These two roots unite to form the spinal nerve.

**Somatic nervous system.** The SNS primarily innervates (supplies with nerves) skeletal muscles and is associated with voluntary movement. Examples of voluntary movement include walking and talking.

**Autonomic nervous system.** In contrast, the ANS innervates glands, smooth muscles, and cardiac muscles. This system is considered involuntary, because it operates without conscious control. Examples of autonomic activities include digestion, heart contraction, and vasoconstriction.

The ANS is further subdivided into the *sympathetic* and *parasympathetic* systems. To a large extent, these subdivisions oppose the action of the other, although in certain instances, they may exhibit independent action. In general, sympathetic nerve fibers produce vasoconstriction, increased heart rate, elevated blood pressure, and slowing of gastrointestinal activity. Sympathetic functions are evident in "fight-or-flight" situations. Blood flow increases in skeletal muscles to prepare an individual to either fight or retreat from a threatening situation. The parasympathetic system generally transmits impulses that bring about vasodilation, a slower heart rate, a decrease in blood pressure, and a return to normal gastrointestinal activity.

 **It is time to review nervous system structures by completing Learning Activity 14–1.**

**Figure 14–3** Cranial nerve distribution.

Cervical nerves

Thoracic nerves

Lumbar nerves

Sacral nerves

Coccygeal nerve

C1
C2
C3
C4
C5
C6
C7
C8
T1
T2
T3
T4
T5
T6
T7
T8
T9
T10
T11
T12
L1
L2
L3
L4
L5
S1
S2
S3
S4
S5
Co

A.

White
matter

Central
canal

Gray
matter

Posterior
root

Posterior root
ganglion

Spinal
nerve

Pia mater

Arachnoid
membrane

Dura mater

Anterior
roots

Subarachnoid
space

Cauda
equina

**Figure 14–4**   Spinal nerves. (A) Spinal cord enlargement

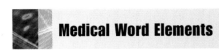

## Medical Word Elements

This section introduces combining forms, suffixes, and prefixes related to the nervous system. Word analyses are also provided.

| Element | Meaning | Word Analysis |
|---|---|---|
| **COMBINING FORMS** | | |
| **cerebr/o** | cerebrum | cerebr/o/tomy (sĕr-ĕ-BRŎT-ō-mē): incision of the cerebrum<br>  *-tomy:* incision |
| **crani/o** | cranium (skull) | crani/o/malacia (krā-nē-ō-mă-LĀ-shē-ă): softening of the cranial bones<br>  *-malacia:* softening |
| **dendr/o** | tree | dendr/oid (DĔN-droyd): resembling a branching tree such as cytoplasmic branches of a neuron<br>  *-oid:* resembling<br>*Dendrons conduct nerve impulses to the cell body.* |
| **encephal/o** | brain | encephal/o/cele (ĕn-SĔF-ă-lō-sēl): herniation of the brain<br>  *-cele:* hernia, swelling<br>*Encephalocele is a condition in which portions of the brain and meninges protrude through a bony midline defect in the skull. It is usually associated with a neural tube defect.* |
| **gangli/o** | ganglion (knot or knotlike mass) | gangli/ectomy (găng-glē-ĔK-tō-mē): excision of a ganglion<br>  *-ectomy:* excision, removal<br>*A ganglion is a mass of nerve cell bodies (gray matter) in the peripheral nervous system.* |
| **gli/o** | glue; neuroglial tissue | gli/oma (glī-Ō-mă): tumor composed of neuroglial or supporting tissue of the nervous system<br>  *-oma:* tumor |
| **lex/o** | word, phrase | dys/lex/ia (dĭs-LĔK-sē-ă): difficulty using and interpreting written forms of communication<br>  *dys-:* bad; painful; difficult<br>  *-ia:* condition<br>*In dyslexia, disability is not associated with vision or intelligence.* |
| **kinesi/o** | movement | brady/kinesia (brăd-ē-kĭ-Nē-sē-ă): slow movement<br>  *brady-:* slow |

*(Continued)*

| Element | Meaning | Word Analysis | (Continued) |
|---|---|---|---|
| **lept/o** | thin, slender | lept/o/mening/o/pathy (lĕp-tō-mĕn-ĭn-GŎP-ă-thē): disease of the leptomeninges<br><br>*mening/o:* meninges (membranes covering brain and spinal cord)<br><br>*-pathy:* disease<br><br>*The leptomeninges include the pia mater and arachnoid, both of which are thin and delicate in structure, as opposed to the dura mater.* | |
| **mening/o**<br><br><br><br>**meningi/o** | meninges (membranes covering brain and spinal cord) | mening/o/cele (mĕn-ĬN-gō-sēl): herniation of the meninges through the skull or spinal column<br><br>*-cele:* hernia, swelling<br><br>meningi/oma (mĕn-ĭn-jē-Ō-mă): slow-growing tumor that originates in the meninges<br><br>*-oma:* tumor | |
| **myel/o** | bone marrow; spinal cord | poli/o/myel/itis (pōl-ē-ō-mī-ĕl-Ī-tĭs): inflammation of the gray matter of the spinal cord<br><br>*poli/o:* gray; gray matter (of brain or spinal cord)<br>*-itis:* inflammation | |
| **narc/o** | stupor; numbness; sleep | narc/o/tic (năr-KŎT-ĭk): relating to or producing stupor or sleep<br><br>*-tic:* pertaining to, relating to<br><br>*Narcotics depress the central nervous system, thus relieving pain and producing sleep.* | |
| **neur/o** | nerve | neur/o/lysis (nū-RŎL-ĭs-ĭs): loosening of adhesions surrounding a nerve<br><br>*-lysis:* separation; destruction; loosening | |
| **sthen/o** | strength | hyper/sthen/ia (hī-pĕr-STHĒ-nē-ă): abnormal strength with excessive tension in all parts of the body<br><br>*hyper-:* excessive, above normal<br>*-ia:* condition | |
| **radicul/o** | nerve root | radicul/algia (ră-dĭk-ū-LĂL-jē-ă): pain in the nerve roots<br>*-algia:* pain | |
| **thec/o** | sheath (usually refers to meninges) | intra/thec/al (ĭn-tră-THĒ-kăl): pertaining to the space within a sheath, especially the meninges<br><br>*intra-:* in, within<br>*-al:* pertaining to, relating to | |
| **thalam/o** | thalamus | thalam/o/tomy (thăl-ă-MŎT-ō-mē): incision of the thalamus to treat intractable pain or psychoses<br><br>*-tomy:* incision | |
| **ton/o** | tension | dys/ton/ia (dĭs-TŌ-nē-ă): any abnormality in muscle tone<br><br>*dys-:* bad; painful; difficult<br>*-ia:* condition<br><br>*Dystonia usually refers to a movement disorder characterized by sustained muscle contractions resulting in a persistently abnormal posture.* | |

| Element | Meaning | Word Analysis |
|---------|---------|---------------|
| **ventricul/o** | ventricle (of heart or brain) | ventricul/o/metry (vĕn-trĭk-ū-LŎM-ĕ-trē): measurement of intraventricular cerebral pressure<br>*-metry:* act of measuring |

## SUFFIXES

| Element | Meaning | Word Analysis |
|---------|---------|---------------|
| **-algesia** | pain | an/algesia (ăn-ăl-JĒ-zē-ă): absence of a normal sense of pain<br>*an-:* without, not |
| **-algia** | | syn/algia (sĭn-ĂL-jē-ă): referred pain<br>*syn-:* union, together, joined |
| **-asthenia** | weakness, debility | my/asthenia (mī-ăs-THĒ-nē-ă): muscular weakness and abnormal fatigue<br>*my:* muscle |
| **-esthesia** | feeling | hyper/esthesia (hī-pĕr-ĕs-THĒ-zē-ă): increased sensitivity to sensory stimuli, such as pain and touch<br>*hyper-:* excessive, above normal |
| **-kinesia** | movement | hyper/kinesia (hī-pĕr-kĭ-NĒ-zē-ă): increased muscular movement and physical activity<br>*hyper-:* excessive, above normal |
| **-lepsy** | seizure | epi/lepsy (ĔP-ĭ-lĕp-sē): any disorder characterized by recurrent seizures<br>*epi-:* above, upon |
| **-paresis** | partial paralysis | hemi/paresis (hĕm-ē-PĂR-ĕ-sĭs): paralysis of one side of the body; also called *hemiplegia*<br>*hemi-:* one-half<br>*When used alone, the term* paresis *means partial paralysis or motor weakness.* |
| **-phasia** | speech | a/phasia (ă-FĀ-zē-ă): impairment in the ability to communicate through speech, writing, or signs because of brain dysfunction<br>*a-:* without, not |
| **-plegia** | paralysis | quadri/plegia (kwŏd-rĭ-PLĒ-jē-ă): paralysis of all four extremities<br>*quadri-:* four |
| **-plexy** | stroke | cata/plexy (KĂT-ă-plĕks-ē): sudden, brief loss of muscle control that commonly results in collapse<br>*cata-:* down<br>*Cataplexy is commonly brought on by extreme emotion, such as surprise, anger, and excitement.* |
| **-taxia** | order, coordination | a/taxia (ă-TĂK-sē-ă): defective muscle coordination, especially when voluntary movements are attempted<br>*a-:* without, not |

*(Continued)*

| Element | Meaning | Word Analysis | (Continued) |
|---|---|---|---|
| **-trophy** | development, nourishment | dys/trophy (DĬS-trō-fē): disorder caused by defective nutrition or metabolism<br><br>*dys-:* bad; painful; difficult | |

**PREFIXES**

| Element | Meaning | Word Analysis | |
|---|---|---|---|
| **contra-** | against | contra/later/al (kŏn-tră-LĂT-ĕr-ăl): pertaining to opposite sides<br><br>*later:* side, to one side<br>*-al:* pertaining to, relating to | |
| **pachy-** | thick | pachy/mening/itis (păk-ē-mĕn-ĭn-JĪ-tĭs): inflammation of the dura mater<br><br>*mening:* meninges (membranes covering brain and spinal cord)<br>*-itis:* inflammation<br><br>*The dura mater is a thick membrane that provides protection for the brain and spinal cord.* | |
| **para-** | near, beside; beyond | para/plegia (păr-ă-PLĒ-jē-ă): paralysis of the lower part of the body and both legs<br><br>*-plegia:* paralysis | |
| **syn-** | union, together, joined | syn/esthesia (sĭn-ĕs-THĒ-zē-ă): stimulation of one sense that causes a perception in one or more different senses<br><br>*-esthesia:* feeling<br><br>*An example of synesthesia is hearing a sound that may also produce a sensation of smell.* | |
| **uni-** | one | uni/later/al (ū-nĭ-LĂT-ĕr-ăl): pertaining to or affecting only one side<br><br>*later:* side, to one side<br>*-al:* pertaining to, relating to | |

 **It is time to review medical word elements by completing Learning Activity 14–2.**

 **Pathology**

Damage to the brain and spinal cord invariably causes signs and symptoms in other parts of the body. Therefore, it is always essential to identify the neurological deficit as involving a muscle, a nerve, the spinal cord, or the brain. Common symptoms for many neurological disorders include headache, insomnia, back or neck pain, weakness, and involuntary movement **(dyskinesia).** Careful observation of the patient during the patient history and physical examination may provide valuable clues about mental status and cognitive and motor ability. Muscle strength, coordination, gait, balance, and reflexes provide additional diagnostic clues. Lumbar punctures provide a sample of CSF for analysis and help identify various types of meningitis and encephalitis. Radiology—especially CT and MRI scans—provide detailed images that can locate cerebrovascular irregularities, lesions, and tumors.

## Bell Palsy

Bell palsy is a facial paralysis caused by a functional disorder of the seventh cranial nerve and any or all of its branches and is associated with herpes virus. It may be unilateral, bilateral, transient, or permanent. Symptoms include weakness (**asthenia**) and numbness of the face, distortion of taste perception, facial disfigurement, and facial spasms. The cornea becomes dry because of an absent blink reflex and commonly leads to corneal infection (**keratitis**). Speech difficulties (**dysphasia**) and pain behind the ear or in the face are also symptoms of this disease. Anti-inflammatory drugs and the application of heat promote circulation and ease pain. Spontaneous recovery can be expected in about 3 to 5 weeks.

## Cerebrovascular Disease

Cerebrovascular disease (CVD) refers to any functional abnormality of the cerebrum caused by disorders of the blood vessels of the brain. CVD is most commonly associated with a stroke, also called *cerebrovascular accident (CVA)*. The three major types of strokes are *ischemic stroke*, *intracerebral hemorrhage*, and *subarachnoid hemorrhage*. The most common type, which accounts for about 80% of all strokes, is ischemic stroke. It is caused by a narrowing of the arteries of the brain or neck (**carotid**), generally due to arteriosclerosis. This narrowing causes insufficient oxygen delivery to the brain tissue and, within a few minutes, the tissue begins to die. An intracerebral hemorrhage is a type of stroke caused by the sudden rupture of an artery within the brain. After the rupture, released blood compresses brain structures and destroys them. In a subarachnoid hemorrhage, blood is released into the space surrounding the brain. This condition is commonly caused by a ruptured aneurysm and is usually fatal.

Signs and symptoms of stroke include weakness in one half of the body (**hemiparesis**), paralysis in one half of the body (**hemiplegia**), inability to speak (**aphasia**), lack of muscular coordination (**ataxia**), stupor, coma, or even death. If the CVA is mild, the patient may experience a brief "blackout," blurred vision, or dizziness and may be unaware of the "minor stroke." Stroke symptoms that resolve within 24 hours are known as a *transient ischemic attack (TIA)*. About one-third of all strokes are preceded by a TIA. A family history of cerebrovascular disease and high blood pressure appears to be a contributing factor to stroke. Treatment involves speech, physical, and occupational therapy and various medications, depending on the type of stroke.

## Seizure Disorders

Chronic or recurring seizure disorders are called *epilepsies*. These disorders involve electrical disturbances (**dysrhythmias**) in the brain that result in abnormal, recurrent, and uncontrolled electrical discharges. Causes of epilepsy include brain injury, congenital anomalies, metabolic disorders, brain tumors, vascular disturbances, and genetic disorders.

Seizures are characterized by sudden bursts of abnormal electrical activity in neurons, resulting in temporary changes in brain function. Two major types of seizures are *partial* and *generalized*. In partial seizures there is a short alteration of consciousness of about 10 to 30 seconds, characterized by repetitive, unusual movements and confusion. In generalized seizures there is a temporary lapse in consciousness, accompanied by rhythmic movement of the eyes, head, or hands, without convulsions.

*Status epilepticus* is a life-threatening emergency that involves the whole cortex. It is diagnosed when a continuous seizure occurs without a pause; that is, without an intervening period of normal brain function. It is characterized by tonic-clonic convulsions that may cause irreversible brain damage or even death. Diagnosis and evaluation commonly rely on *electroencephalography* and *magnetoencephalography* to locate the affected area of the brain. Epilepsy is controlled by antiepileptic medications.

## Parkinson Disease

Parkinson disease, also called "shaking palsy," is a progressive neurological disorder affecting the portion of the brain responsible for controlling movement. As neurons degenerate, the patient develops uncontrollable nodding of the head, decreased speed of movement **(bradykinesia, hypokinesia),** tremors, large joint stiffness, and a shuffling gait. Muscle rigidity causes facial expressions to appear fixed and masklike with unblinking eyes. Sometimes the patient exhibits "pill rolling," in which he or she inadvertently rubs the thumb against the index finger.

In patients with Parkinson disease, dopamine, a neurotransmitter that facilitates the transmission of impulses at synapses, is lacking in the brain. Management involves the administration of L-dopa, which can cross the blood-brain barrier. L-dopa is converted in the brain to dopamine. Even so, this treatment only reduces symptoms; it is not a cure for Parkinson disease.

## Multiple Sclerosis

Multiple sclerosis (MS) is a progressive, degenerative disease of the CNS. MS is characterized by inflammation, hardening and, finally, loss of myelin **(demyelination)** throughout the spinal cord and brain. As myelin deteriorates, the transmission of electrical impulses from one neuron to another is impeded. In effect, the conduction pathway develops "short circuits."

Signs and symptoms of MS include tremors, muscle weakness, and bradykinesia. Occasionally, visual disturbances exist. During remissions, symptoms temporarily disappear, but progressive hardening of myelin areas leads to other attacks. Ultimately, most voluntary motor control is lost and the patient becomes bedridden. Death occurs anywhere from 7 to 30 years after the onset of the disease. Young adults, usually women, between ages 20 and 40 are the most common victims of MS. The etiology of the disease is unclear, but autoimmune disease or a slow viral infection is believed to be the most probable cause.

## Alzheimer Disease

Alzheimer disease is a progressive neurological disorder that causes memory loss and serious mental deterioration. Small lesions called *plaques* develop in the cerebral cortex and disrupt the passage of electrochemical signals between cells. The clinical manifestations of Alzheimer disease include memory loss and cognitive decline. There is also a decline in social skills and ability to carry out activities of daily living. Most patients undergo personality, emotional, and behavioral changes. As the disease progresses, loss of concentration and increased fatigue, restlessness, and anxiety are common. Alzheimer disease was once considered rare but is now identified as a leading cause of senile dementia. Although there is no specific treatment, moderate relief has been associated with medications that prevent a breakdown of brain chemicals required for neurotransmission.

## Mental Illness

Mental illness includes an array of psychological disorders, syndromes, and behavioral patterns that cause alterations in mood, behavior, and thinking. (See Table 14–2.) Its forms range from mild to profound. For example, anxiety may manifest as a slight apprehension or uneasiness lasting a few days to a more severe form, involving intense fears lasting for months and even years.

*Psychosis* refers to a serious mental disorder commonly characterized by false beliefs despite overwhelming evidence to the contrary **(delusions).** The psychotic patient typically "hears voices" and "sees visions" in the absence of an actual stimulus **(hallucinations).** The patient's speech is usually incoherent and disorganized and behavior is erratic.

*Neurosis* is a mental disorder caused by an emotion experienced in the past that overwhelmingly interferes or affects a present emotion. For example, a child bitten by a dog may show irrational fear of animals as an adult. Many mental disorders are forms of neuroses, including irrational fears **(phobias),** exaggerated emotional and reflexive behaviors **(hysterias),** or irrational, uncontrolled performance of ritualistic actions for fear of a dire consequence **(obsessive compulsive disorders).**

Research and education have removed much of the stigma attached to mental illness. Today, mental illness is becoming a more recognizable and treatable disorder. Many psychological disorders can be effectively treated or managed by family physicians, school psychologists, marriage counselors, family counselors, and even support groups such as grief support groups and Alcoholics Anonymous.

Diagnosis and treatment of serious mental disorders usually require the skills of a medical specialist called a *psychiatrist.* In the capacity of a physician, the psychiatrist is licensed to prescribe medications and perform medical procedures not available to those who do not hold a medical license. Psychiatrists commonly work in association with *clinical psychologists,* who are individuals trained in evaluating human behavior, intelligence, and personality.

## Table 14-2    COMMON TERMS ASSOCIATED WITH MENTAL ILLNESS

This table lists common terms or disorders associated with mental illness along with their definitions.

| Term | Definition |
| --- | --- |
| affective disorder | Psychological disorder in which the major characteristic is an abnormal mood, usually mania or depression |
| anorexia nervosa | Eating disorder characterized by a refusal to maintain adequate weight for age and height and an all-consuming desire to remain thin |
| anxiety | Psychological "worry" disorder characterized by excessive pondering or thinking "what if…" <br> *Feelings of worry, dread, lack of energy, and a loss of interest in life are common signs associated with anxiety.* |
| attention-deficit hyperactivity disorder (ADHD) | Disorder affecting children and adults characterized by impulsiveness, overactivity, and the inability to remain focused on a task |
| bipolar disorder | Mental disorder that causes unusual shifts in mood, emotion, energy, and ability to function; also called *manic-depressive illness* |
| bulimia nervosa | Eating disorder characterized by binging (overeating) and purging (vomiting or use of laxatives) |
| depression | Mood disorder associated with sadness, despair, discouragement, and, commonly, feelings of low self-esteem, guilt, and withdrawal |
| mania | Mood disorder characterized by mental and physical hyperactivity, disorganized behavior, and hyper-elevated mood |
| panic attack | Sudden, profound, overwhelming feeling of fear that comes without warning and is not attributable to any immediate danger <br> *A key symptom of a panic attack is the fear of its recurrence.* |

## Oncology

Intracranial tumors can arise from any structure within the cranial cavity, including the pituitary and pineal glands, cranial nerves, and the arachnoid and pia mater **(leptomeninges).** However, most intracranial tumors originate directly in brain tissue. In addition, all of these tissues may be the site of metastatic spread from primary malignancies that occur outside of the nervous system. Metastatic tumors of the cranial cavity tend to exhibit growth characteristics similar to those of the primary malignancy but tend to grow more slowly than the parent tumor. Metastatic tumors of the cranial cavity are usually easier to remove than primary intracranial tumors.

Primary intracranial tumors are commonly classified according to histological type and include those that originate in neurons and those that develop in glial tissue. Signs and symptoms of intracranial tumors include headaches, especially upon arising in the morning, during coughing episodes, and upon bending or sudden movement. Occasionally, the optic disc in the back of the eyeball swells **(papilledema)** because of increased intracranial pressure. Personality changes are common and include depression, anxiety, and irritability.

Computed tomography (CT) scans and magnetic resonance imaging (MRI) help establish a diagnosis but are not definitive. Surgical removal relieves pressure and confirms or rules out malignancy. Even after surgery, most intracranial tumors require radiation therapy (RT) as a second line of treatment. Chemotherapy, when added to RT, provides the best chance for survival and quality of life.

## Diagnostic, Symptomatic, and Related Terms

This section introduces diagnostic, symptomatic, and related terms and their meanings. Word analyses for selected terms are also provided.

| Term | Definition |
| --- | --- |
| **agnosia** <br> ăg-NŌ-zē-ă <br><br> *a-:* without, not <br> *gnos:* knowing <br> *-ia:* condition | Inability to comprehend auditory, visual, spacial, olfactory, or other sensations even though the sensory sphere is intact <br><br> *The type of agnosia is usually identified by the sense or senses affected, such as visual agnosia. Agnosia is common in parietal lobe tumors.* |
| **asthenia** <br> ăs-THĒ-nē-ă <br><br> *a-:* without, not <br> *sthen:* strength <br> *-ia:* condition | Weakness, debility, or loss of strength <br><br> *Asthenia is a characteristic of multiple sclerosis.* |
| **ataxia** <br> ă-TĂK-sē-ă <br><br> *a-:* without, not <br> *tax:* order, coordination <br> *-ia:* condition | Lack of muscle coordination in the execution of voluntary movement <br><br> *Ataxia may be the result of head injury, stroke, MS, alcoholism, or a variety of hereditary disorders.* |
| **aura** <br> AW-ră | Premonitory awareness of an approaching physical or mental disorder; peculiar sensation that precedes seizures |

| Term | Definition |
|------|------------|
| **autism**<br>AW-tĭzm | Mental disorder chracterized by extreme withdrawal and an abnormal absorption in fantasy, usually accompanied by an inability to communicate even on a basic level<br><br>*A person with autism may engage in repetitive behavior, such as rocking or repeating words.* |
| **cerebral palsy**<br>sĕ-RĒ-brăl PAWL-zē<br><br>*cerebr:* cerebrum<br>*-al:* pertaining to, relating to | Self-limiting paralysis due to developmental defects in the brain or trauma during the birth process |
| **clonic spasm**<br>KLŎN-ĭk SPĂZM | Alternate contraction and relaxation of muscles |
| **closed head trauma**<br>TRAW-mă | Injury to the head in which the dura mater remains intact and brain tissue is not exposed<br><br>*In closed head trauma, the injury site may occur at the impact site where the brain hits the inside of the skull (coup), or at the rebound site where the opposite side of the brain strikes the skull (contrecoup).* |
| **coma**<br>KŌ-mă | Abnormally deep unconsciousness with absence of voluntary response to stimuli |
| **concussion**<br>kŏn-KŬSH-ŭn | Transient loss of consciousness as a result of trauma to the head<br><br>*Delayed symptoms of concussion may include headache, nausea, vomiting, and blurred vision.* |
| **dementia**<br>dĭ-MĔN-shē-ă<br><br>*de-:* cessation<br>*ment:* mind<br>*-ia:* condition | Broad term that refers to cognitive deficit, including memory impairment |
| **dyslexia**<br>dĭs-LĔK-sē-ă<br><br>*dys-:* bad; painful; difficult<br>*lex:* word, phrase<br>*-ia:* condition | Inability to learn and process written language despite adequate intelligence, sensory ability, and exposure |
| **Guillain-Barré syndrome**<br>gē-YĂ băr-RĀ SĬN-drōm | Condition of acute polyneuritis with progressive muscle weakness in extremities<br><br>*Guillain-Barré syndrome occurs most commonly in people ages 30 to 50 with spontaneous and complete recovery in about 95% of cases.* |
| **herpes zoster**<br>HĔR-pēz ZŎS-tĕr | Painful, acute infectious disease of the posterior root ganglia of only a few segments of the spinal or cranial nerves; also called *shingles*<br><br>*Herpes zoster is caused by the same organism (varicella-zoster) that causes chickenpox in children. The disease is self-limiting and usually resolves in 10 days to 5 weeks.* |

*(Continued)*

| Term | Definition | (Continued) |
|------|------------|-------------|

| Term | Definition |
|------|------------|
| **Huntington chorea**<br>HŬNT-ing-tŭn kō-RE-ă | Inherited disease of the CNS that usually has its onset in people between ages 30 and 50<br><br>*Huntington chorea is characterized by quick, involuntary movements; speech disturbances; and mental deterioration.* |
| **hydrocephalus**<br>hi-drō-SĔF-ă-lŭs | Accumulation of fluid in the ventricles of the brain, causing thinning of brain tissue and separation of cranial bones |
| **lethargy**<br>LĔTH-ăr-jē | Abnormal activity or lack of response to normal stimuli; also called *sluggishness* |
| **neurosis**<br>nū-RŌ-sĭs<br><br>*neur:* nerve<br>*-osis:* abnormal condition; increase (used primarily with blood cells) | Unconscious conflict that produces anxiety and other symptoms and leads to maladaptive use of defense mechanisms |
| **psychosis**<br>si-KŌ-sĭs<br><br>*psych:* mind<br>*-osis:* abnormal condition; increase (used primarily with blood cells) | Major emotional disorder where contact with reality is lost to the point that the individual is incapable of meeting challenges of daily life |
| **spina bifida**<br>SPĪ-nă BĬ-fĭ-dă | Defect in which the neural tube (tissue that forms the brain and spinal cord in the fetus) fails to close during embryogenesis<br><br>*Spina bifida is a serious birth defect. Forms of spina bifida include meningomyelocele, meningocele, and occulta. (See Figure 14–5.)* |
| **meningocele**<br>mĕn-ĬN-gō-sēl<br><br>*mening/o:* meninges (membranes covering brain and spinal cord)<br>*-cele:* hernia, swelling | Form of spina bifida in which the spinal cord develops properly but the meninges protrude through the spine |
| **myelomeningocele**<br>mi-ĕ-lō-mĕn-ĬN-gō-sēl<br><br>*myel/o:* bone marrow; spinal cord<br>*mening/o:* meninges (membranes covering brain and spinal cord)<br>*-cele:* hernia, swelling | Most severe form of spina bifida where the spinal cord and meninges protrude through the spine |

| Term | Definition |
|------|------------|
| **occulta**<br>ŏ-KŬL-tă | Form of spina bifida where one or more vertebrae are malformed and the spinal cord is covered with a layer of skin |

**Figure 14–5** Spina bifida.

| Term | Definition |
|------|------------|
| **paraplegia**<br>păr-ă-PLĒ-jē-ă<br><br>*para-:* near, beside; beyond<br>*-plegia:* paralysis | Paralysis of the lower portion of the trunk and both legs usually as a result of injury or disease of the spine |
| **paresthesia**<br>păr-ĕs-THĒ-zē-ă | Sensation of numbness, prickling, tingling, or heightened sensitivity<br><br>*Paresthesia can be caused by disorders affecting the central nervous system, such as stroke, transient ischemic attack, multiple sclerosis, transverse myelitis, and encephalitis.* |
| **poliomyelitis**<br>pōl-ē-ō-mi-ĕl-Ī-tĭs<br><br>*poli/o:* gray; gray matter (of brain or spinal cord)<br>*myel:* bone marrow; spinal cord<br>*-itis:* inflammation | Inflammation of the gray matter of the spinal cord caused by a virus, commonly resulting in spinal and muscle deformity and paralysis<br><br>*Through the Global Polio Eradication Initiative of 1988, the incidence of polio has decreased worldwide by 99%.* |
| **quadriplegia**<br>kwŏd-rĭ-PLĒ-jē-ă<br><br>*quadri-:* four<br>*-plegia:* paralysis | Paralysis of all four extremities and usually the trunk |
| **Reye syndrome**<br>RĪ SĬN-drōm | Acute encephalopathy and fatty infiltration of the brain, liver and, possibly, the pancreas, heart, kidney, spleen, and lymph nodes; usually seen in children younger than age 15 who had an acute viral infection<br><br>*Mortality in Reye syndrome may be as high as 80%. The use of aspirin by children experiencing chickenpox or influenza may induce Reye syndrome.* |

*(Continued)*

| Term | Definition | (Continued) |
|---|---|---|
| **sciatica**<br>si-ĂT-ĭ-kă | Severe pain in the leg along the course of the sciatic nerve felt at the base of the spine, down the thigh, and radiating down the leg due to a compressed nerve | |
| **syncope**<br>SĬN-kō-pē | Temporary loss of consciousness due to the sudden decline of blood flow to the brain; also called *fainting* | |
|   **vasovagal**<br>  văs-ō-VĀ-găl | Syncope due to a drop in blood pressure brought on by the response of the nervous system to abrupt emotional stress, pain, or trauma | |
| **transient ischemic attack (TIA)**<br>TRĂN-zē-ĕnt ĭs-KĒ-mĭk | Temporary interference with blood supply to the brain lasting from a few minutes to a few hours<br><br>*Symptoms of TIA may include numbness or weakness in the extremities, especially on one side of the body; confusion or difficulty in talking or understanding speech; visual impairment; dizziness; loss of balance; and difficulty walking.* | |

 **It is time to review pathological, diagnostic, symptomatic, and related terms by completing Learning Activity 14–3.**

 ## Diagnostic and Therapeutic Procedures

This section introduces procedures used to diagnose and treat nervous disorders. Descriptions are provided as well as pronunciations and word analyses for selected terms.

| Procedure | Description |
|---|---|
| **DIAGNOSTIC PROCEDURES** | |
| **Clinical** | |
| **electroencephalography (EEG)**<br>ē-lĕk-trō-ĕn-sĕf-ă-LŎG-ră-fē<br><br>  *electr/o:* electricity<br>  *encephal/o:* brain<br>  *-graphy:* process of recording | Recording of electrical activity in the brain, whose cells emit distinct patterns of rhythmic electrical impulses<br><br>*Different wave patterns on the EEG are associated with normal and abnormal waking and sleeping states and help diagnose such conditions as tumors, infections, and seizure disorders.* |
| **electromyography (EMG)**<br>ē-lĕk-trō-mi-ŎG-ră-fē<br><br>  *electr/o:* electricity<br>  *my/o:* muscle<br>  *-graphy:* process of recording | Recording of electrical signals (action potentials) that occur in a muscle when it is at rest and during contraction to assess nerve damage<br><br>*In EMG, an electrode inserted into a muscle records the impulses and displays them on a monitor called an* oscilloscope. |

| Procedure | Description |
|-----------|-------------|
| **lumbar puncture**<br>LŬM-băr PŬNK-chūr | Needle puncture of the spinal cavity to extract spinal fluid for diagnostic purposes, introduce anesthetic agents into the spinal canal, or remove fluid to allow other fluids (such as radiopaque substances) to be injected; also called *spinal puncture* and *spinal tap* |
| **magnetoencephalography (MEG)**<br>măg-nĕt-ō-ĕn-cĕf-ă-LŎG-ră-fē | Noninvasive test that records electromagnetic activity produced as neurons discharge and maps their pathway through the brain<br><br>*MEG is performed in seizure disorders because it can pinpoint active regions in the brain and trace their movement from region to region. A helmet that contains magnetic sensors tracks the impulses and records them.* |
| **nerve conduction velocity (NCV)**<br>NĔRV kŏn-DŬK-shŭn vĕ-LŎ-sĭ-tē | Test that measures the speed at which impulses travel through a nerve<br><br>*In NCV, one electrode stimulates a nerve while other electrodes, placed over different areas of the nerve, record an electrical signal (action potential) as it travels through the nerve. This test is used for diagnosing muscular dystrophy and neurological disorders that destroy myelin.* |

## Laboratory

| Procedure | Description |
|-----------|-------------|
| **cerebrospinal fluid (CSF) analysis**<br>sĕr-ē-brō-SPĪ-năl, ă-NĂL-ĭ-sĭs<br><br>   *cerebr/o:* cerebrum<br>   *spin:* spine<br>   *-al:* pertaining to, relating to | Series of chemical, microscopic, and microbial tests used to diagnose disorders of the central nervous system, including viral and bacterial infections, tumors, and hemorrhage |

## Radiographic

| Procedure | Description |
|-----------|-------------|
| **angiography**<br>ăn-jē-ŎG-ră-fē<br><br>   *angi/o:* vessel (usually blood or lymph)<br>   *-graphy:* process of recording | Radiography of the blood vessels after introduction of a contrast medium<br><br>*Angiography is used to visualize vascular abnormalities. The contrast medium may be injected into an artery or vein or administered through a catheter inserted in a peripheral artery, run through the vessel, and positioned at a visceral site.* |
|    **cerebral**<br>   sĕr-Ē-brăl<br><br>     *cerebr/o:* cerebrum<br>     *-al:* pertaining to, relating to | Angiography of blood vessels of the brain after injection of a contrast medium; also called *cerebral arteriography*<br><br>*Vascular tumors, aneurysms, and occlusions are identified using cerebral angiography. In addition, abscesses, nonvascular tumors, and hematomas are commonly identified because they distort the normal vascular image.* |
| **myelography**<br>mī-ĕ-LŎG-ră-fē<br><br>   *myel/o:* bone marrow; spinal cord<br>   *-graphy:* process of recording | Diagnostic radiological examination of the spinal canal, nerve roots, and spinal cord after injection of contrast medium into the spinal canal<br><br>*Myelography is usually performed in conjunction with a CT scan and when an MRI is not possible because the patient has a pacemaker or other implantable device.* |

*(Continued)*

| Procedure | Description | (Continued) |
|---|---|---|

| **scan** | Term used to describe a computerized image by modality (such as *computed tomography, magnetic resonance,* and *nuclear*) or by structure (such as *thyroid, bone,* or *brain*) |
|---|---|
| **brain** | Diagnostic procedure using radioisotope imaging to localize and identify intracranial masses, lesions, tumors, or infarcts |
| | *Because radioactive material concentrates in rapidly growing cells, a brain scan is used to identify brain tumors and evaluate the progress of treatment.* |
| **computed tomography (CT)** kŏm-PŪ-tĕd tō-MŎG-ră-fē  *tom/o:* to cut  *-graphy:* process of recording | Imaging technique that rotates an x-ray emitter around the area to be scanned and measures the intensity of transmitted rays from different angles |
| **positron emission tomography (PET)** PŎZ-ĭ-trŏn ē-MĬSH-ŭn tō-MŎG-ră-fē | Scan using computed tomography to record the positrons (positively charged particles) emitted from a radiopharmaceutical and produce a cross-sectional image of metabolic activity in body tissues to determine the presence of disease |
| | *PET is especially useful in scanning the brain and nervous system to diagnose disorders that involve abnormal tissue metabolism, such as schizophrenia, brain tumors, epilepsy, stroke, and Alzheimer disease. The images are produced using colors that indicate degrees of metabolism or blood flow. The highest rates appear red; lower rates appear yellow, then green; and the lowest rates appear blue. (See Figure 4–4F.)* |
| **ultrasonography** ŭl-tră-sŏn-ŎG-ră-fē  *ultra-:* excess, beyond  *son/o:* sound  *-graphy:* process of recording | Image produced by using high-frequency sound waves (ultrasound) and displaying the reflected "echoes" on a monitor; also called *ultrasound, sonography, echo,* and *echogram* |
| **echoencephalography** ĕk-ō-ĕn-sĕf-ă-LŎG-ră-fē  *echo-:* repeated sound  *encephal/o:* brain  *-graphy:* process of recording | Ultrasound technique used to study the intracranial structures of the brain and, especially, diagnose conditions that cause a shift in the midline structures of the brain |

### THERAPEUTIC PROCEDURES

#### Surgical

| **cryosurgery** kri-ō-SĔR-jĕr-ē | Technique that exposes abnormal tissue to extreme cold to destroy it |
|---|---|
| | *Cryosurgery is sometimes used to destroy malignant tumors of the brain.* |

| Procedure | Description |
|-----------|-------------|
| **stereotaxic radiosurgery**<br>stĕr-ē-ō-TĂK-sĭk rā-dē-ō-SŬR-jĕr-ē | Precise method of locating and destroying sharply circumscribed lesions on specific, tiny areas of pathological tissue in deep-seated structures of the central nervous system; also called *stereotaxy* or *stereotactic surgery*<br><br>*Stereotaxic radiosurgery is used in the treatment of seizure disorders, aneurysms, brain tumors, and many other neuropathological conditions and is performed without a surgical incision. The site to be worked on is localized with three-dimensional coordinates, and methods of destroying lesions include heat, cold, and radiation.* |
| **thalamotomy**<br>thăl-ă-MŎT-ō-mē<br><br>  *thalam/o:* thalamus<br>  *-tomy:* incision | Partial destruction of the thalamus to treat intractable pain, involuntary movements, or emotional disturbances<br><br>*Thalamotomy produces few neurological deficits or changes in personality.* |
| **tractotomy**<br>trăk-TŎT-ō-mē | Transection of a nerve tract in the brainstem or spinal cord<br>*Tractotomy is sometimes used to relieve intractable pain.* |
| **trephination**<br>trĕf-ĭn-Ā-shŭn | Technique that cuts a circular opening into the skull to reveal brain tissue and decrease intracranial pressure |
| **vagotomy**<br>vā-GŎT-ō-mē | Interruption of the function of the vagus nerve to relieve peptic ulcer<br><br>*Vagotomy is performed when ulcers in the stomach and duodenum do not respond to medication or changes in diet.* |

## Pharmacology

Neurological agents are used to relieve or eliminate pain, suppress seizures, control tremors, and reduce muscle rigidity. Hypnotics, a class of drugs used as sedatives, depress central nervous system (CNS) function to relieve agitation and induce sleep. Anesthetics are capable of producing a complete or partial loss of feeling and are used for surgery. Psychotherapeutic agents alter brain chemistry to treat mental illness. These drugs are used as mood stabilizers in various mental disorders. They also reduce symptoms of depression and treat attention deficit hyperactivity disorder and narcolepsy. (See Table 14–3.)

## Table 14-3 · DRUGS USED TO TREAT NEUROLOGICAL AND PSYCHIATRIC DISORDERS

This table lists common drug classifications used to treat neurological and psychiatric disorders, their therapeutic actions, and selected generic and trade names.

| Classification | Therapeutic Action | Generic and Trade Names |
|---|---|---|
| **Neurological** | | |
| **analgesics** | Relieve or eliminate pain<br><br>*Nonnarcotic and nonsteroidal anti-inflammatory drugs (NSAIDs), such as Bayer and Vioxx, are used to treat mild aches and pain. Moderate to severe pain is commonly treated with narcotic analgesics, such as Demerol. Because they are addictive in nature, narcotic analgesics require a prescription.* | **aspirin**<br>ĂS-pĕr-ĭn<br>*Bayer, Bufferin, Ecotrin*<br>**acetaminophen**<br>ă-sē-tă-MĬN-ō-fĕn<br>*Tylenol, Panadol, Tempra*<br>**rofecoxib**<br>rō-fĕ-CŌKS-ĭb<br>*Vioxx*<br>**meperidine**<br>mĕ-PĔR-ĭ-dēn<br>*Demerol* |
| **anesthetics** | Produce partial or complete loss of sensation, with or without loss of consciousness<br><br>*Anesthetics may be classified as general or local.* | **lidocaine**<br>LĪ-dō-kān<br>*Xylocaine*<br>**nitrous oxide**<br>NĪ-trŭs ŎK-sĭd<br>*N₂O* |
| **general** | Act upon the brain to produce complete loss of feeling with loss of consciousness<br><br>*General anesthetics are commonly used for surgical procedures and include Nembutal, Diprivan, and Versed.* | **pentobarbital**<br>pĕn-tō-BĂR-bĭ-tăl<br>*Nembutal*<br>**propofol**<br>PRŌ-pō-fŏl<br>*Diprivan* |
| **local** | Act upon nerves or nerve tracts and affect a local area only<br><br>*Local anesthetics include Xylocaine and Novocain.* | **procaine**<br>PRŌ-kān<br>*Novocain* |
| **anticonvulsants** | Suppress or control seizures by stabilizing the neuron membrane and reducing its excitability<br><br>*Anticonvulsants are used to prevent or control partial and generalized epileptic seizures.* | **carbamazepine**<br>kăr-bă-MĂZ-ĕ-pēn<br>*Tegretol*<br>**valproate**<br>văl-PRŌ-āt<br>*Depakote*<br>**lamotrigine**<br>lă-MŌ-tri-jēn<br>*Lamictal* |
| **antiparkinsonian agents** | Reduce the signs and symptoms associated with Parkinson disease by increasing dopamine in the brain<br><br>*Antiparkinsonian agents control tremors and muscle rigidity.* | **levodopa**<br>lē-vō-DŌ-pă<br>*L-dopa, Larodopa, Dopar*<br>**levodopa/carbidopa**<br>kăr-bĭ-DŌ-pă<br>*Sinemet, Sinemet CR* |

**Table 14–3** DRUGS USED TO TREAT NEUROLOGICAL AND PSYCHIATRIC DISORDERS

| Classification | Therapeutic Action | Generic and Trade Names |
|---|---|---|
| hypnotics | Depress central nervous system (CNS) functions and promote sedation and sleep<br><br>*Hypnotics may be nonbarbiturates or barbiturates. Nonbarbiturate hypnotics (such as Restoril) carry a low risk of addiction; barbiturate hypnotics (such as Seconal) carry a higher risk of addiction.* | **secobarbital**<br>sē-kō-BĂR-bĭ-tŏl<br>*Seconal*<br>**temazepam**<br>tĕ-MĂZ-ĕ-păm<br>*Restoril* |
| **Psychiatric** | | |
| antipsychotics | Treat hallucinations, delusions, agitation, and paranoia and symptoms associated with schizophrenia<br><br>*The first antipsychotics, known as neuroleptics (such as Thorazine and Haldol), caused numerous adverse effects. Newer medications called atypical antipsychotics (such as Zyprexa and Risperdal) have fewer adverse effects. In addition to psychotic disorders, antipsychotics are used to treat agitation associated with post-traumatic stress disorder and dementia.* | **clozapine**<br>CLŌ-ză-pēn<br>*Clozaril*<br>**haloperidol**<br>hă-lō-PĔR-ĭ-dŏl<br>*Haldol*<br>**olanzapine**<br>ō-LĂN-ză-pēn<br>*Zyprexa*<br>**risperidone**<br>rĭs-PĔR-ĭ-dōn<br>*Risperdal* |
| antidepressants | Treat multiple symptoms of depression<br><br>*Antidepressants fall under different classifications and some are also used to treat anxiety and pain.* | **paroxetine**<br>pă-RŎK-sĕ-tēn<br>*Paxil*<br>**fluoxetine**<br>floo-ŎK-sĕ-tēn<br>*Prozac*<br>**amitriptyline**<br>ăm-ĭ-TRĬP-tĭ-lēn<br>*Elavil* |
| psychostimulants | Treat narcolepsy and attention-deficit hyperactivity disorder (ADHD) in children and adults<br><br>*Psychostimulants used to treat ADHD are mainly amphetamines. Amphetamines reduce the symptoms of restlessness, emotional lability, and impulsive behavior and may increase attention span without overstimulation.* | **dextroamphetamine**<br>dĕks-trō-ăm-FĔT-ă-mēn<br>*Dexedrine*<br>**methylphenidate**<br>mĕth-ĭl-FĔN-ĭ-dāt<br>*Ritalin* |

## Abbreviations

This section introduces nervous system-related abbreviations and their meanings.

| Abbreviation | Meaning |
|---|---|
| AD | Alzheimer disease |
| ALS | amyotrophic lateral sclerosis; also called *Lou Gehrig disease* |
| ANS | autonomic nervous system |
| BEAM | brain electrical activity mapping |
| CNS | central nervous system |
| CP | cerebral palsy |
| CSF | cerebrospinal fluid |
| CT scan, CAT scan | computed tomography scan |
| CVA | cerebrovascular accident |
| EEG | electroencephalogram; electroencephalography |
| ICP | intracranial pressure |
| LOC | loss of consciousness |
| LP | lumbar puncture |
| MEG | magnetoencephalography |
| MRA | magnetic resonance angiogram; magnetic resonance angiography |
| MRI | magnetic resonance imaging |
| MS | musculoskeletal; multiple sclerosis; mental status; mitral stenosis |
| NCV | nerve conduction velocity |
| PET | positron emission tomography |
| SNS | sympathetic nervous system |
| TIA | transient ischemic attack |

**It is time to review procedures, pharmacology, and abbreviations by completing Learning Activity 14–4.**

## LEARNING ACTIVITIES

The activities that follow provide a review of the nervous system terms introduced in this chapter. Complete each activity and review your answers to evaluate your understanding of the chapter.

# Learning Activity 14–1

## Identifying structures of the brain

*Label the following illustration using the terms listed below.*

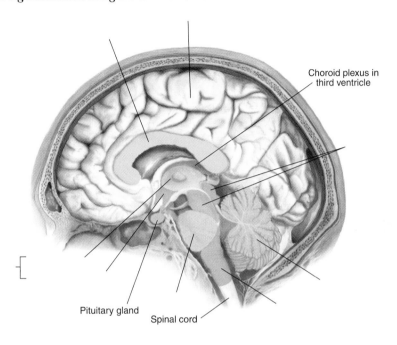

Choroid plexus in third ventricle

Pituitary gland

Spinal cord

cerebellum

cerebrum

corpus callosum

diencephalon (interbrain)

frontal lobe

hypothalamus

medulla

midbrain (mesencephalon)

occipital lobe

parietal lobe

pons

temporal lobe

thalamus

Check your answers by referring to Figure 14–2 on page 424. Review material that you did not answer correctly.

## Building medical words

*Use* **encephal/o** *(brain) to build words that mean:*

1. disease of the brain _____
2. herniation of the brain _____
3. radiography of the brain _____

*Use* **cerebr/o** *(cerebrum) to build words that mean:*

4. disease of the cerebrum _____
5. inflammation of the cerebrum

*Use* **crani/o** *(cranium [skull]) to build words that mean:*

6. herniation (through the) cranium _____
7. instrument for measuring the skull _____

*Use* **neur/o** *(nerve) to build words that mean:*

8. pain in a nerve _____
9. specialist in the study of the nervous system _____
10. crushing a nerve _____

*Use* **myel/o** *(bone marrow; spinal cord) to build words that mean:*

11. herniation of the spinal cord _____
12. paralysis of the spinal cord _____

*Use* **psych/o** *(mind) to build words that mean:*

13. pertaining to the mind _____
14. abnormal condition of the mind _____

*Use the suffix* **-kinesia** *(movement) to build words that mean:*

15. movement that is slow _____
16. movement that is painful or difficult _____

*Use the suffix* **-plegia** *(paralysis) to build words that mean:*

17. paralysis of one half (of the body) _____
18. paralysis of four (limbs) _____

*Use the suffix* **-phasia** *(speech) to build words that mean:*

19. difficult speech _____
20. lacking or without speech _____

*Build surgical terms that mean:*

21. destruction of a nerve _____

22. incision of the skull _____

23. surgical repair of the skull _____

24. suture of a nerve _____

25. incision of the brain _____

✓ Check your answers in Appendix A. Review material that you did not answer correctly.

**CORRECT ANSWERS** _____ × 4 = _____ **% SCORE**

# Learning Activity 14–3

## Matching pathological, diagnostic, symptomatic, and related terms

*Match the following terms with the definitions in the numbered list.*

| | | |
|---|---|---|
| Alzheimer disease | dysrhythmias | paraplegia |
| asthenia | hemiparesis | Parkinson disease |
| autism | Guillain-Barré syndrome | poliomyelitis |
| bipolar disorder | leptomeningitis | shingles |
| bulimia nervosa | lethargy | stroke |
| clonic spasm | multiple sclerosis | transient ischemic attack (TIA) |
| concussion | phobias | |

1. _____ weakness in one half of the body

2. _____ electrical disturbances in the brain

3. _____ pathological condition associated with the formation of small plaques in the cerebral cortex

4. _____ eating disorder characterized by binging and purging

5. _____ alternate contraction and relaxation of muscles

6. _____ acute polyneuritis with progressive muscle weakness in extremities

7. _____ type of neurosis characterized by irrational fears

8. _____ mental disorder that causes unusual shifts in mood, emotion, and energy

9. _____ inflammation of the arachnoid and pia mater

10. _____ weakness, debility, or loss of strength

11. _____ disease caused by the same organism that causes chickenpox in children

12. _____ abnormal activity or lack of response to normal stimuli; sluggishness

13. _____ paralysis of the lower portion of the trunk and both legs

14. _____ disease that causes inflammation of the gray matter of the spinal cord

15. _____ disease in which the brain fails to receive an adequate supply of oxygen

16. _____ denoting stroke symptoms that resolve within 24 hours

17. _____ severe seizure characterized by spastic, involuntary muscle contraction, and, sometimes, loss of consciousness

18. _____ disease characterized by head nodding, bradykinesia, tremors, and shuffling gait

19. _____ disease characterized by demyelination in the spinal cord and brain

20. _____ loss of consciousness caused by trauma to the head

✓ Check your answers in Appendix A. Review any material that you did not answer correctly.

**CORRECT ANSWERS** _____ × 5 = _____ **% SCORE**

## Learning Activity 14–4

## Matching procedures, pharmacology, and abbreviations

_Match the following terms with the definitions in the numbered list._

| | | |
|---|---|---|
| _analgesics_ | _electromyography_ | _PET_ |
| _antipsychotics_ | _encephalography_ | _psychostimulants_ |
| _cerebral angiography_ | _general anesthetics_ | _tractotomy_ |
| _cryosurgery_ | _hypnotics_ | _trephination_ |
| _CSF analysis_ | _myelography_ | |
| _echoencephalography_ | _NVC_ | |

1. _____ tests the speed at which impulses travel through a nerve

2. _____ treat narcolepsy and attention-deficit hyperactivity disorder (ADHD) in children and adults

3. _____ treat hallucinations, delusions, agitation, paranoia, and symptoms associated with schizophrenia

4. _____ act upon the brain to produce complete loss of feeling with loss of consciousness

5. _____ ultrasound technique used to study the intracranial structures of the brain

6. _____ technique that employs extreme cold to destroy tissue

7. _____ radiological examination of the spinal canal, nerve roots, and spinal cord

8. _____ visualization of the cerebrovascular system after injection of radiopaque dye

9. _____ laboratory test used to diagnose viral and bacterial infections, tumors, and hemorrhage

10. _____ recording of electrical signals when a muscle is at rest and during contraction to assess nerve damage

11. _____ agents that relieve or eliminate pain

12. _____ scan using computed tomography to record the positrons emitted from a radiopharmaceutical

13. _____ transection of a nerve tract in the brainstem or spinal cord

14. _____ agents that depress central nervous system (CNS) functions and promote sedation and sleep

15. _____ cutting a circular opening into the skull to reveal brain tissue and decrease intracranial pressure

✓ Check your answers in Appendix A. Review any material that you did not answer correctly.

**CORRECT ANSWERS** _____ × **6.67** = _____ **% SCORE**

# MEDICAL RECORD ACTIVITIES

The two medical records included in the activities that follow use common clinical scenarios to show how medical terminology is used to document patient care. Complete the terminology and analysis sections for each activity to help you recognize and understand terms related to the nervous system.

## Medical Record Activity 14–1

### Subarachnoid hemorrhage

#### Terminology

The terms listed in the chart come from the medical record *Subarachnoid Hemorrhage* that follows. Use a medical dictionary such as *Taber's Cyclopedic Medical Dictionary*, the appendices of this book, or other resources to define each term. Then review the pronunciations for each term and practice by reading the medical record aloud.

| Term | Definition |
|------|------------|
| **aneurysm**<br>ĂN-ū-rĭzm | |
| **cerebral MRI** | |
| **cisterna subarachnoidalis**<br>sĭs-TĔR-nă sŭb-ă-răk-NOYD-ă-lĭs | |
| **CSF** | |
| **CT scan** | |
| **hydrocephalus**<br>hī-drō-SĔF-ă-lŭs | |
| **lumbar puncture**<br>LŬM-băr PŬNK-chūr | |
| **meningismus**<br>mĕn-ĭn-JĬS-mŭs | |
| **occipital**<br>ŏk-SĬP-ĭ-tăl | |
| **R/O** | |
| **subarachnoid**<br>sŭb-ă-RĂK-noyd | |

### SUBARACHNOID HEMORRHAGE

**HISTORY OF PRESENT ILLNESS:** The patient is a 61-year-old woman with a history of developing sudden onset of "extremely severe headaches" while swimming. She had associated neck pain, occipital pain, nausea, and vomiting.

A CT scan was obtained that showed blood in the cisterna subarachnoidalis consistent with subarachnoid hemorrhage. The patient also had mild acute hydrocephalus. Neurologically, the patient was found to be within normal limits. A cerebral MRI was performed and no aneurysm was noted. The patient was hospitalized on 7/5/xx. On 7/7/xx, she had sudden worsening of her headache associated with nausea and vomiting. Also, she was noted to have meningismus on examination. A lumbar puncture was performed to R/O possible rebleed. At the time of the lumbar puncture, CSF in four tubes was read as consistent with recurrent subarachnoid hemorrhage. A repeat MRI was performed without evidence of an aneurysm.

**PROCEDURE:** On 7/16/xx, the patient underwent repeat MRI, which again showed no aneurysm. The patient was deemed stable for discharge on 7/16/xx.

**ACTIVITY:** She was instructed to avoid any type of activity that could result in raised pressure in the head. The patient was advised that she should undergo no activity more vigorous than walking.

**DISCHARGE DIAGNOSIS:** Subarachnoid hemorrhage

## Analysis

**Review the medical record *Subarachnoid Hemorrhage* to answer the following questions.**

1. In what part of the head did the patient feel pain?

   _____

2. What imaging tests were performed, and what was the finding in each test?

   _____

3. How does meningismus differ from meningitis?

   _____

4. Did the lumbar puncture rule out or confirm a second subarachnoid hemorrhage?

   _____

# Medical Record Activity 14-2

## Consultation report: Acute onset paraplegia

### Terminology

The terms listed in the chart come from the medical record *Consultation Report: Acute Onset Paraplegia* that follows. Use a medical dictionary such as *Taber's Cyclopedic Medical Dictionary*, the appendices of this book, or other resources to define each term. Then review the pronunciations for each term and practice by reading the medical record aloud.

| Term | Definition |
| --- | --- |
| **abscess** <br> ĂB-sĕs | |
| **acute** <br> ă-KŪT | |
| **clonidine** <br> KLŌ-nĭ-dēn | |
| **epidural** <br> ĕp-ĭ-DOO-răl | |
| **fluoroscopy** <br> floo-ŏr-ŎS-kō-pē | |
| **infarct** <br> ĬN-fărkt | |
| **L2-3** | |
| **lumbar** <br> LŬM-băr | |
| **methadone** <br> MĔTH-ă-dōn | |
| **myelitis** <br> mī-ĕ-LĪ-tĭs | |
| **paraplegia** <br> păr-ă-PLĒ-jē-ă | |
| **paresthesia** <br> păr-ĕs-THĒ-zē-ă | |
| **subarachnoid** <br> sŭb-ă-RĂK-noyd | |
| **T10-11** | |
| **transverse** <br> trăns-VĔRS | |

## CONSULTATION REPORT: ACUTE ONSET PARAPLEGIA

**DATE OF CONSULTATION:** 4/14/xx

**HISTORY OF PRESENT ILLNESS:** This is a 41-year-old, right-handed, white female with a history of low back pain for the past 15 to 20 years after falling at work. She has had four subsequent lumbar surgeries, with the most recent in July 20xx. She was admitted to the hospital for pain management. The patient had a subarachnoid catheter placement for pain control and management, placed 4/10/xx, at the L2–3 level with the catheter placed at the T10–11 level. This was followed by trials of clonidine for hypertension and methadone for pain control, with bladder retention noted after clonidine administration. Upon catheter removal the patient noted the subacute onset of paresis, paresthesias, and pain in the legs approximately $2\frac{1}{2}$ to 3 hours later. We were consulted neurologically for assessment of the lower extremity weakness.

**IMPRESSION AND PLAN:** The patient has symptoms of acute onset paraplegia. Differential diagnoses include a subarachnoid hemorrhage, epidural abscess, and transverse myelitis. The patient will be placed on I.V. steroids with compression stockings for lymphedema should physical therapy be cleared by cardiology for manipulation of that region. Documentation of spinal fluid will be obtained under fluoroscopy. Her glucose and blood pressures must be carefully monitored.

## Analysis

Review the medical record *Consultation Report: Acute Onset Paraplegia* to answer the following questions.

1. What was the original cause of the patient's current problems and what treatments were provided?

   _____

2. Why was the patient admitted to the hospital?

   _____

3. What intravenous medications did the patient receive and why was each given?

   _____

4. What was the cause of bladder retention?

   _____

5. What occurred after the catheter was removed?

   _____

6. What three disorders were listed in the differential diagnosis?

   _____

# Chapter

# 15

# Special Senses

## CHAPTER OUTLINE

## OBJECTIVES

*Upon completion of this chapter, you will be able to:*

■ Locate and describe the structures of the eye and ear.

■ Recognize, pronounce, spell, and build words related to the special senses.

■ Describe pathological conditions, diagnostic and therapeutic procedures, and other terms related to the special senses.

- Explain pharmacology related to the treatment of eye and ear disorders.
- Demonstrate your knowledge of this chapter by completing the learning and medical record activities.

 **Key Terms**

This section introduces important terms associated with the special senses and their definitions. Word analyses are also provided.

| Term | Definition |
|------|------------|
| **accommodation**<br>ă-kŏm-ō-DĀ-shŭn | Adjustment of the eye for various distances so that the image falls on the retina of the eye |
| **acuity**<br>ă-KŪ-ĭ-tē | Clearness or sharpness of a sensory function |
| **adnexa**<br>ăd-NĔK-să | Tissues or structures in the body adjacent to or near a related structure<br>*The adnexa of the eye include the extraocular muscles, orbits, eyelids, conjunctiva, and lacrimal apparatus.* |
| **articulate**<br>ăr-TĬK-ū-lāt | To join or connect together loosely to allow motion between the parts |
| **gustation**<br>gŭs-TĀ-shŭn | Sense and act of tasting foods, beverages, or other substances |
| **humor**<br>HŪ-mor | Any fluid or semifluid of the body |
| **labyrinth**<br>LĂB-ĭ-rĭnth | Series of intricate communicating passages<br>*The labyrinth of the ear includes the cochlea, semicircular canals, and vestibule.* |
| **olfaction**<br>ŏl-FĂK-shŭn | The act and sense of smelling<br>*The sense of smell depends on airborne chemicals that stimulate receptors located in the deep nasal cavity. It not only warns of danger (such as from smoke or caustic chemicals) but may also influence mood, memory, emotions, and even the functioning of the immune and endocrine systems.* |
| **ossicle**<br>ŎS-ĭ-kŭl | Any small bone, especially one of the three bones of the ear |
| **photopigment**<br>fō-tō-PĬG-mĕnt | Light-sensitive pigment in the retinal cones and rods that absorbs light and initiates the visual process; also called *visual pigment* |
| **slit lamp** | Microscope with a specialized light that allows magnification of eye structures—especially the lens, cornea, and iris—and, with additional attachments, the vitreous humor and retina |
| **tunic**<br>TŪ-nĭk | A layer or coat of tissue; also called *membrane layer*<br>*The fibrous, vascular, and sensory tunics are the three tunics of the eyeball.* |

## Anatomy and Physiology

General sensations perceived by the body include touch, pressure, pain, and temperature. These sensations are not identified with any specific site of the body. Specific sensations include smell **(olfaction),** taste **(gustation),** vision, hearing **(audition),** and balance. Each sensation is connected to a specific organ or structure in the body. (For a discussion of olfaction, see Chapter 7, Respiratory System, and for a discussion of gustation, see Chapter 6, Digestive System.) This chapter presents information on the sense of vision provided by the eye and senses of hearing and equilibrium provided by the ear.

## Eye

The eye is a globe-shaped organ composed of three distinct **tunics,** or layers: the fibrous tunic, the vascular tunic, and the sensory tunic. (See Figure 15–1.)

### Fibrous Tunic

The outermost layer of the eyeball, the fibrous tunic, serves as a protective coat for the more sensitive structures beneath. It includes the (1) **sclera** and the (2) **cornea.** The sclera, or "white of the eye," provides strength, shape, and structure to the eye. As the sclera passes in front of the eye, it bulges forward to become the cornea. Rather than being opaque, the cornea is transparent, allowing light to enter the interior of the eye. The cornea is one of the few body

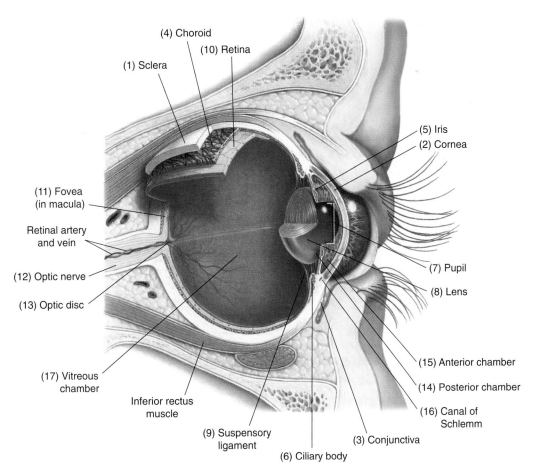

**Figure 15–1** Eye structures.

structures that does not contain capillaries and must rely on eye fluids for nourishment. A thin membrane, the (3) **conjunctiva,** covers the outer surface of the eye and lines the eyelids.

## Vascular Tunic

The middle layer of the eyeball, the vascular tunic, is also known as the *uvea.* The uvea consists of the choroid, iris, and ciliary body. The (4) **choroid** provides the blood supply for the entire eye. It contains pigmented cells that prevent extraneous light from entering the inside of the eye. An opening in the choroid allows the optic nerve to enter the inside of the eyeball. The anterior portion of the choroid contains two modified structures, the (5) **iris** and the (6) **ciliary body.** The iris is a colored, contractile membrane whose perforated center is called the (7) **pupil.** The iris regulates the amount of light passing through the pupil to the interior of the eye. As environmental light increases, the pupil constricts and as light decreases, the pupil dilates. The ciliary body is a circular muscle that produces aqueous humor. The ciliary body is attached to a capsular bag that holds the (8) **lens** by the (9) **suspensory ligaments.** As the ciliary muscle contracts and relaxes, it alters the shape of the lens making it thicker or thinner. These changes in shape allow the eye to focus on an image, a process called **accommodation.**

## Sensory Tunic

The innermost sensory tunic is the delicate, double-layered (10) **retina.** It consists of a thin, outer *pigmented layer* lying over the choroid and a thick, inner *nervous layer,* or visual portion. The retina is responsible for the reception and transmission of visual impulses to the brain. It has two types of visual receptors called *rods* and *cones.* Rods function in dim light and produce black-and-white vision. Cones function in bright light and produce color vision. The (11) **fovea** is in the center of the macula. All of its receptors are cones that lie very close to each other. It provides the greatest **acuity** for color vision. When the eye focuses on an object, light rays from that object are directed to the fovea.

## Other Structures

Rods and cones contain a chemical called **photopigment,** or *visual pigment.* As light strikes the photopigment, a chemical change occurs that stimulates rods and cones. The chemical changes produce impulses that are transmitted through the (12) **optic nerve** to the brain, where they are interpreted as vision. Both the optic nerve and blood vessels of the eye enter at the (13) **optic disc.** Its center is referred to as the *blind spot* because the area has neither rods nor cones for vision.

One of two major fluids (**humors**) of the eye is **aqueous humor.** It is found in the (14) **posterior chamber** and (15) **anterior chamber** and provides nourishment for the lens and the cornea. Aqueous humor is continually produced by the ciliary body and is drained from the eye through a small opening called the (16) **canal of Schlemm.** If aqueous humor fails to drain from the eye at the rate at which it is produced, a condition called *glaucoma* results. The second major humor of the eye is **vitreous humor,** a jellylike substance that fills the interior of eye, the (17) **vitreous chamber.** The vitreous humor, lens, and aqueous humor are the refractive structures of the eye. They bend light rays, focusing them sharply on the retina. If any one of these structures does not function properly, vision is impaired.

The **adnexa** of the eye include all supporting structures of the eye globe. Six muscles control the movement of the eye: the superior, inferior, lateral, and medial rectus muscles and the superior and inferior oblique muscles. These muscles coordinate the eyes so that they move in a synchronized manner.

Two movable folds of skin constitute the eyelids, each with eyelashes that protect the front of the eye. (See Figure 15–2.) The (1) **conjunctiva** lines the inner surface of the eyelids and the cornea. Lying superior and to the outer edge of each eye are the (2) **lacrimal glands,** which produce tears that bathe and lubricate the eyes. The tears collect at the inner edges of the eyes, the *canthi* (singular, *canthus*), and pass through pinpoint openings, the (3) **lacrimal canals,** to the mucous membranes that line the inside of the (4) **nasal cavity.**

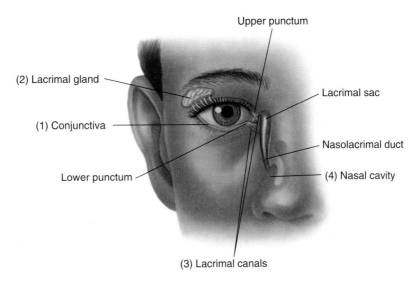

Upper punctum

(2) Lacrimal gland

Lacrimal sac

(1) Conjunctiva

Nasolacrimal duct

Lower punctum

(4) Nasal cavity

(3) Lacrimal canals

**Figure 15–2**    Lacrimal apparatus.

## Ear

The ear is the sense receptor organ for hearing and equilibrium. Hearing is a function of the cochlea; the semicircular canals and vestibule control equilibrium.

### Hearing

The ear consists of three major sections: the outer or **external ear,** the middle ear or **tympanic cavity,** and the inner ear or **labyrinth.** (See Figure 15–3.) Each of these sections transmits sound waves differently. The external ear conducts sound waves through air; the middle ear, through bone; and the inner ear, through fluid. This series of transmissions ultimately generates impulses that are sent to and interpreted by the brain as sound.

   An (1) **auricle** (or **pinna**) collects waves traveling through air and channels them to the (2) **external auditory canal,** also called the *ear canal.* The ear canal is a slender tube lined with glands that produce a waxy secretion called **cerumen.** Its stickiness traps tiny foreign particles and prevents them from entering the deeper areas of the canal. The (3) **tympanic membrane** (also called the *tympanum* or *eardrum*) is a flat, membranous structure drawn over the end of the ear canal. Sound waves entering the ear canal strike against the tympanic membrane, causing it to vibrate. Its movement causes movement of the three smallest bones of the body, collectively called the *ossicles.* These tiny articulating bones, the (4) **malleus** (hammer), the (5) **incus** (anvil), and the (6) **stapes** (stirrups), are located within the tympanic cavity and form a coupling between the tympanic membrane and the (7) **cochlea,** the first structure of the inner ear. The malleus is attached to the eardrum and **articulates** with the incus. The stapes articulates with the incus and is attached to cochlea. The cochlea is a snail-shaped structure, filled with a fluid called perilymph. Its inner surfaces are lined with a highly sensitive hearing structure called the *organ of Corti,* which contains tiny nerve endings called the *hair cells.* A membrane-covered opening on the external surface of the cochlea called the (8) **oval window** provides a place for attachment of the stapes. The movement of the ossicles in the middle ear causes the stapes to exert a gentle pumping action against the oval window. The pumping action forces the perilymph to disturb the hair cells, generating impulses that are transmitted to the brain by way of the auditory nerve, where they are interpreted as sound. The (9) **eustachian tube** connects the middle ear to the pharynx. It equalizes pressure on the outer and inner surfaces of the eardrum. When sudden pressure changes occur, pressure can be equalized on either side of the tympanic membrane by deliberate swallowing.

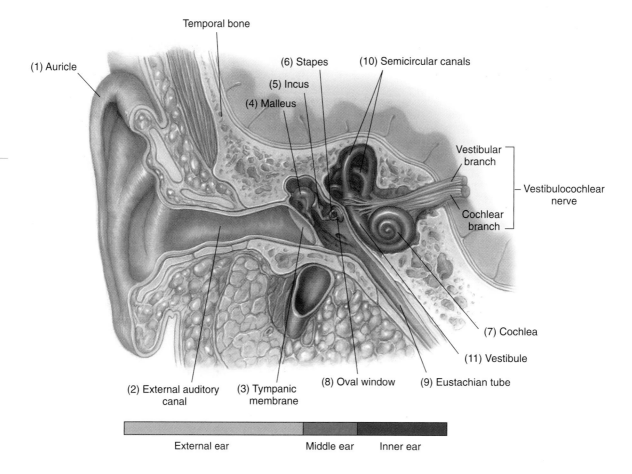

**Figure 15–3**  Ear structures.

## Equilibrium

The inner ear consists of a system of fluid-filled tubes and sacs as well as the nerves that connect these structures to the brain. Because of its mazelike design, it is referred to as the *labyrinth*. The labyrinth, which rests inside the bone of the skull, includes not only the cochlea (the organ devoted to hearing) but also the vestibular system, which is devoted to the control of balance and eye movements. The vestibular system contains the (10) **semicircular canals** and the (11) **vestibule.** The vestibule joins the cochlea and the semicircular canals. Many complex structures located in this maze are responsible for maintaining both **static** and **dynamic equilibrium.** Static equilibrium refers to the orientation of the body relative to gravity. It allows an individual to maintain posture and orientation while at rest. Dynamic equilibrium refers to maintaining body position in response to movement.

 **It is time to review eye and ear anatomy by completing Learning Activities 15–1 and 15–2.**

## Medical Word Elements

This section introduces combining forms, suffixes, and prefixes related to the special senses. Word analyses are also provided.

| Element | Meaning | Word Analysis |
|---|---|---|
| **COMBINING FORMS** | | |
| **Eye** | | |
| **ambly/o** | dull, dim | ambly/opia (ăm-blē-Ō-pē-ă): reduction or dimness of vision<br>*-opia:* vision |
| **aque/o** | water | aque/ous (Ā-kwē-ŭs): pertaining to water<br>*-ous:* pertaining to, relating to |
| **blephar/o** | eyelid | blephar/o/ptosis (blĕf-ă-rō-TŌ-sĭs): drooping of the upper eyelid<br>*-ptosis:* prolapse, downward displacement |
| **choroid/o** | choroid | choroid/o/pathy (kō-roy-DŎP-ă-thē): any disease of the choroid<br>*-pathy:* disease |
| **core/o** | pupil | core/o/meter (kō-rē-ŎM-ĕ-tĕr): instrument for measuring the pupil<br>*-meter:* instrument for measuring |
| **pupill/o** | | pupill/o/graphy (pū-pĭ-LŎG-ră-fē): process of recording movement of the pupil<br>*-graphy:* process of recording |
| **conjunctiv/o** | conjunctiva | conjunctiv/al (kŏn-jŭnk-TĪ-văl): pertaining to the conjunctiva<br>*-al:* pertaining to, relating to |
| **corne/o** | cornea | corne/al (KOR-nē-ăl): pertaining to the cornea<br>*-al:* pertaining to, relating to |
| **kerat/o** | horny tissue; hard; cornea | kerat/o/tomy (kĕr-ă-TŎT-ō-mē): incision of the cornea<br>*-tomy:* incision |
| **cycl/o** | ciliary body of eye; circular, cycle | cycl/o/plegia (sī-klō-PLĒ-jē-ă): paralysis of the ciliary body<br>*-plegia:* paralysis |

*(Continued)*

| Element | Meaning | Word Analysis | *(Continued)* |
|---|---|---|---|
| **dacry/o** | tear; lacrimal apparatus (duct, sac, or gland) | dacry/oma (dăk-rē-Ō-mă): tumorlike swelling due to obstruction of the lacrimal duct<br><br>*-oma:* tumor | |
| **lacrim/o** | | lacrim/o/tome (LĂK-rĭ-mō-tōm): instrument used for incising the lacrimal sac or duct<br><br>*-tome:* instrument to cut | |
| **dacryocyst/o** | lacrimal sac | dacryocyst/o/ptosis (dăk-rē-ō-sĭs-tŏp-TŌ-sĭs): prolapse of the lacrimal sac<br><br>*-ptosis:* prolapse, downward displacement | |
| **glauc/o** | gray | glauc/oma (glaw-KŌ-mă): increased intraocular pressure that destroys the retina and optic nerve if not treated<br><br>*-oma:* tumor<br><br>*Poor blood flow to the back of the eye causes the optic nerve to appear pale gray, hence the name* glaucoma. | |
| **goni/o** | angle | goni/o/scopy (gŏ-nē-ŌS-kŏ-pē): examination of the angle and drainage area of the eye<br><br>*-scopy:* visual examination<br><br>*Gonioscopy is used to differentiate the two forms of glaucoma (open- and closed-angle).* | |
| **irid/o** | iris | irid/o/plegia (ĭr-ĭd-ō-PLĒ-jē-ă): paralysis of the sphincter of the iris<br><br>*-plegia:* paralysis | |
| **ocul/o** | eye | ocul/o/myc/osis (ŏk-ū-lō-mī-KŌ-sĭs): fungal infection of the eye or its parts<br><br>*myc:* fungus<br>*-osis:* abnormal condition; increase (used primarily with blood cells) | |
| **ophthalm/o** | | opthalm/o/logist (ŏf-thăl-MŌL-ō-jĭst): physician specializing in treating disorders of the eye<br><br>*-logist:* specialist in study of | |
| **opt/o** | eye, vision | opt/o/kinet/ic (ŏp-tō-kĭ-NĔT-ĭk): pertaining to the twitching movement of the eyes, as in nystagmus<br><br>*kinet:* movement<br>*-ic:* pertaining to, relating to | |
| **optic/o** | | optic/al (ŎP-tĭ-kăl): pertaining to the eye or vision<br><br>*-al:* pertaining to, relating to | |
| **phac/o** | lens | phac/o/cele (FĂK-ō-sēl): displacement of the crystalline lens into the interior chamber of the eye<br><br>*-cele:* hernia, swelling | |

| Element | Meaning | Word Analysis |
|---|---|---|
| **phot/o** | light | phot/o/phobia (fō-tō-FŌ-bē-ă): abnormal intolerance and sensitivity to light<br>*-phobia:* fear |
| **presby/o** | old age | presby/opia (prĕz-bē-Ō-pē-ă): loss of accommodation of the crystalline lens associated with the aging process<br>*-opia:* vision |
| **retin/o** | retina | retin/osis (rĕt-ĭ-NŌ-sĭs): any degenerative process of the retina not associated with inflammation<br>*-osis:* abnormal condition; increase (used primarily with blood cells) |
| **scler/o** | hardening; sclera (white of eye) | scler/o/malacia (sklĕ-rō-mă-LĀ-shē-ă): softening of the sclera<br>*-malacia:* softening |
| **scot/o** | darkness | scot/oma (skō-TŌ-mă): islandlike blind spot in the visual field<br>*-oma:* tumor |
| **vitr/o** | vitreous body (of eye) | vitr/ectomy (vĭ-TRĔK-tō-mē): removal of the contents of the vitreous chamber and replacing with sterile saline<br>*-ectomy:* excision, removal<br>*The removal of the vitreous allows surgical procedures that would otherwise be impossible, including repair of macular holes and tears in the retina.* |

### Ear

| Element | Meaning | Word Analysis |
|---|---|---|
| **audi/o** | hearing | audi/o/meter (aw-dē-ŎM-ĕ-tĕr): instrument used to measure hearing<br>*-meter:* instrument for measuring |
| **aur/o** | ear | bi/aur/al (bī-AW-răl): pertaining to both ears<br>*bi-:* two<br>*-al:* pertaining to, relating to |
| **ot/o** | | ot/o/py/o/rrhea (ō-tō-pī-ō-RĒ-ă): discharge of pus from the ear<br>*py/o:* pus<br>*-rrhea:* discharge, flow |
| **labyrinth/o** | labyrinth (inner ear) | labyrinth/o/tomy (lăb-ĭ-rĭn-THŎT-ō-mē): incision of the labyrinth<br>*-tomy:* incision |
| **mastoid/o** | mastoid process | mastoid/ectomy (măs-toyd-ĔK-tō-mē): removal of the mastoid process<br>*-ectomy:* excision, removal |

*(Continued)*

| Element | Meaning | Word Analysis | (Continued) |
|---|---|---|---|
| **salping/o** | tubes (usually fallopian or eustachian [auditory] tubes) | salping/o/scope (săl-PĬNG-gō-skōp): instrument to examine the eustachian tubes<br>*-scope:* instrument to view or examine | |
| **staped/o** | stapes | staped/ectomy (stā-pĕ-DĔK-tō-mē): excision of the stapes to improve hearing, especially in cases of otosclerosis<br>*-ectomy:* excision, removal | |
| **myring/o** | tympanic membrane (eardrum) | myring/o/myc/osis (mĭr-ĭn-gō-mĭ-KŌ-sĭs): inflammation of the tympanic membrane as a result of a fungal infection<br>*myc:* fungus<br>*-osis:* abnormal condition; increase (used primarily with blood cells) | |
| **tympan/o** | | tympan/o/stomy (tĭm-pă-NŎS-tō-mē): forming an opening in the tympanic membrane, usually for tube insertion<br>*-stomy:* forming an opening (mouth) | |

**SUFFIXES**

| Element | Meaning | Word Analysis | |
|---|---|---|---|
| **-opia** | vision | dipl/opia (dĭp-LŌ-pē-ă): double vision<br>*dipl-:* double, twofold | |
| **-opsia** | | heter/opsia (hĕt-ĕr-ŎP-sē-ă): inequality of vision in the two eyes<br>*heter-:* different | |
| **-tropia** | turning | eso/tropia (ĕs-ō-TRŌ-pē-ă): marked turning inward of the eyes; also called *convergent strabismus*<br>*eso-:* inward | |
| **-acusia** | hearing | an/acusia (ăn-ă-KŪ-sē-ă): deafness<br>*an-:* without, not | |
| **-cusis** | hearing | presby/cusis (prĕz-bĭ-KŪ-sĭs): progressive hearing loss due to the aging process<br>*presby:* old age | |

**PREFIXES**

| Element | Meaning | Word Analysis | |
|---|---|---|---|
| **exo-** | outside, outward | exo/tropia (ĕks-ō-TRŌ-pē-ă): abnormal turning outward of one or both eyes; also called *divergent strabismus*<br>*-tropia:* turning | |
| **hyper-** | excessive, above normal | hyper/opia (hī-pĕr-Ō-pē-ă): farsightedness<br>*-opia:* vision | |

 **It is time to review medical word elements by completing Learning Activity 15–3.**

## Pathology

For diagnosis, treatment, and management of visual disorders, the medical services of a specialist may be warranted. *Ophthalmology* is the medical specialty concerned with disorders of the eye. The physician who treats these disorders is called an *ophthalmologist*. *Optometrists* either work with ophthalmologists in a medical practice or practice independently. Optometrists are not medical doctors, but are doctors of optometry (OD). They diagnose vision problems and eye disease, prescribe eyeglasses and contact lenses, and prescribe drugs to treat eye disorders. Although they cannot perform surgery, they commonly provide preoperative and postoperative care.

For diagnosis, treatment, and management of hearing disorders, the medical services of a specialist may be warranted. *Otolaryngology* is the medical specialty concerned with disorders of the ear, nose, and throat. The physician who treats these disorders is called an *otolaryngologist*. Many otolaryngologists employ *audiologists*. Audiologists are allied health care professionals who work with patients that have hearing, balance, and related problems. They perform hearing examinations, evaluate hearing loss, clean and irrigate the ear canal, fit and dispense hearing aids or other assistive devices, and provide audiological rehabilitation, including auditory training and instruction in speech or lip reading.

## Eye Disorders

Eye disorders include not only visual deficiencies associated with refractive errors, but also disorders of associated structures, such as the eye muscles, nerves, and blood vessels. A complete examination of the eye and its **adnexa** is necessary to identify the source of any disorder. Most ocular examinations begin by recording visual acuity and visual field. Then the eyelids, pupils, cornea, and lacrimal structures are examined and intraocular pressure is assessed as well. If infection is detected, it must be located and treated by testing eye and nasal discharge cultures and performing CT scans of the sinuses. Occasionally, the patient may be referred for dental examination to determine if abscesses in the mouth are the source of infection. Family history is important because many eye disorders have a genetic predisposition, including glaucoma. Common eye disorders include errors of refraction, cataracts, glaucoma, strabismus, and macular degeneration.

### Errors of Refraction

An error of refraction **(ametropia)** exists when light rays fail to focus sharply on the retina. This may be due to a defect in the lens, cornea, or the shape of the eyeball. If the eyeball is too long, the image falls in front of the retina, causing nearsightedness **(myopia).** (See Figure 15–4.) In farsightedness **(hyperopia, hypermetropia),** the opposite of myopia, the eyeball is too short and the image falls behind the retina. A form of farsightedness is **presbyopia,** a defect associated with the aging process. The onset of presbyopia usually occurs between ages 40 and 45. Distant objects are seen clearly, but near objects are not in proper focus. In another form of ametropia called *astigmatism,* the cornea or lens has a defective curvature. This curvature causes light rays to diffuse over a large area of the retina, rather than being sharply focused.

Corrective lenses usually compensate for the various types of ametropia. An alternative to corrective lenses is laser-assisted *in situ* keratomileusis (LASIK) surgery. This procedure permanently changes the shape of the cornea. A small incision is made in the cornea to produce a flap. The flap is lifted to the side while a laser reshapes the underlying corneal tissue. At the completion of the procedure, the corneal flap is replaced. The procedure usually takes less than 15 minutes. However, not all people are candidates for this surgery. Some

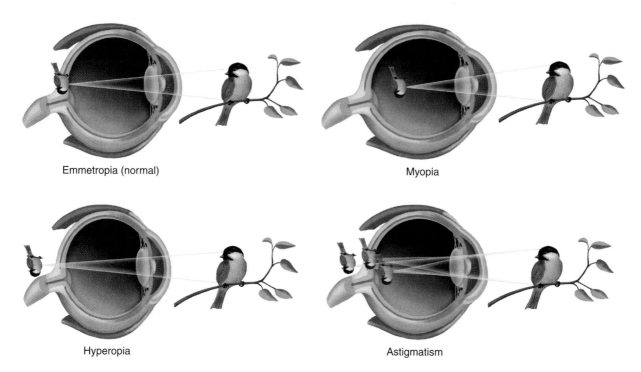

Emmetropia (normal)

Myopia

Hyperopia

Astigmatism

**Figure 15–4**    Refraction of eye.

medical conditions, certain medications, or the shape and structure of the eye may preclude this procedure as a viable alternative to corrective lenses.

## Cataracts

Cataracts are opacities that form on the lens and impair vision. These opacities are commonly produced by protein that slowly builds up over time until vision is lost. The most common form of cataract is age related. More than one-half of Americans older than 65 are affected. Congenital cataracts found in children are usually a result of genetic defects or maternal rubella during the 1st trimester of pregnancy. This rare form of cataract is treated in the same manner as age-related cataract. The usual treatment is removal of the clouded lens by emulsifying it using ultrasound or a laser probe **(phacoemulsification).** (See Figure 15–5.) An artificial, bendable *intraocular lens* (IOL) is then inserted into the capsule. Once in position, the

Artificial lens

Lens capsule

Cataract removal

Artificial lens insertion

**Figure 15–5**    Phacoemulsification.

lens unfolds. The surgery is usually performed using a topical anesthetic, and the incision normally does not require stitches. This is one of the safest and most effective surgical procedures performed in medicine.

## Glaucoma

Glaucoma is characterized by increased intraocular pressure caused by the failure of aqueous humor to drain from the eye through a tiny duct called the *canal of Schlemm*. The increased pressure on the optic nerve destroys it, and vision is permanently lost.

Although there are various forms of glaucoma, all of them eventually lead to blindness unless the condition is detected and treated in its early stages. Glaucoma may occur as a primary or congenital disease or secondary to other causes, such as injury, infection, surgery, or prolonged topical corticosteroid use. Primary glaucoma can be chronic or acute. The chronic form is also called *open-angle, simple,* or *wide-angle glaucoma*. The acute form is called *angle-closure* or *narrow-angle glaucoma*. Chronic glaucoma may produce no symptoms except gradual loss of peripheral vision over a period of years. Headaches, blurred vision, and dull pain in the eye may also be present. Cupping of the optic discs may be noted on ophthalmoscopic examination. Acute glaucoma is accompanied by extreme ocular pain, blurred vision, redness of the eye, and dilation of the pupil. Nausea and vomiting may also occur. If untreated, acute glaucoma causes complete and permanent blindness within 2 to 5 days.

Glaucoma is diagnosed by **tonometry,** a screening test that measures intraocular pressure by determining the resistance of the eyeball to indentation by an applied force. A slit lamp with a high-intensity beam is used to examine the external surface and internal segments of the eye after administration of a local anesthetic. Devices such as a *tonometer,* which measures intraocular pressure, and a *gonioscope,* which visualizes the anterior chamber angle, expand the scope of the examination. (See Figure 15–6.) Several methods of tonometry are available, but the one that is considered most accurate is *applanation tonometry*. Numbing drops are used and the test is pain-free. Treatment for glaucoma includes medications that cause the pupils to constrict **(miotics),** which permits aqueous humor to escape from the eye, thereby relieving pressure. If miotics are ineffective, surgery may be necessary.

**Figure 15–6**   Applanation tonometry using a slit lamp to measure intraocular pressure (courtesy of Richard H. Koop, MD).

## Strabismus

Strabismus, also called *heterotropia* or *tropia*, is a condition in which one eye is misaligned with the other and the eyes do not focus simultaneously when viewing an object. This misalignment may be in any direction—inward **(esotropia)**, outward **(exotropia)**, up, down, or any combination of these. The deviation may be a constant condition or may arise intermittently with stress, exhaustion, or illness. (See Figure 15–7.) In normal vision, each eye views an image from a somewhat different vantage point, thus transmitting a slightly different image to the brain. The result is binocular perception of depth or three-dimensional space, a phenomenon known as *stereopsis*. Strabismus commonly causes a loss of stereopsis. In children, strabismus is commonly but not always associated with "lazy-eye syndrome" **(amblyopia).** Vision is suppressed in the "lazy" eye so that the child uses only the "good" eye for vision. The vision pathway fails to develop in the "lazy" eye.

There is a critical period during which amblyopia must be corrected, usually before age 6. If not detected and treated early in life, amblyopia can cause a permanent loss of vision in the affected eye, with associated loss of stereopsis. Treatment for strabismus depends on the cause. It commonly consists of covering the normal eye, forcing the child to use the deviated one. Eye exercises and corrective lenses may be prescribed, or surgical correction may be necessary.

## Macular Degeneration

Macular degeneration is the deterioration of the macula, the most sensitive portion of the retina. The macula is responsible for central, or "straight-ahead" vision required for reading, driving, detail work, and recognizing faces. (See Figure 15–8.) Although deterioration of the macula is associated with the toxic effects of some drugs, the most common type is age-related macular degeneration (ARMD, or AMD). ARMD is a leading cause of visual loss in the United States. The disease is unpredictable and progresses differently in each individual.

So far, two forms of ARMD have been identified: wet and dry. The less common but more severe form is wet, or *neovascular* ARMD. It affects about 10% of those afflicted with the disease. Small blood vessels form under the macula. Blood and other fluids leak from these vessels and destroy the visual cells, leading to severe loss of central vision and permanent visual impair-

**Figure 15–7**  Types of strabismus.

Normal macula                    Macular degeneration

Normal vision                      Central vision loss

**Figure 15–8**   Macular degeneration.

ment. If identified in its early stages, laser surgery can be employed to destroy the newly form-ing vessels. This treatment is called *laser photocoagulation*. It is successful in about one-half of the patients with wet ARMD. However, the effects of the procedure commonly do not last and new vessels begin to form.

The more common form of the disease is dry ARMD. Small yellowish deposits called *drusen* develop on the macula and interfere with central vision. Drusen are dried retinal pigment epithelial cells that form granules on the macula. Although some vision is lost, this form of the disease rarely leads to total blindness. Patients with dry ARMD are encour-aged to see their ophthalmologist frequently and perform a simple at-home test that iden-tifies visual changes that may indicate the development of the more serious neovascular ARMD.

## Ear Disorders

Common signs and symptoms of ear disorders include hearing loss, earache, vertigo, and tinni-tus. Hearing tests are important in diagnosing hearing loss as well as aiding in localizing the source and nature of the hearing deficiency. In addition, many infections of the nose and throat refer pain to the ear. Therefore, an examination of the nose and throat is usually essential in identifying the cause of ear pain. Common ear disorders include otitis media and otosclerosis.

## Otitis Media

**Otitis media** is an inflammation of the middle ear. This infection may be caused by a virus or bacterium. However, the most common culprit is *Streptococcus pneumoniae.* Otitis media is found most commonly in infants and young children, especially in the presence of an upper respiratory infection (URI). Symptoms may include earache and draining of pus from the ear **(otopyorrhea).** In its most severe form, otitis media may lead to infection of the mastoid process **(mastoiditis)** or inflammation of brain tissue near the middle ear **(otoencephalitis).** Recurrent episodes of otitis media may cause scarring of the tympanic membrane, leading to hearing loss. Treatment consists of bed rest, medications to relieve pain **(analgesics),** and antibiotics. Occasionally, an incision of the eardrum **(myringotomy, tympanotomy)** may be necessary to relieve pressure and promote drainage.

The main treatment for children with recurrent infection is the use of pressure-equalizing tubes (PE tubes) that are passed through the tympanic membrane. These tubes help drain fluid from the middle ear.

## Otosclerosis

**Otosclerosis** is a disorder characterized by an abnormal hardening **(ankylosis)** of bones of the middle ear that causes hearing loss. The ossicle most commonly affected is the stapes, the bone that attaches to the oval window of the cochlea. The formation of a spongy growth at the footplate of the stapes decreases its ability to move the oval window, resulting in hearing loss. Occasionally, the patient perceives a ringing sound **(tinnitus)** within the ear, along with dizziness and a progressive loss of hearing, especially of low tones. Development of otosclerosis is typically closely tied to genetic factors; if one or both parents have the disorder, the child is at high risk for developing the disease. Surgical correction involves removing part of the stapes **(stapedectomy,** or more commonly **stapedotomy)** and implanting of a prosthetic device that allows sound waves to pass to the inner ear. The procedure requires only a local anesthetic and usually lasts only 45 minutes. Hearing is immediately restored.

## Oncology

Two major neoplastic diseases account for more than 90% of all primary intraocular diseases: *retinoblastoma,* found primarily in children, and *melanoma,* found primarily in adults. Most retinoblastomas tend to be familial. The cell involved is the retinal neuron. Vision is impaired, and, in about 30% of patients, the disease is found in both eyes **(bilateral).** Melanoma may occur in the orbit, the bony cavity of the eyeball, the iris, or the ciliary body, but it arises most commonly in the pigmented cells of the choroid. The disease is usually asymptomatic until there is a hemorrhage into the anterior chamber. Any discrete, fleshy mass on the iris should be examined by an ophthalmologist. If malignancy occurs in the choroid, it usually appears as a brown or gray mushroom-shaped lesion.

Treatment for retinoblastoma usually involves the removal of the affected eye(s) **(enucleation),** followed by radiation. In melanoma where the lesion is on the iris, an iridectomy is performed. For melanoma of the choroid, enucleation is necessary. Many eye tumors are noninvasive and are not necessarily life threatening.

**Diagnostic, Symptomatic, and Related Terms**

This section introduces diagnostic, symptomatic, and related terms and their meanings. Word analyses for selected terms are also provided.

| Term | Definition |
|---|---|
| **EYE** | |
| **achromatopsia**<br>ă-krō-mă-TŎP-sē-ă<br><br>*a-:* without, not<br>*chromat:* color<br>*-opsia:* vision | Severe congenital deficiency in color perception; also called *complete color blindness* |
| **chalazion**<br>kă-LĀ-zē-ŏn | Small, hard tumor developing on the eyelid, somewhat similar to a sebaceous cyst |
| **conjunctivitis**<br>kŏn-jŭnk-tĭ-VĪ-tĭs<br><br>*conjunctiv:* conjunctiva<br>*-itis:* inflammation | Inflammation of the conjunctiva with vascular congestion, producing a red or pink eye; may be secondary to viral, chlamydial, bacterial, or fungal infections or allergy |
| **convergence**<br>kŏn-VĔR-jĕnts | Medial movement of the two eyeballs so that they are both directed at the object being viewed |
| **diopter**<br>dī-ŎP-tĕr | Measurement of refractive error<br><br>*A negative diopter value signifies an eye with myopia and a positive diopter value signifies an eye with hyperopia.* |
| **ectropion**<br>ĕk-TRŌ-pē-ŏn | Eversion, or outward turning, of the edge of the lower eyelid |
| **emmetropia**<br>ĕm-ĕ-TRŌ-pē-ă | Normal condition of the eye in refraction in which, when the eye is at rest, parallel rays focus exactly on the retina |
| **entropion**<br>ĕn-TRŌ-pē-ŏn | Inversion, or inward turning, of the edge of the lower eyelid |
| **epiphora**<br>ĕ-PĬF-ō-ră | Abnormal overflow of tears<br><br>*Epiphora is sometimes caused by obstruction of the tear ducts.* |
| **exophthalmos**<br>ĕks-ŏf-THĂL-mŏs | Protrusion of one or both eyeballs<br><br>*Common causes of exophthalmos include hyperactive thyroid, trauma, and tumor.* |
| **hordeolum**<br>hor-DĒ-ō-lŭm | Localized, circumscribed, inflammatory swelling of one of the several sebaceous glands of the eyelid, generally caused by a bacterial infection; also called *sty* |

*(Continued)*

| Term | Definition | (Continued) |
|------|------------|-------------|
| **metamorphopsia**<br>mĕt-ă-mor-FOP-sē-ă<br><br>*meta-:* change; beyond<br>*morph:* form, shape, structure<br>*-opsia:* vision | Visual distortion of objects<br><br>*Metamorphopsia is commonly associated with errors of refraction, retinal disease, choroiditis, detachment of the retina, and tumors of the retina or choroid.* | |
| **nyctalopia**<br>nĭk-tă-LO-pē-ă<br><br>*nyctal:* night<br>*-opia:* vision | Inability to see well in dim light; also called *night blindness*<br><br>*Common causes of nyctalopia include cataracts, vitamin A deficiency, certain medications, and hereditary causes.* | |
| **nystagmus**<br>nĭs-TĂG-mŭs | Involuntary eye movements that appear jerky and may reduce vision or be associated with other, more serious conditions that limit vision | |
| **papilledema**<br>păp-ĭl-ĕ-DĒ-mă | Edema and hyperemia of the optic disc usually associated with increased ocular pressure resulting from intracranial pressure; also called *choked disc* | |
| **photophobia**<br>fō-tō-FO-bē-ă<br><br>*phot/o:* light<br>*-phobia:* fear | Unusual intolerance and sensitivity to light<br><br>*Photophobia commonly occurs in such diseases as meningitis, inflammation of the eyes, measles, and rubella.* | |
| **presbyopia**<br>prĕz-bē-Ō-pē-ă<br><br>*presby:* old age<br>*-opia:* vision | Loss of accommodation of the crystalline lens associated with the aging process<br><br>*During the aging process, proteins in the lens become harder and less elastic and muscle fibers surrounding the lens lose strength. These changes cause a decreased ability to focus, especially at close range.* | |
| **retinopathy**<br>rĕt-ĭn-ŎP-ă-thē<br><br>*retin/o:* retina<br>*-pathy:* disease | Any disorder of retinal blood vessels | |
| **diabetic**<br>dī-ă-BĔT-ĭk | Disorder that occurs in patients with diabetes and is manifested by small hemorrhages, edema, and formation of new vessels on the retina, leading to scarring and eventual loss of vision | |
| **trachoma**<br>trā-KO-mă | Chronic, contagious form of conjunctivitis common in the southwestern United States that typically leads to blindness | |
| **visual field**<br>VĬZH-ū-ăl | Area within which objects may be seen when the eye is in a fixed position | |

### EAR

| | | |
|------|------------|-------------|
| **anacusis**<br>ăn-ă-KŪ-sĭs<br><br>*an-:* without, not<br>*-acusis:* hearing | Deafness; also called *anacusia*<br><br>*Anacusis may be unilateral or bilateral. Hearing loss should not be confused with anacusis, which refers to the complete inability to hear and is commonly congenital.* | |

| Term | Definition |
|---|---|
| **conduction impairment**<br>kŏn-DŬK-shŭn | Blocking of sound waves as they are conducted through the external and middle ear (conduction pathway) |
| **labyrinthitis**<br>lăb-ĭ-rĭn-THĪ-tĭs<br><br>*labyrinth:* labyrinth (inner ear)<br>*-itis:* inflammation | Inflammation of the inner ear that usually results from an acute febrile process<br><br>*Labyrinthitis may lead to progressive vertigo.* |
| **Ménière disease**<br>mĕn-ē-ĀR | Disorder of the labyrinth that leads to progressive loss of hearing<br><br>*Ménière disease is characterized by vertigo, sensorineural hearing loss, and tinnitus.* |
| **otitis externa**<br>ō-TĪ-tĭs ĕks-TĔR-nă<br><br>*ot:* ear<br>*-itis:* inflammation | Infection of the external auditory canal<br><br>*Common causes of otitis externa include exposure to swimming pool water (swimmer's ear), bacterial or fungal infections, seborrhea, eczema, and chronic conditions such as allergies.* |
| **presbyacusis**<br>prĕz-bē-ă-KŪ-sĭs<br><br>*presby:* old age<br>*-acusis:* hearing | Impairment of hearing resulting from old age; also called *presbyacusia*<br><br>*In presbyacusis, patients are generally able to hear low tones but ability to hear higher tones is lost. This condition usually affects speech perception, especially in the presence of background noise, as in a restaurant or a large crowd. This type of hearing loss is irreversible.* |
| **pressure-equalizing (PE) tubes** | Tubes that are inserted through the tympanic membrane, commonly to treat chronic otitis media; also called *tympanostomy tubes* or *ventilation tubes*<br><br>*The average period that PE tubes remain in the ear is about 9 months, at which time they fall out on their own. If they do not fall out, they are removed surgically, usually by age 5 or 6.* |
| **tinnitus**<br>tĭn-Ī-tŭs | Perception of ringing, hissing, or other sounds in the ears or head when no external sound is present<br><br>*Tinnitus may be caused by a blow to the head, ingestion of large doses of aspirin, anemia, noise exposure, stress, impacted wax, hypertension, and certain types of medications and tumors.* |
| **vertigo**<br>VĔR-tĭ-gō | Hallucination of movement, or a feeling of spinning or dizziness<br><br>*Vertigo may be caused by a variety of disorders, including Ménière disease and labyrinthitis.* |

 **It is time to review pathological, diagnostic, symptomatic, and related terms by completing Learning Activity 15–4.**

## Diagnostic and Therapeutic Procedures

This section introduces procedures used to diagnose and treat eye and ear disorders. Descriptions are provided as well as pronunciations and word analyses for selected terms.

| Procedure | Description |
|---|---|
| **DIAGNOSTIC PROCEDURES** | |
| Clinical | |
| **audiometry**<br>aw-dē-ŎM-ĕ-trē<br><br>*audi/o:* hearing<br>*-metry:* act of measuring | Measurement of hearing acuity at various sound wave frequencies<br><br>*In audiometry, pure tones of controlled intensity are delivered through earphones to one ear at a time while the patient indicates if the tone was heard. The minimum intensity (volume) required to hear each tone is graphed.* |
| **caloric stimulation test** | Test that uses different temperatures to assess the vestibular portion of the nerve of the inner ear (acoustic nerve) to determine if nerve damage is the cause of vertigo<br><br>*In the caloric stimulation test, cold and warm water are separately introduced into each ear while electrodes, placed around the eye, record nystagmus. Eyes move in a predictable pattern when the water is introduced, except with acoustic nerve damage.* |
| **electronystagmography**<br>ē-lĕk-trō-nĭs-tăg-MŎG-ră-fē | Method of assessing and recording eye movements by measuring the electrical activity of the extraocular muscles<br><br>*In electronystagmography, electrodes are placed above, below, and to the side of each eye. A ground electrode is placed on the forehead. The electrodes record eye movement relative to the position of the ground electrode.* |
| **ophthalmodynamometry**<br>ŏf-thăl-mō-di-nă-MŎM-ĕ-trē | Measurement of the blood pressure of the retinal vessels<br><br>*Ophthalmodynamometry is a screening test used to determine reduction of blood flow in the carotid artery.* |
| **tonometry**<br>tōn-ŎM-ĕ-trē<br><br>*ton/o:* tension<br>*-metry:* act of measuring | Evaluation of intraocular pressure by measuring the resistance of the eyeball to indentation by an applied force<br><br>*Tonometry is used to detect glaucoma. Several kinds of tonometers can be used. The applanation method of tonometry uses a sensor to depress the cornea and is considered the most accurate method of tonometry.* |
| **visual acuity test**<br>ă-KŪ-i-tē | Part of an eye examination that determines the smallest letters that can be read on a standardized chart at a distance of 20′<br><br>*Visual acuity is expressed as a fraction. The top number refers to the distance from the chart (usually 20′) and the bottom number indicates the distance at which a person with normal eyesight could read the same line. For example 20/40 indicates that the patient correctly read letters at 20′ that could be read by a person with normal vision at 40′.* |

| Procedure | Description |
|---|---|
| **Endoscopic** | |
| **gonioscopy**<br>gō-nē-ŎS-kō-pē<br><br>*goni/o:* angle<br>*-scopy:* visual examination | Examination of the angle of the anterior chamber of the eye to determine ocular motility and rotation and diagnose and manage glaucoma |
| **ophthalmoscopy**<br>ŏf-thăl-MŎS-kō-pē<br><br>*ophthalm/o:* eye<br>*-scopy:* visual examination | Visual examination of the interior of the eye using a handheld instrument called an *ophthalmoscope,* which has various adjustable lenses for magnification and a light source to illuminate the interior of the eye<br><br>*Ophthalmoscopy is used to detect eye disorders as well as disorders of other organs that cause changes in the eye.* |
| **otoscopy**<br>ō-TŎS-kŏ-pē<br><br>*ot/o:* ear<br>*-scopy:* visual examination | Visual examination of the external auditory canal and the tympanic membrane using an otoscope |
| **pneumatic**<br>nū-MĂT-ĭk | Procedure that assesses the ability of the tympanic membrane to move in response to a change in air pressure<br><br>*In pneumatic otoscopy, a tight seal is created in the ear canal and then a very slight positive pressure and then a negative pressure is applied by squeezing and releasing a rubber bulb attached to the pneumatic otoscope. The fluctuation in air pressure causes movement of a normal tympanic membrane.* |
| **retinoscopy**<br>rĕt-ĭn-ŎS-kō-pē<br><br>*retin/o:* retina<br>*-scopy:* visual examination | Evaluation of refractive errors of the eye by projecting a light into the eyes and determining the movement of reflected light rays<br><br>*Retinoscopy is especially important in determining errors of refraction in babies and small children who cannot be refracted by traditional methods.* |
| **Radiographic** | |
| **dacryocystography**<br>dăk-rē-ō-sĭs-TŎG-ră-fē<br><br>*dacryocyst/o:* lacrimal sac<br>*-graphy:* process of recording | Radiographic imaging procedures of the nasolacrimal (tear) glands and ducts<br><br>*Dacryocystography is performed for excessive tearing (epiphora) to determine the cause of hypersecretion of the lacrimal gland or obstruction in the lacrimal passages.* |
| **fluorescein angiography**<br>floo-RĔS-ēn ăn-jē-ŎG-ră-fē<br><br>*angio:* vessel (usually blood or lymph)<br>*-graphy:* process of recording | Assesses blood vessels and their leakage in and beneath the retina by injecting a colored dye (fluorescein) and allowing it to circulate while photographs of the intraocular circulation are recorded<br><br>*Fluorescein angiography facilitates the in vivo study of the retinal circulation and is particularly useful in the management of diabetic retinopathy and macular degeneration, two leading causes of blindness.* |

*(Continued)*

| Procedure | Description | (Continued) |
|---|---|---|

## THERAPEUTIC PROCEDURES

### Clinical

| Procedure | Description |
|---|---|
| **orthoptic training**<br>or-THŎP-tĭk<br>TRĀ-nĭng<br><br>  *orth:* straight<br>  *opt:* eye, vision<br>  *-ic:* pertaining to, relating to | Exercises intended to improve eye movements or visual tracking that use training glasses, prism glasses, or tinted or colored lenses |

### Surgical

| Procedure | Description |
|---|---|
| **blepharectomy**<br>blĕf-ă-RĔK-tō-mē<br><br>  *blephar:* eyelid<br>  *-ectomy:* excision, removal | Excision of a lesion on the eyelid |
| **blepharoplasty**<br>BLĔF-ă-rō-plăs-tē<br><br>  *blephar/o:* eyelid<br>  *-plasty:* surgical repair | Cosmetic surgery that removes fatty tissue called "bags" above and below the eye, which commonly form as a result of the aging process or excessive exposure to the sun |
| **cochlear implant**<br>KŎK-lē-ăr  ĬM-plănt<br><br>  *cochle:* cochlea<br>  *-ar:* pertaining to, relating to | Artificial hearing device that produces useful hearing sensations by electrically stimulating nerves inside the inner ear; also called *bionic ear* |
| **cyclodialysis**<br>sī-klō-dī-ĂL-ĭ-sĭs<br><br>  *cycl/o:* ciliary body of eye;<br>  circular, cycle<br>  *dia:* through, across<br>  *-lysis:* separation; destruction;<br>  loosening | Formation of an opening between the anterior chamber and the suprachoroidal space for the draining of aqueous humor in glaucoma |
| **enucleation**<br>ē-nū-klē-Ā-shŭn | Removal of the eyeball from the orbit<br><br>*Enucleation is performed to treat cancer of the eye when the tumor is large and fills most of the structure.* |
| **evisceration**<br>ē-vĭs-ĕr-Ā-shŭn | Removal of the contents of the eye while leaving the sclera and cornea<br><br>*Evisceration is performed when the blind eye is painful or unsightly. The eye muscles are left intact, and a prothesis is fitted over the shell.* |

| Procedure | Description |
|---|---|
| **keratotomy**<br>kĕr-ă-TŎT-ō-mē<br><br>*kerat/o:* horny tissue; hard; cornea<br>*-tomy:* incision<br>**radial** | Incision of the cornea<br><br>Surgical treatment for nearsightedness<br>*In radial keratotomy, hairline radial incisions of the outer portion of the cornea allow it to flatten, thus correcting nearsightedness.* |
| **mastoid antrotomy**<br>MĂS-toyd<br>ăn-TRŎT-ō-mē | Surgical opening of a cavity within the mastoid process |
| **otoplasty**<br>Ō-tō-plăs-tē<br><br>*ot/o:* ear<br>*-plasty:* surgical repair | Corrective surgery for a deformed or excessively large or small pinna<br>*Otoplasty is also performed to rebuild new ears for those who lost them through burns or other trauma or were born without them.* |
| **phacoemulsification**<br>făk-ō-ē-MŬL-si-fĭ-kā-shŭn | Method of treating cataracts by using ultrasonic waves to disintegrate the cloudy lens, which is then aspirated and removed |
| **sclerostomy**<br>sklē-RŎS-tō-mē<br><br>*scler/o:* hardening; sclera (white of eye)<br>*-stomy:* forming an opening (mouth) | Surgical formation of an opening in the sclera<br>*Sclerostomy is commonly performed in conjunction with surgery for glaucoma.* |
| **tympanoplasty**<br>tĭm-păn-ō-PLĂS-tē<br><br>*tympan/o:* tympanic membrane (eardrum)<br>*-plasty:* surgical repair | Reconstruction of the eardrum, commonly due to a perforation; also called *myringoplasty* |

 **Pharmacology**

Disorders of the eyes and ears are commonly treated with instillation of drops onto the surface of the eye or into the cavity of the ear. The eyes and ears are commonly irrigated with liquid solution to remove foreign objects and to provide topical applications of medications. Pharmacological agents used to treat eye disorders include antibiotics for bacterial eye infections, beta blockers and carbonic anhydrase inhibitors for glaucoma, and ophthalmic decongestants and moisturizers for irritated eyes. Mydriatics and miotics are used, not only to treat eye disorders but also to dilate (mydriatics) and contract (miotics) the pupil during eye examinations. Ear medications include antiemetics to relieve nausea associated with inner ear infections, products to loosen and remove wax buildup in the ear canal, and local anesthetics to relieve pain associated with ear infections. (See Table 15–1.)

## Table 15–1    DRUGS USED TO TREAT SENSORY DISORDERS

This table lists common drug classifications used to treat eye and ear disorders, their therapeutic actions, and selected generic and trade names.

| Classification | Therapeutic Action | Generic and Trade Names |
|---|---|---|
| **Eye** | | |
| **antibiotics, ophthalmic** | Inhibit the growth of microorganisms that infect the eye<br><br>*Ophthalmic antibiotics are dispensed as topical ointments and solutions to treat various bacterial eye infections such as conjunctivitis (pinkeye).* | **erythromycin base**<br>ĕ-rith-rō-MI-sĭn<br> *Del-Mycin, Ilotycin Ophthalmic, Staticin* |
| **antiglaucoma agents** | Treat glaucoma<br><br>*Antiglaucoma agents include beta blockers and carbonic anhydrase inhibitors. Beta blockers block the production of aqueous humor to decrease intraocular pressure and are administered topically as eyedrops. Carbonic anhydrase inhibitors decrease the production of aqueous humor by blocking the enzyme carbonic anhydrase and are given orally.* | **betaxolol**<br>bĕ-TĂK-sō-lŏl<br> *Kerlone*<br>**timolol**<br>TĬ-mō-lŏl<br> *Betimol, Blocadren, Timoptic*<br>**acetazolamide**<br>ăs-ĕt-ă-ZŌL-ă-mĭd<br> *AK-Zol, Dazamide, Diamox* |
| **mydriatics** | Dilate the pupil (mydriasis) and paralyze the muscles of accommodation (cycloplegia)<br><br>*Mydriatics dilate the eye for internal examination and to treat inflammatory conditions of the uveal tract and iris.* | **atropine sulfate**<br>ĂT-rō-pēn SŬL-fāt<br> *Atropine-Care Ophthalmic, Atropisol Ophthalmic* |
| **ophthalmic decongestants** | Constrict the small arterioles of the eye, decreasing redness and relieving conjunctival congestion<br><br>*Ophthalmic decongestants are over-the-counter products that temporarily relieve the itching and minor irritation commonly associated with allergy.* | **tetrahydrozoline**<br>tĕt-ră-hĭ-DRŎZ-ō-lēn<br> *Murine, Visine* |
| **ophthalmic moisturizers** | Soothe dry eyes due to environmental irritants and allergens<br><br>*Ophthalmic moisturizers are administered topically and may also be used to facilitate ophthalmoscopic examination in gonioscopy and ophthalmoscopy.* | **buffered isotonic solutions**<br>BŬ-fĕrd ī-sō-TŎN-ĭk sō-LŪ-shŭnz<br> *Akwa Tears, Refresh Plus, Moisture Eyes* |

## Table 15–1    DRUGS USED TO TREAT SENSORY DISORDERS

| Classification | Therapeutic Action | Generic and Trade Names |
|---|---|---|
| **Ear** | | |
| **antiemetics** | Treat and prevent nausea, vomiting, dizziness, and vertigo by reducing the sensitivity of the inner ear to motion or inhibiting stimuli from reaching the part of the brain that triggers nausea and vomiting<br><br>*Antiemetics are commonly used to treat symptoms of labyrinthitis and vestibular neuritis, which irritate the inner ear and may cause vertigo.* | **meclizine**<br>MĔK-lĭ-zēn<br>*Antivert, Antrizine, Bonine, Meni-D* |
| **otic analgesics** | Provide temporary relief from pain and inflammation associated with otic disorders<br><br>*Otic analgesics may be prescribed for otitis media, otitis externa, and swimmer's ear. Some otic analgesics are also wax emulsifiers.* | **antipyrine and benzocaine**<br>ăn-tĭ-PĪ-rēn, BĔN-zō-kān<br>*Allergan Ear Drops, A/B Otic* |
| **wax emulsifiers** | Loosen and help remove impacted cerumen (ear wax)<br><br>*When excessive wax blocks the canal and causes pain or loss of hearing, the physician may wash it out, vacuum it out, or remove it with special instruments. Alternatively, the physician may recommend various wax emulsifying drops to aid in wax removal.* | **carbamide peroxide**<br>KĂR-bă-mĭd pĕr-ŎK-sīd<br>*Debrox Drops, Murine Ear Drops* |

## Abbreviations

This section introduces abbreviations related to the eye and ear along with their meanings.

| Abbreviation | Meaning |
|---|---|
| **EYE** | |
| **Acc** | accommodation |
| **ARMD, AMD** | age-related macular degeneration |
| **Ast** | astigmatism |
| **D** | diopter (lens strength) |
| **Em** | emmetropia |
| **EOM** | extraocular movement |

*(Continued)*

| Abbreviation | Meaning | (Continued) |
|---|---|---|
| IOL | intraocular lens | |
| IOP | intraocular pressure | |
| mix astig | mixed astigmatism | |
| Myop | myopia | |
| *OD | right eye | |
| OD | Doctor of Optometry | |
| *OS | left eye | |
| *OU | both eyes together | |
| PERRLA | pupils equal, round, and reactive to light and accommodation | |
| RK | radial keratotomy | |
| SICS | small incision cataract surgery | |
| ST | esotropia | |
| VA | visual acuity | |
| VF | visual field | |
| XT | exotropia | |
| **EAR** | | |
| AC | air conduction | |
| *AD | right ear | |
| *AS | left ear | |
| *AU | both ears | |
| BC | bone conduction | |
| ENT | ears, nose, and throat | |
| NIHL | noise-induced hearing loss | |
| PE tube | pressure-equalizing tube (placed in the eardrum) | |

*Although these abbreviations are currently found in medical records and clinical notes, the Joint Commission on Accreditation of Healthcare Organizations (JCAHO) requires their discontinuance. Instead, write out the meanings.

 **It is time to review procedures, pharmacology, and abbreviations by completing Learning Activity 15–5.**

# LEARNING ACTIVITIES

The activities that follow provide review of the special senses terms introduced in this chapter. Complete each activity and review your answers to evaluate your understanding of the chapter.

## Learning Activity 15–1

### Identifying eye structures

*Label the following illustration using the terms listed below.*

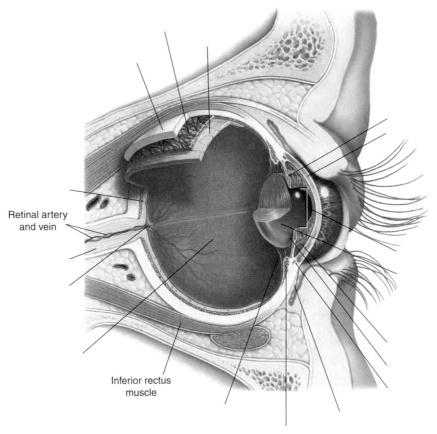

Retinal artery and vein

Inferior rectus muscle

| | | |
|---|---|---|
| *anterior chamber* | *fovea* | *pupil* |
| *canal of Schlemm* | *iris* | *retina* |
| *choroid* | *lens* | *sclera* |
| *ciliary body* | *optic disc* | *suspensory ligaments* |
| *conjunctiva* | *optic nerve* | *vitreous chamber* |
| *cornea* | *posterior chamber* | |

 Check your answers by referring to Figure 15–1 on page 459. Review material that you did not answer correctly.

Learning Activity 15–2

## Identifying ear structures

*Label the following illustration using the terms listed below.*

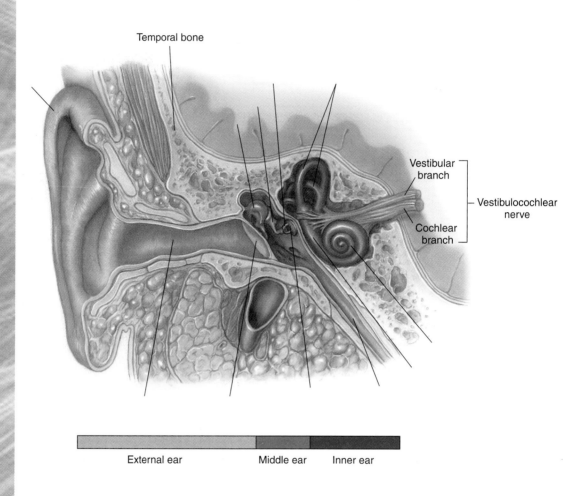

Temporal bone

Vestibular branch

Vestibulocochlear nerve

Cochlear branch

External ear    Middle ear    Inner ear

| | | |
|---|---|---|
| *auricle* | *incus* | *stapes* |
| *cochlea* | *malleus* | *tympanic membrane* |
| *eustachian tube* | *oval window* | *vestibule* |
| *external auditory canal* | *semicircular canals* | |

✓ Check your answers by referring to Figure 15–3 on page 462. Review material that you did not answer correctly.

## Learning Activity 15–3

### Building medical words

---

*Use **ophthalm/o** (eye) to build words that mean:*

1. paralysis of the eye _____
2. study of the eye _____

*Use **pupill/o** (pupil) to build a word that means:*

3. examination of the pupil _____

*Use **kerat/o** (cornea) to build words that mean:*

4. softening of the cornea _____
5. instrument for measuring the cornea _____

*Use **scler/o** (sclera) to build words that mean:*

6. inflammation of the sclera _____
7. softening of the sclera _____

*Use **irid/o** (iris) to build words that mean:*

8. paralysis of the iris _____
9. herniation of the iris _____

*Use **retin/o** (retina) to build words that mean:*

10. disease of the retina _____
11. inflammation of the retina _____

*Use **blephar/o** (eyelid) to build words that mean:*

12. paralysis of the eyelid _____
13. prolapse of the eyelid _____

*Use **ot/o** (ear) to build a word that means:*

14. flow of pus from the ear _____

*Use **audi/o** (hearing) to build a word that means:*

15. instrument for measuring hearing _____

*Use **myring/o** (tympanic membrane [eardrum]) to build a word that means:*

16. instrument for cutting the eardrum _____

*Use the suffix -opia (vision) to build words that mean:*

17. dim or dull vision _____

18. excessive (far-sighted) vision _____

*Use the suffix -acusis (hearing) to build words that mean:*

19. without hearing _____

20. excessive (sensitivity to) hearing _____

*Build surgical words that mean:*

21. removal of the stapes _____

22. incision of the labyrinth _____

23. removal of the mastoid process _____

24. surgical repair of the eardrum _____

25. incision of the cornea _____

Check your answers in Appendix A. Review material that you did not answer correctly.

**CORRECT ANSWERS** _____ × 4 = _____ **% SCORE**

Learning Activity 15–4

## Matching pathological, diagnostic, symptomatic, and related terms

*Match the following terms with the definitions in the numbered list.*

| | | |
|---|---|---|
| *achromatopsia* | *epiphora* | *retinoblastoma* |
| *amblyopia* | *exotropia* | *strabismus* |
| *anacusis* | *gonioscopy* | *tinnitus* |
| *cataract* | *Ménière disease* | *tonometer* |
| *chalazion* | *neovascular* | *vertigo* |
| *diopter* | *nyctalopia* | *visual field* |
| *enucleation* | *otitis externa* | |

1. _____ opacity that forms on the lens and impairs vision
2. _____ complete color blindness
3. _____ inability to see well in dim light
4. _____ examination that determines the angle where the cornea meets the iris
5. _____ deafness
6. _____ infection of the external auditory canal
7. _____ measurement of refractive errors
8. _____ instrument that measures the internal pressure of the eye
9. _____ area in which objects are seen when the eye is in a fixed position
10. _____ abnormal overflow of tears
11. _____ a condition in which one eye is misaligned with the other eye; also called *heterotropia*
12. _____ disorder of the labyrinth that leads to progressive hearing loss
13. _____ refers to the wet form of macular degeneration
14. _____ feeling of dizziness or spinning
15. _____ outward deviation of the eye
16. _____ removal of the eye
17. _____ tumor of the eyelid
18. _____ "lazy-eye" syndrome
19. _____ neoplastic disease of the eye found primarily in children
20. _____ perception of ringing in the ears with no external stimuli

✓ Check your answers in Appendix A. Review any material that you did not answer correctly.

**CORRECT ANSWERS** _____ × 5 = _____ % **SCORE**

Learning Activity 15–5

## Matching procedures, pharmacology, and abbreviations

*Match the following terms with the definitions in the numbered list.*

| | | | |
|---|---|---|---|
| *audiometry* | *evisceration* | *ophthalmoscopy* | *ST* |
| *beta blockers* | *fluorescein angiography* | *otic analgesics* | *tonometry* |
| *caloric stimulation test* | *gonioscopy* | *otoplasty* | *visual acuity test* |
| *cochlear implant* | *mydriatics* | *otoscopy* | *wax emulsifiers* |
| *enucleation* | *ophthalmic decongestants* | *radial keratotomy* | *XT* |

1. _____ test that uses different temperatures to assess the vestibular portion of the nerve

2. _____ visual examination of the interior of the eye

3. _____ artificial device that produces hearing sensations by electrically stimulating nerves inside the inner ear

4. _____ assesses blood vessels and retinal circulation using a colored dye while photographs are taken

5. _____ corrective surgery for excessively large, small, or deformed ears

6. _____ agents that dilate the pupils and paralyze the eye muscles of accommodation

7. _____ measurement of the intraocular pressure for detecting glaucoma

8. _____ determines the smallest letters that can be read on a standardized chart

9. _____ removal of the contents of the eyeball, leaving the sclera and cornea

10. _____ antiglaucoma agents that block the production of aqueous humor

11. _____ loosen and help remove impacted cerumen

12. _____ removal of the entire eyeball from its orbit

13. _____ esotropia

14. _____ constrict small arterioles of the eye to decrease redness and conjunctival congestion

15. _____ exotropia

16. _____ procedure used in diagnosing and managing glaucoma

17. _____ visual examination of the external auditory canal

18. _____ measurement of hearing acuity at various frequencies

19. _____ surgical treatment for nearsightedness that uses small incisions to flatten the cornea

20. _____ provide temporary relief from earache

✓ Check your answers in Appendix A. Review any material that you did not answer correctly.

**CORRECT ANSWERS** _____ × 5 = _____ **% SCORE**

# MEDICAL RECORD ACTIVITIES

The two medical records included in the following activities use common clinical scenarios to show how medical terminology is used to document patient care. Complete the terminology and analysis sections for each activity to help you recognize and understand terms related to the eye and ear.

## Medical Record Activity 15-1

### Retained foreign bodies

#### Terminology

The terms listed in the chart come from the medical record *Retained Foreign Bodies* that follows. Use a medical dictionary such as *Taber's Cyclopedic Medical Dictionary*, the appendices of this book, or other resources to define each term. Then review the pronunciations for each term and practice by reading the medical record aloud.

| Term | Definition |
|------|------------|
| **bilateral** <br> bī-LĂT-ĕr-ăl | |
| **cerumen** <br> sĕ-ROO-mĕn | |
| **perforation** <br> pĕr-fō-RĀ-shŭn | |
| **supine** <br> sū-PĪN | |
| **tympanostomy** <br> tĭm-pă-NŎS-tō-mē | |

### RETAINED FOREIGN BODIES

**PREOPERATIVE DIAGNOSIS:** Foreign body, ears

**POSTOPERATIVE DIAGNOSIS:** Foreign body, ears

**ANESTHESIA:** General

**OPERATIVE INDICATIONS:** The patient is a 9-year-old girl who presents with bilateral retained tympanostomy tubes. The tubes had been placed for more than 2.5 years.

**OPERATIVE FINDINGS:** Retained tympanostomy tubes, bilateral

**PROCEDURE:** Removal of foreign bodies from ears with placement of paper patches.

The risks and alternatives were explained to the mother, and she consented to the surgery. In the supine position under satisfactory general anesthesia via mask, the patient was draped in a routine fashion.

The operating microscope was used to inspect the right ear. A previously placed tympanostomy tube was found to be in position and was surrounded with hard cerumen. The cerumen and the tube were removed, resulting in a very large perforation. The edges of the perforation were freshened sharply with a pick, and a paper patch was applied. The patient tolerated the surgery very well, and was sent to recovery.

## Analysis

**Review the medical record _Retained Foreign Bodies_ to answer the following questions.**

1. Did the patient's surgery involve one or both ears?

   _____

2. What was the nature of the foreign body in the patient's ears?

   _____

3. What ear structure was involved?

   _____

4. What instrument was used to locate the tubes?

   _____

5. What was the material in which the tubes were embedded?

   _____

# Medical Record Activity 15-2

## Phacoemulsification and lens implant

### Terminology

The terms listed in the chart come from the medical record *Phacoemulsification and Lens Implant* that follows. Use a medical dictionary such as *Taber's Cyclopedic Medical Dictionary*, the appendices of this book, or other resources to define each term. Then review the pronunciations for each term and practice by reading the medical record aloud.

| Term | Definition |
|------|------------|
| **anesthesia**<br>ăn-ĕs-THĒ-zē-ă | |
| **blepharostat**<br>BLĔF-ă-rō-stăt | |
| **capsulorrhexis**<br>kăp-sū-lō-RĔK-sĭs | |
| **cataract**<br>KĂT-ă-răkt | |
| **conjunctival**<br>kŏn-jŭnk-TĪ-văl | |
| **diopter**<br>dī-ŎP-tĕr | |
| **intravenous**<br>ĭn-tră-VĒ-nŭs | |
| **keratome**<br>KĔR-ă-tōm | |
| **peritomy**<br>pĕr-ĬT-ō-mē | |
| **phacoemulsification**<br>făk-ō-ē-MŬL-sĭ-fĭ-kā-shŭn | |
| **posterior chamber**<br>pŏs-TĒ-rē-or CHĀM-bĕr | |
| **retrobulbar block**<br>rĕt-rō-BŬL-băr BLŎK | |
| **sutures**<br>SŪ-chūrz | |
| **TobraDex**<br>TŌ-bră-dĕks | |

## PHACOEMULSIFICATION AND LENS IMPLANT

**PREOPERATIVE DIAGNOSIS:** Right eye cataract

**POSTOPERATIVE DIAGNOSIS:** Right eye cataract

**PROCEDURE:** Phacoemulsification, Rt eye, with posterior chamber lens implantation.

This 68-year-old male was brought to the operating suite on 8/4/xx as an outpatient. Intravenous anesthesia and retrobulbar block to the right eye were administered. The rt eye was prepped in the usual manner. A blepharostat was inserted and a surgical microscope was positioned. Conjunctival peritomy was performed. Using a keratome, the anterior chamber was entered at the 12 o'clock position. A capsulorrhexis was performed. The cataract was removed by phacoemulsification.

After confirming the 20.5 diopters on the package, the implant was easily inserted into the capsular bag. The wound was observed and shown to be fluid tight. The incision required no sutures. TobraDex ointment was applied and a sterile patch was taped into place. The patient was monitored until stable. Postoperative care was reviewed, and he was released with instructions to return to the office the following day.

## Analysis

**Review the medical record *Phacoemulsification and Lens Implant* to answer the following questions.**

1. What technique was used to destroy the cataract?

   _____

2. In what portion of the eye was the implant placed?

   _____

3. What anesthetics were used for surgery?

   _____

4. What was the function of the blepharostat?

   _____

5. What was the function of the keratome?

   _____

6. Where was the implant inserted?

   _____

# Answer Key

# CHAPTER 1 — Basic Elements of a Medical Word

## LEARNING ACTIVITY 1–1

### Understanding medical word elements

**Fill in the following blanks to complete the sentences correctly.**

1. root, combining form, suffix, and prefix.
2. teach

**Identify the following statements as true or false. If false, rewrite the statement correctly in the space provided.**

3. False—A combining vowel is usually an "o."
4. False—A combining form links a suffix that begins with a consonant.
5. True
6. True
7. False—To define a medical word, first define the suffix or the end of the word. Second, define the first part of the word. Third, define the middle of the word.
8. True

**Underline the word root in each of following combining forms.**

9. <u>splen</u>/o
10. <u>hyster</u>/o
11. <u>enter</u>/o
12. <u>neur</u>/o
13. <u>ot</u>/o
14. <u>dermat</u>/o
15. <u>hydr</u>/o

## LEARNING ACTIVITY 1–2

### Identifying word roots and combining forms

**Underline the word roots in the following terms.**

1. <u>nephr</u>itis
2. <u>arthr</u>odesis
3. <u>phleb</u>otomy
4. <u>dent</u>ist
5. <u>gastr</u>ectomy
6. <u>chondr</u>itis
7. <u>hepat</u>oma
8. <u>cardi</u>ologist
9. <u>gastr</u>ia
10. <u>oste</u>oma

**Underline the elements below that are combining forms.**

11. nephr
12. <u>cardi/o</u>
13. arthr
14. <u>oste/o</u>/arth
15. <u>cholangi/o</u>

## LEARNING ACTIVITY 1–3

### Identifying suffixes and prefixes

**Analyze each term and write the element from each that is a suffix.**

1. -tomy
2. -scope
3. -itis
4. -itis
5. -ectomy

**Analyze each term and write the element from each that is a prefix.**

6. micro-
7. hyper-
8. macro-
9. intra-
10. a-

## LEARNING ACTIVITY 1–4

### Defining and building medical words

Use the three basic steps to define the following words.

| Term | Definition |
|------|------------|
| 1. **gastritis**<br>găs-TRĪ-tĭs | inflammation of the stomach |
| 2. **nephritis**<br>nĕf-RĪ-tĭs | inflammation of the kidneys |
| 3. **gastrectomy**<br>găs-TRĔK-tō-mē | excision of the stomach |
| 4. **osteoma**<br>ŏs-tē-Ō-mă | tumor of bone |
| 5. **hepatoma**<br>hĕp-ă-TŌ-mă | tumor of the liver |
| 6. **hepatitis**<br>hĕp-ă-TĪ-tĭs | inflammation of the liver |

**Write the number for the rule that applies to each listed term as well as a short summary of the rule.**

| Term | Rule | Summary of the Rule |
|------|------|---------------------|
| 7. **arthr/itis**<br>ăr-THRĪ-tĭs | 1 | A WR links a suffix that begins with a vowel. |
| 8. **scler/osis**<br>sklĕ-RŌ-sĭs | 1 | A WR links a suffix that begins with a vowel. |
| 9. **arthr/o/centesis**<br>ăr-thrō-sĕn-TĒ-sĭs | 2 | A CF links a suffix that begins with a consonant. |
| 10. **colon/o/scope**<br>kō-LŎN-ō-skōp | 2 | A CF links a suffix that begins with a consonant. |
| 11. **chondr/itis**<br>kŏn-DRĪ-tĭs | 1 | A WR links a suffix that begins with a vowel. |
| 12. **chondr/oma**<br>kŏn-DRŌ-mă | 1 | A WR links a suffix that begins with a vowel. |
| 13. **oste/o/chondr/itis**<br>ŏs-tē-ō-kŏn-DRĪ-tĭs | 3 | A CF links multiple roots to each other. This rule holds true even if the next word root begins with a vowel. |
| | 1 | A WR links a suffix that begins with a vowel. |
| 14. **muscul/ar**<br>MŬS-kū-lăr | 1 | A WR links a suffix that begins with a vowel. |
| 15. **oste/o/arthr/itis**<br>ŏs-tē-ō-ăr-THRĪ-tĭs | 3 | A CF links multiple roots to each other. This ŏs-tē-ō-ăr-rule holds true even if the next word root begins with a vowel. |
| | 1 | A WR links a suffix that begins with a vowel. |

## LEARNING ACTIVITY 1–5

### Understanding pronunciations

Review the pronunciation guidelines (located inside the front cover of this book) and then underline the correct answer in each of the following statements.

1. macron
2. breve
3. long
4. short
5. k
6. n
7. is
8. eye
9. second
10. separate

# CHAPTER 2 — Suffixes

## LEARNING ACTIVITY 2–1

### Completing and building surgical words

1. episiotomy
2. colectomy
3. arthrocentesis
4. splenectomy
5. colostomy
6. osteotome
7. tympanotomy
8. tracheostomy
9. mastectomy
10. lithotomy
11. hemorrhoidectomy
12. colostomy
13. colectomy
14. osteotome
15. arthrocentesis
16. lithotomy
17. mastectomy
18. tympanotomy
19. tracheostomy
20. splenectomy

## LEARNING ACTIVITY 2–2

### Completing and building more surgical words

1. arthrodesis
2. rhinoplasty
3. tenoplasty
4. myorrhaphy
5. mastopexy
6. cystorrhaphy
7. osteoclasis
8. lithotripsy
9. enterolysis
10. neurotripsy
11. rhinoplasty
12. arthrodesis
13. myorrhaphy
14. mastopexy
15. cystorrhaphy
16. tenoplasty
17. osteoclasis
18. lithotripsy
19. enterolysis
20. neurotripsy

## LEARNING ACTIVITY 2–3

### Selecting a surgical suffix

1. lithotripsy
2. arthrocentesis
3. splenectomy
4. colostomy
5. dermatome
6. tracheostomy
7. lithotomy
8. mastectomy
9. hemorrhoidectomy
10. tracheotomy
11. mastopexy
12. colectomy
13. gastrorrhaphy
14. hysteropexy
15. rhinoplasty
16. arthrodesis
17. osteoclasis
18. neurolysis
19. myorrhaphy
20. tympanotomy

## LEARNING ACTIVITY 2–4

### Selecting diagnostic, pathological, and related suffixes

1. hepatoma
2. neuralgia
3. bronchiectasis
4. carcinogenesis
5. dermatosis
6. nephromegaly
7. otorrhea
8. hysterorrhexis

9. blepharospasm
10. cystocele
11. hemorrhage
12. lithiasis
13. hemiplegia
14. myopathy
15. dysphagia
16. osteomalacia
17. aphasia
18. leukemia
19. erythropenia
20. pelvimetry

## LEARNING ACTIVITY 2–5

### Building pathological and related words

1. bronchiectasis
2. cholelith
3. carcinogenesis
4. osteomalacia
5. hepatomegaly
6. cholelithiasis

7. hepatocele
8. neuropathy
9. dermatosis
10. hemiplegia
11. dysphagia
12. aphasia
13. cephalalgia
14. blepharospasm
15. hyperplasia, hypertrophy

## LEARNING ACTIVITY 2–6

### Selecting adjective, noun, and diminutive suffixes

1. thoracic
2. gastric, gastral
3. bacterial
4. aquatic
5. axillary
6. cardiac, cardial
7. spinal, spinous

8. membranous
9. internist
10. leukemia
11. sigmoidoscopy
12. alcoholism
13. senilism
14. allergist
15. mania
16. arteriole
17. ventricle
18. venule

## LEARNING ACTIVITY 2–7

### Forming plural words

| Singular | Plural | Rule |
|---|---|---|
| 1. diagnosis | diagnoses | Drop *is* and add *es.* |
| 2. fornix | fornices | Drop *ix* and add *ices.* |
| 3. vertebra | vertebrae | Retain *a* and add *e.* |
| 4. keratosis | keratoses | Drop *is* and add *es.* |
| 5. bronchus | bronchi | Drop *us* and add *i.* |
| 6. spermatozoon | spermatozoa | Drop *on* and add *a.* |
| 7. septum | septa | Drop *um* and add *a.* |
| 8. coccus | cocci | Drop *us* and add *i.* |
| 9. ganglion | ganglia | Drop *on* and add *a.* |
| 10. prognosis | prognoses | Drop *is* and add *es.* |
| 11. thrombus | thrombi | Drop *us* and add *i.* |
| 12. appendix | appendices | Drop *ix* and add *ices.* |
| 13. bacterium | bacteria | Drop *um* and add *a.* |
| 14. testis | testes | Drop *is* and add *es.* |
| 15. nevus | nevi | Drop *us* and add *i.* |

# CHAPTER 3 — Prefixes

## LEARNING ACTIVITY 3–1

### Identifying and defining prefixes

| Word | Definition of Prefix |
|---|---|
| 1. inter/dental | *between* |
| 2. hypo/dermic | under, below, deficient |
| 3. epi/dermis | above, upon |
| 4. retro/version | backward, behind |
| 5. sub/lingual | under, below |
| 6. trans/vaginal | through, across |
| 7. infra/costal | under, below |
| 8. post/natal | after, behind |
| 9. quadri/plegia | four |
| 10. hyper/calcemia | excessive, above normal |
| 11. primi/gravida | first |
| 12. micro/scope | small |
| 13. tri/plegia | three |
| 14. poly/dipsia | many, much |

| Word | Definition of Prefix |
|---|---|
| 15. ab/duction | from, away from |
| 16. an/esthesia | without, not |
| 17. macro/cyte | large |
| 18. intra/muscular | in, within |
| 19. supra/pelvic | above, excessive, superior |
| 20. dia/rrhea | through, across |
| 21. circum/duction | around |
| 22. ad/duction | toward |
| 23. peri/odontal | around |
| 24. brady/cardia | slow |
| 25. tachy/pnea | rapid |
| 26. dys/tocia | bad, painful, difficult |
| 27. eu/pnea | good, normal |
| 28. hetero/graft | different |
| 29. mal/nutrition | bad |
| 30. pseudo/cyesis | false |

## LEARNING ACTIVITY 3–2

### Matching prefixes of position, number and measurement, and direction

1. retroversion
2. hypodermic
3. prenatal
4. subnasal
5. postoperative
6. intercostal
7. pseudocyesis
8. periodontal
9. diarrhea
10. ectogenous
11. suprarenal
12. hemiplegia
13. quadriplegia
14. macrocyte
15. polyphobia

## LEARNING ACTIVITY 3–3

### Matching other prefixes

1. dyspepsia
2. heterosexual
3. panarthritis
4. antibacterial
5. bradycardia
6. malnutrition
7. amastia
8. anesthesia
9. eupnea
10. syndactylism
11. tachycardia
12. contraception
13. homosexual
14. dystocia
15. homograft

# CHAPTER 4 — Body Structure

## LEARNING ACTIVITY 4–3

### Matching body cavity, spine, and directional terms

1. h.  ventral cavity that contains digestive, reproductive, and excretory structures
2. k.  movement toward the median plane
3. j.  part of the spine known as the neck
4. b.  tailbone
5. m.  away from the surface of the body; internal
6. f.  turning outward
7. l.  away from the head; toward the tail or lower part of a structure
8. i.  turning inward or inside out

9. n.  part of the spine known as the loin
10. a.  pertaining to the sole of the foot
11. o.  near the back of the body
12. e.  lying horizontal with face downward

13. g.  nearer to the center (trunk of the body)
14. d.  toward the surface of the body
15. c.  ventral cavity that contains heart, lungs, and associated structures

## LEARNING ACTIVITY 4–4

### Matching word elements

1. kary/o
2. dist/o
3. -graphy
4. -gnosis
5. leuk/o
6. viscer/o
7. jaund/o
8. hist/o
9. -genesis
10. infra-
11. ultra-
12. caud/o
13. dors/o
14. poli/o
15. eti/o
16. morph/o
17. xer/o
18. idi/o
19. ad-
20. somat/o

## LEARNING ACTIVITY 4–5

### Matching diagnostic and therapeutic terms and procedures

1. radiology
2. Doppler
3. ultrasonography
4. thoracoscopy
5. punch biopsy
6. endoscopy
7. nuclear scan
8. fluoroscopy
9. morbid
10. radionuclide
11. febrile
12. resection
13. suppurative
14. cauterize
15. ablation

## MEDICAL RECORD ACTIVITY 4–1

### Radiologic consultation: Cervical and lumbar spine

1. Why was the x-ray film taken of the cervical spine?
   *To determine cervical curvature*
2. Did the patient appear to have experienced any type of recent injury to the spine?
   *No, there was no evidence of recent body disease or injury.*
3. What cervical vertebrae form the atlantoaxial joint?
   *The first cervical vertebra (atlas) and the second cervical vertebra (axis)*
4. Was the odontoid process fractured?
   *No, the odontoid process was intact.*
5. What did the radiologist believe was the possible cause of the minimal scoliosis?
   *Muscle spasm*

## MEDICAL RECORD ACTIVITY 4–2

### Radiographic consultation: Injury of left wrist and hand

1. What is the abbreviation for anteroposterior?
   *AP*
2. What caused the soft tissue deformity?
   *Fracture caused damage to surrounding tissue.*
3. Why was an AP view of the humerus taken?
   *To determine whether the elbow was fractured*
4. Where are the left wrist fractures located?
   *The distal shafts of the radius and ulna*
5. Did the radiologist take any side views of the left elbow?
   *Single view of the left elbow was obtained in the lateral projection.*

# CHAPTER 5 — Integumentary System

## LEARNING ACTIVITY 5–2

### Building medical words

1. adipoma, lipoma
2. adipocele, lipocele
3. adipoid, lipoid
4. adipocyte, lipocyte
5. dermatitis
6. dermatotome
7. onychoma
8. onychomalacia
9. onychosis
10. onychomycosis
11. onychocryptosis
12. onychopathy
13. trichopathy
14. trichomycosis
15. dermatology
16. dermatologist
17. adipectomy, lipectomy
18. onychectomy
19. onychotomy
20. dermatoplasty, dermoplasty

## LEARNING ACTIVITY 5–4

### Matching burn and oncology terms

1. i.  redness of skin
2. e.  no evidence of primary tumor
3. h.  cancerous; may be life-threatening
4. g.  heals without scar formation
5. f.  determines degree of abnormal cancer cells compared with normal cells
6. a.  develops from keratinizing epidermal cells
7. b.  noncancerous
8. j.  primary tumor size, small with minimal invasion
9. c.  no evidence of metastasis
10. d.  extensive damage to underlying connective tissue

## LEARNING ACTIVITY 5–5

### Matching diagnostic, symptomatic, procedure, and pharmacology terms

1. pediculosis
2. vitiligo
3. tinea
4. scabies
5. impetigo
6. urticaria
7. chloasma
8. ecchymosis
9. petechiae
10. alopecia
11. antifungals
12. fulguration
13. corticosteroids
14. dermabrasion
15. parasiticides
16. keratolytics
17. intradermal test
18. patch test
19. autograft
20. xenograft

## MEDICAL RECORD ACTIVITY 5–1

### Pathology report of skin lesion

1. In the specimen section, what does "skin on dorsum left wrist" mean?
   *Skin was obtained from the back or posterior surface of the left wrist.*
2. What was the inflammatory infiltrate?
   *Lymphocytic inflammatory infiltrate in the papillary dermis*
3. What was the pathologist's diagnosis for the left forearm?
   *Nodular and infiltrating basal cell carcinoma near the elbow*
4. Provide a brief description of Bowen disease, the pathologist's diagnosis for the left wrist.
   *Bowen disease is a form of intraepidermal carcinoma (squamous cell), characterized by red-brown scaly or crusted lesions that resemble a patch of psoriasis or dermatitis.*

## MEDICAL RECORD ACTIVITY 5–2

### Patient referral letter: Onychomycosis

1. What pertinent disorders were identified in the past medical history?
   *History of hypertension and cancer*
2. What pertinent surgery was identified in the past surgical history?
   *Mastectomy*
3. Did the doctor identify any problems in the vascular system or nervous system?
   *Vascular and neurological systems were intact.*

4. What was the significant finding in the laboratory results?
   *Alkaline phosphatase was elevated.*
5. What treatment did the doctor employ for the onychomycosis?
   *Debridement and medication or Sporanox PulsePak*
6. What did the doctor recommend regarding the abnormal laboratory finding?
   *The doctor recommended a repeat of the liver enzymes in approximately 4 weeks.*

# CHAPTER 6 — Digestive System

### LEARNING ACTIVITY 6–3

**Building medical words**

1. esophagodynia, esophagalgia
2. esophagospasm
3. esophagostenosis
4. gastritis
5. gastrodynia, gastralgia
6. gastropathy
7. jejunectomy
8. duodenal
9. ileitis
10. jejunoileal
11. enteritis
12. enteropathy
13. colitis
14. colorectal
15. coloenteritis, enterocolitis
16. coloptosis
17. colopathy
18. proctostenosis, rectostenosis
19. rectocele, proctocele
20. proctoplegia, proctoparalysis
21. cholecystitis
22. cholelithiasis
23. hepatoma
24. hepatomegaly
25. pancreatitis

### LEARNING ACTIVITY 6–4

**Building surgical words**

1. gingivectomy
2. glossectomy
3. esophagoplasty
4. gastrectomy
5. gastrojejunostomy
6. esophagectomy
7. gastroenterocolostomy
8. enteroplasty
9. enteropexy
10. choledochorrhaphy
11. colostomy
12. hepatopexy
13. proctoplasty, rectoplasty
14. cholecystectomy
15. choledochoplasty

### LEARNING ACTIVITY 6–5

**Matching pathological, diagnostic, symptomatic, and related terms**

1. hematemesis
2. dysphagia
3. fecalith
4. halitosis
5. anorexia
6. dyspepsia
7. cirrhosis
8. cachexia
9. obstipation
10. lesion

## LEARNING ACTIVITY 6–6

### Matching procedures, pharmacology, and abbreviations

1. pc, pp
2. bilirubin
3. emetics
4. bid
5. choledochoplasty
6. lower GI series
7. gastroscopy
8. stomatoplasty
9. intubation
10. anastomosis
11. stool guaiac
12. endoscopy
13. laxatives
14. antacids
15. ultrasonography
16. liver function tests
17. qid
18. stat
19. proctosigmoidoscopy
20. upper GI series

## MEDICAL RECORD ACTIVITY 6–1

### GI evaluation

1. While referring to Figure 6–3, describe the location of the gallbladder in relation to the liver.
   *Posterior and inferior portion of the right lobe of the liver*
2. Why did the patient undergo the cholecystectomy?
   *To treat cholecystitis and cholelithiasis*
3. List the patient's prior surgeries.
   *Tonsillectomy, appendectomy, and cholecystectomy*
4. How does the patient's most recent postoperative episode of discomfort (pain) differ from the initial pain she described?
   *Continuous deep right-sided pain, which took a crescendo pattern and then a decrescendo pattern—the initial pain was intermittent and sharp.*

## MEDICAL RECORD ACTIVITY 6–2

### Esophagogastroduodenoscopy with biopsy

1. What caused the hematemesis?
   *Etiology was unknown. Inflammation of the mucosa in the stomach and duodenum was noted.*
2. What procedures were carried out to determine the cause of bleeding?
   *During x-ray tomography using the videoendoscope, biopsies were taken of the stomach and duodenum. It was also noted that previously the patient had esophageal varices.*
3. How much blood did the patient lose during the procedure?
   *None*
4. Were there any ulcerations or erosions found during the exploratory procedure that might account for the bleeding?
   *No*
5. What type of sedation was used during the procedure?
   *Demerol and Versed administered intravenously*
6. What did the doctors find when they examined the stomach and duodenum?
   *Diffuse and punctate erythema*

# CHAPTER 7 — Respiratory System

## LEARNING ACTIVITY 7–2

### Building medical words

1. rhinorrhea
2. rhinitis
3. laryngoscopy
4. laryngitis
5. laryngostenosis
6. bronchiectasis
7. bronchopathy
8. bronchospasm
9. pneumothorax
10. pneumonitis
11. pulmonologist
12. pulmonary, pulmonic
13. dyspnea
14. bradypnea
15. tachypnea
16. apnea
17. rhinoplasty
18. thoracocentesis, thoracentesis
19. pulmonectomy, pneumonectomy
20. tracheostomy

## LEARNING ACTIVITY 7–3

### Matching pathological, diagnostic, symptomatic, and related terms

1. atelectasis
2. empyema
3. surfactant
4. consolidation
5. ascites
6. anosmia
7. hypoxemia
8. tubercles
9. apnea
10. emphysema
11. compliance
12. epistaxis
13. pulmonary edema
14. rale, crackle
15. deviated nasal septum
16. coryza
17. pneumoconiosis
18. pleurisy
19. stridor
20. pertussis

## LEARNING ACTIVITY 7–4

### Matching procedures, pharmacology, and abbreviations

1. lung scan
2. polysomnography
3. resection of lung
4. antral lavage
5. antihistamines
6. antitussives
7. sweat test
8. oximetry
9. AFB
10. aerosol therapy
11. decongestants
12. Mantoux test
13. ABGs
14. expectorants
15. throat culture
16. pulmonary function studies
17. laryngoscopy
18. septoplasty
19. pneumonectomy
20. rhinoplasty

## MEDICAL RECORD ACTIVITY 7–1

### Respiratory evaluation

1. What symptom caused the patient to seek medical help?
   *Shortness of breath*
2. What was the patient's previous history?
   *Difficult breathing, high blood pressure, chronic obstructive pulmonary disease, and peripheral vascular disease*
3. What were the findings of the physical examination?
   *Bilateral wheezes and rhonchi heard anteriorly and posteriorly*

4. What changes were noted from the previous film?
   *Interstitial vascular congestion with possible superimposed inflammatory change and some pleural reactive change*
5. What is the present Dx?
   *Acute exacerbation of chronic obstructive pulmonary disease; heart failure; hypertension; peripheral vascular disease*
6. What new diagnosis was made that did not appear in the previous medical history?
   *Heart failure*

## MEDICAL RECORD ACTIVITY 7–2

### Chronic interstitial lung disease

1. When did the patient notice SOB?
   *With activity*
2. Other than the respiratory system, what other body systems are identified in the history of present illness?
   *Cardiovascular, urinary, and nervous system*
3. What were the findings regarding the neck?
   *Supple and no evidence of thyromegaly or adenomegaly*
4. What was the finding regarding the spine?
   *Mild kyphosis without scoliosis*

5. What appears to be the likely cause of the chronic interstitial lung disease?
   *Combination of pulmonary fibrosis and heart failure*
6. Define the following abbreviations: ABGs, $Po_2$, $Pco_2$, and pH.
   *ABGs, arterial blood gasses; $Po_2$, partial pressure of oxygen; $Pco_2$, carbon dioxide partial pressure; pH, degree of alkalinity and acidity*
7. What is the therapeutic action of Lasix?
   *Diuretic*

# CHAPTER 8 — Cardiovascular System

## LEARNING ACTIVITY 8–2

### Building medical words

1. atheroma
2. atherosclerosis
3. phlebitis
4. phlebothrombosis
5. venous
6. venospasm
7. cardiologist
8. cardiorrhexis
9. cardiotoxic
10. cardiomegaly
11. angiomalacia
12. angioma
13. thrombogen, thrombogenesis
14. thrombosis
15. aortostenosis
16. aortography
17. cardiocentesis
18. arteriorrhaphy
19. embolectomy
20. thrombolysis

## LEARNING ACTIVITY 8–3

### Matching pathological, diagnostic, symptomatic, and related terms

1. infarct
2. angina
3. incompetent
4. vegetations
5. varices
6. bruit
7. catheter
8. palpitation
9. lumen
10. aneurysm
11. embolus
12. arrhythmia
13. arrest
14. thrombolysis
15. stent
16. hypertension
17. hyperlipidemia
18. primary
19. secondary
20. perfusion

## LEARNING ACTIVITY 8–4

### Matching procedures, pharmacology, and abbreviations

1. Holter monitor test
2. echocardiography
3. coronary angiography
4. nitrates
5. statins
6. diuretics
7. cardiac enzyme studies
8. scintigraphy
9. stress test
10. ligation and stripping
11. commissurotomy
12. arterial biopsy
13. catheter ablation
14. embolization
15. angioplasty
16. PTCA
17. CABG
18. atherectomy
19. venipuncture
20. thrombolysis

## MEDICAL RECORD ACTIVITY 8–1

### Acute myocardial infarction

1. How long had the patient experienced chest pain before she was seen in the hospital?
   *Approximately 2 hours*
2. Did the patient have a previous history of chest pain?
   *Yes*
3. What are the cardiac enzymes that are tested to confirm the diagnosis of MI?
   *Tropinin T, tropinin I, creatine, creatinine kinase*
4. Initially, what medications were administered to stabilize the patient?
   *Streptokinase and heparin*
5. During the current admission, what part of the heart was damaged?
   *The lateral front side of the heart (anterior of heart)*
6. Was the location of damage to the heart for this admission the same as for the initial MI?
   *No, in the earlier admission, the damage was to the lower part of the heart.*

## MEDICAL RECORD ACTIVITY 8–2

### Operative report: Rule out temporal arteritis

1. Why was the right temporal artery biopsied?
   *Rule out arteritis*
2. In what position was the patient placed?
   *Supine*
3. What was the incision area?
   *Right preauricular area*

4. How was the temporal artery described in the report?
   *Palpable*
5. How was the dissection carried out?
   *Down through the subcutaneous tissue and superficial fascia*
6. What was the size of the specimen?
   *Approximately 1.5 cm*

# CHAPTER 9 — Blood, Lymph, and Immune Systems

## LEARNING ACTIVITY 9–2

### Building medical words

1. erythrocytosis
2. leukocytosis
3. lymphocytosis
4. reticulocytosis
5. erythropenia
6. leukopenia
7. thrombocytopenia, thrombopenia
8. lymphocytopenia
9. hemopoiesis, hematopoiesis
10. leukopoiesis, leukocytopoiesis
11. thrombocytopoiesis
12. immunologist
13. immunology
14. splenocele
15. splenolysis
16. splenectomy
17. thymectomy
18. thymolysis
19. splenotomy
20. splenopexy

## LEARNING ACTIVITY 9–3

### Matching pathological, diagnostic, symptomatic, and related terms

1. exacerbations
2. hemoglobinopathy
3. bacteremia
4. hemostasis
5. active
6. Kaposi sarcoma
7. normocytic
8. lymphadenopathy
9. immunocompromised
10. hemophilia
11. infectious mononucleosis
12. myelogenous
13. passive
14. artificial
15. hemolysis
16. hematoma
17. graft rejection
18. anisocytosis
19. titer
20. septicemia

## LEARNING ACTIVITY 9–4

### Matching procedures, pharmacology, and abbreviations

1. aspiration
2. hematocrit
3. Monospot
4. anticoagulants
5. WBC
6. homologous
7. lymphangiectomy
8. RBC indices
9. Shilling
10. lymphadenography
11. autologous
12. hemostatics
13. RBC
14. thrombolytics
15. differential

## MEDICAL RECORD ACTIVITY 9–1

### Discharge summary: Sickle cell crisis

1. What blood product was administered to the patient?
   *Two units of packed red blood cells*
2. Why was this blood product given to the patient?
   *The patient was anemic due to sickle cell anemia.*

## MEDICAL RECORD ACTIVITY 9–2

### Discharge summary: PCP and HIV

1. How do you think the patient acquired the HIV infection?
   *Through her husband, who died of HIV*
2. What were the two diagnoses of the husband?
   *Multifocal leukoencephalopathy (PMN) and Kaposi sarcoma*

3. Why was a CT scan performed on the patient?
   *To determine the cause of abdominal pain*
4. What were the three findings of the CT scan?
   *Ileus in the small bowel, dilated small bowel loops, and abnormal enhancement pattern in the kidney*
5. Why should the patient see his regular doctor?
   *To follow up on the renal abnormality*

3. What four disorders in the medical history are significant for HIV?
   *Several episodes of diarrhea, sinusitis, thrush, and vaginal candidiasis*
4. What was the x-ray finding?
   *Diffuse lower lobe infiltrates*
5. What two procedures are going to be performed to confirm the diagnosis of PCP pneumonia?
   *Bronchoscopy and alveolar lavage*

# CHAPTER 10 — Musculoskeletal System

## LEARNING ACTIVITY 10–4

### Building medical words

1. osteocytes
2. ostealgia, osteodynia
3. osteoarthropathy
4. osteogenesis
5. cervical
6. cervicobrachial
7. cervicofacial
8. myelocele
9. myelosarcoma
10. myelomalacia
11. myeloid
12. suprasternal
13. sternoid
14. chondroblast
15. arthritis
16. osteoarthritis
17. pelvimeter
18. myospasm
19. myopathy
20. myorrhexis
21. phalangectomy
22. thoracotomy
23. vertebrectomy
24. arthrodesis
25. myoplasty

## LEARNING ACTIVITY 10–5

### Matching pathological, diagnostic, symptomatic, and related terms

1. subluxation
2. rickets
3. spondylolisthesis
4. claudication
5. muscular dystrophy
6. talipes
7. sequestrum
8. myasthenia gravis
9. prosthesis
10. ganglion cyst
11. hypotonia
12. Ewing sarcoma
13. greenstick fracture
14. kyphosis
15. osteoporosis
16. scoliosis
17. chondrosarcoma
18. comminuted fracture
19. spondylitis
20. gout
21. hematopoiesis
22. pyogenic
23. necrosis
24. ankylosis
25. phantom limb

## LEARNING ACTIVITY 10–6

### Matching procedures, pharmacology, and abbreviations

1. myelography
2. open reduction
3. gold salts
4. CTS
5. laminectomy
6. arthrography
7. arthrodesis
8. amputation
9. HNP
10. salicylates
11. arthroscopy
12. sequestrectomy
13. ACL
14. relaxants
15. closed reduction

## MEDICAL RECORD ACTIVITY 10–1

### Right knee arthroscopy and medial meniscectomy

1. Describe the meniscus and identify its location.
   *The meniscus is the curved, fibrous cartilage in the knees and other joints.*
2. What is the probable cause of the tear in the patient's meniscus?
   *The continuous pressure on the knees from jogging on a hard surface, such as the pavement*
3. What does normal ACL and PCL refer to in the report?
   *The anterior and posterior cruciate ligaments appeared to be normal.*
4. Explain the McMurray sign test.
   *Rotation of the tibia on the femur is used to determine injury to meniscal structures. An audible click during manipulation of tibia with the leg flexed is an indication that the meniscus has been injured.*
5. Because Lachman and McMurray tests were negative (normal), why was the surgery performed?
   *The medial compartment of the knee showed an inferior surface posterior and midmedial meniscal tear that was flipped up on top of itself. The surgeon resected the tear, and the remaining meniscus was contoured back to a stable rim.*

## MEDICAL RECORD ACTIVITY 10–2

### Radiographic consultation: Tibial diaphysis nuclear scan

1. Where was the pain located?
   *Middle 1/3 of the left tibia*
2. What medication was the patient taking for pain and did it provide relief?
   *He finds no relief with NSAIDs.*
3. How was the blood flow to the affected area described by the radiologist?
   *There is focal, increased blood flow and blood pooling.*
4. How was the radiotracer accumulation described?
   *The radiotracer accumulated within the left mid-posterior tibial diaphysis was delayed.*
5. What will be the probable outcome with continued excessive repetitive stress?
   *The rate of resorption will exceed the rate of bone replacement.*
6. What will happen if resorption continues to exceed replacement?
   *A stress fracture will occur.*

# CHAPTER 11 — Genitourinary System

## LEARNING ACTIVITY 11–3

### Building medical words

1. nephrolith
2. nephropyosis, pyonephrosis
3. hydronephrosis, nephrohydrosis
4. pyelectasis, pyelectasia
5. pyelopathy
6. ureterectasis, ureterectasia
7. ureterolith
8. cystitis
9. cystoscope
10. vesicocele
11. vesicoprostatic
12. urethrostenosis
13. urethrotome
14. urography
15. uropathy
16. dysuria
17. oliguria

18. orchidopathy, orchiopathy
19. orchialgia, orchiodynia, orchidalgia
20. balanorrhea
21. orchidectomy, orchiectomy

22. balanoplasty
23. vasectomy
24. pyelotomy
25. cystopexy

## LEARNING ACTIVITY 11–4

### Matching pathological, diagnostic, symptomatic, and related terms

1. urgency
2. fistula
3. anorchism
4. anuria
5. azotemia
6. orchiopexy
7. benign prostatic hypertrophy
8. hesitancy

9. oliguria
10. nephrotic syndrome
11. phimosis
12. sterility
13. epispadias
14. aspermia
15. pyuria
16. herniorrhaphy
17. nocturia
18. enuresis
19. hydrocele
20. balanitis

## LEARNING ACTIVITY 11–5

### Matching procedures, pharmacology, and abbreviations

1. KUB
2. semen analysis
3. cystoscopy
4. antibiotics
5. C&S
6. diuretics

7. urethrotomy
8. ESWL
9. peritoneal dialysis
10. resection
11. vasectomy
12. orchiectomy
13. circumcision
14. androgens
15. potassium supplements

## MEDICAL RECORD ACTIVITY 11–1

### Operative report: Ureterocele

1. Why did the doctor perform a cystoscopy?
   *To examine the bladder*
2. What was the name and size of the urethral sound used in the procedure?
   *#26 French Van Buren*

3. What is the function of the urethral sound?
   *Dilate the urethra*
4. In what direction was the ureterocele incised?
   *Longitudinally*
5. Was fulguration required? Why or why not?
   *Fulguration was not required because there was no bleeding.*

## MEDICAL RECORD ACTIVITY 11–2

### Operative report: Extracorporeal shockwave lithotripsy

1. What previous procedures were performed on the patient?
   *ESWL and double-J stent placement*
2. Why is this current procedure being performed?
   *To fragment the remaining calculus and remove the double-J stent*

3. What imaging technique was used for positioning the patient to ensure that the shockwaves would strike the calculus?
   *Fluoroscopy*
4. In what position was the patient placed in the cystoscopy suite?
   *Dorsal lithotomy*
5. How was the double-J stent removed?
   *Using grasping forceps and removing it as the scope was withdrawn*

# CHAPTER 12 — Female Reproductive System

## LEARNING ACTIVITY 12–3

### Building medical words

1. gynecopathy
2. gynecologist
3. cervicovaginitis
4. cervicovesical
5. colposcope
6. colposcopy
7. vaginitis
8. vaginocele
9. hysteromyoma
10. hysteropathy
11. hysterosalpingography
12. metrorrhagia
13. parametritis
14. uterocele
15. uterocervical
16. uterovesical
17. oophoritis
18. oophorosalpingitis
19. salpingocele
20. salpingography
21. oophoropexy, ovariopexy
22. hystero-oophorectomy
23. episiorrhaphy, perineorrhaphy
24. hysterosalpingo-oophorectomy
25. amniocentesis

## LEARNING ACTIVITY 12–4

### Matching pathological, diagnostic, symptomatic, and related terms

1. pyosalpinx
2. primipara
3. gestation
4. chancre
5. retroversion
6. congenital
7. dystocia
8. atresia
9. Down syndrome
10. pruritus vulvae
11. asymptomatic
12. metrorrhagia
13. menarche
14. leiomyoma
15. oligomenorrhea
16. parturition
17. eclampsia
18. viable
19. condylomas
20. primigravida

## LEARNING ACTIVITY 12–5

### Matching procedures, pharmacology, and abbreviations

1. Pap test
2. hysterosalpingography
3. amniocentesis
4. antifungals
5. colpocleisis
6. D&C
7. total abdominal hysterectomy (TAH)
8. tubal ligation
9. OCPs
10. laparoscopy
11. episiotomy
12. ultrasonography
13. chorionic villus sampling
14. estrogens
15. oxytocins
16. cryocautery
17. IUD
18. cordocentesis
19. lumpectomy
20. prostaglandins

## MEDICAL RECORD ACTIVITY 12–1

### Primary herpes 1 infection

1. Did the patient have any discharge? If so, describe it.
   *A brownish discharge*
2. What type of discomfort was the patient experiencing around the vulvar area?
   *She was experiencing severe itching (pruritus) and pain.*
3. Has the patient been taking her oral contraceptive pills regularly?
   *Yes*
4. Where was the viral culture obtained?
   *Ulcerlike lesion on the right labia*
5. Even though her partner used a condom, how do you think the patient became infected with herpes?
   *She probably got infected from the cold sore when having oral-genital sex.*

## MEDICAL RECORD ACTIVITY 12–2

### Menometrorrhagia

1. How many pregnancies did this woman have? How many viable infants did she deliver?
   *Two pregnancies and one viable birth*
2. What is a therapeutic abortion?
   *An abortion performed when the pregnancy endangers the mother's mental or physical health or when the fetus has a known condition incompatible with life*
3. Why did the physician propose to perform a hysterectomy?
   *Patient desires definitive treatment for menometrorrhagia and has declined palliative treatment*

4. What is a vaginal hysterectomy?
   *Surgical removal of the uterus through the vagina*
5. Does the surgeon plan to remove one or both ovaries and fallopian tubes?
   *The surgeon plans to perform a bilateral (relates to two sides) salpingo-oophorectomy.*
6. Why do you think the physician will use the laparoscope to perform the hysterectomy?
   *To permit visualization of the abdominal cavity as the ovaries and fallopian tubes are removed through the vagina*

# CHAPTER 13 — Endocrine System

## LEARNING ACTIVITY 13–2

### Building medical words

1. hyperglycemia
2. hypoglycemia
3. glycogenesis
4. pancreatitis
5. pancreatolysis
6. pancreatopathy
7. thyroiditis
8. thyromegaly
9. parathyroidectomy
10. adrenalectomy

## LEARNING ACTIVITY 13–3

### Matching pathological, diagnostic, symptomatic, and related terms

1. virile
2. myxedema
3. diuresis
4. hirsutism
5. cretinism
6. insulin
7. Addison disease
8. exophthalmic goiter
9. hyperkalemia
10. pheochromocytoma
11. type 1 diabetes
12. hyponatremia
13. glycosuria
14. Cushing syndrome
15. type 2 diabetes

## LEARNING ACTIVITY 13–4

### Matching procedures, pharmacology, and abbreviations

1. FBS
2. RAIU
3. corticosteroids
4. growth hormone
5. thyroid scan
6. $T_4$
7. oral antidiabetics
8. GTT
9. antithyroids
10. protein-bound iodine
11. $T_3$
12. magnetic resonance imaging (MRI)
13. exophthalmometry
14. computed tomography (CT) scan
15. Humulin

**MEDICAL RECORD ACTIVITY 13–1**

**Hyperparathyroidism**

1. What is an adenoma?
   *Benign tumor of a gland*
2. What does the physician suspect caused the patient's hyperparathyroidism?
   *Possible parathyroid adenoma*

3. What type of laboratory findings revealed parathyroid disease?
   *Elevated calcium level*
4. What is hypercalciuria?
   *Excessive amount of calcium in the urine*
5. If the patient smoked 548 packs of cigarettes per year, how many packs did she smoke in an average day?
   *Approximately 1.5 packs per day*

**MEDICAL RECORD ACTIVITY 13–2**

**Diabetes mellitus**

1. How long has this patient been experiencing voracious eating?
   *For the past 10 days*
2. Was the patient's obesity due to overeating or metabolic imbalance?
   *Overeating*

3. Why did the doctor experience difficulty in examining the patient's abdomen?
   *Because she was so obese*
4. Was the patient's blood glucose above or below normal on admission?
   *Above normal*
5. What is the reference range for fasting blood glucose?
   *The range for fasting blood glucose is 70/110 mg/dL.*

# CHAPTER 14 — Nervous System

**LEARNING ACTIVITY 14–2**

**Building medical words**

1. encephalopathy
2. encephalocele
3. encephalography
4. cerebropathy
5. cerebritis
6. craniocele
7. craniometer
8. neuralgia, neurodynia
9. neurologist
10. neurotripsy
11. myelocele
12. myeloplegia
13. psychotic, psychic
14. psychosis
15. bradykinesia
16. dyskinesia
17. hemiplegia
18. quadriplegia
19. dysphasia
20. aphasia
21. neurolysis
22. craniotomy
23. cranioplasty
24. neurorrhaphy
25. encephalotomy

**LEARNING ACTIVITY 14–3**

**Matching pathological, diagnostic, symptomatic, and related terms**

1. hemiparesis
2. dysrhythmias
3. Alzheimer disease
4. bulimia nervosa
5. clonic spasm
6. Guillain-Barré syndrome
7. phobias
8. bipolar disorder
9. leptomeningitis
10. asthenia
11. shingles
12. lethargy
13. paraplegia
14. poliomyelitis
15. stroke
16. transient ischemic attack (TIA)
17. concussion
18. Parkinson disease
19. multiple sclerosis
20. autism

## LEARNING ACTIVITY 14–4

### Matching procedures, pharmacology, and abbreviations

1. NVC
2. psychostimulants
3. antipsychotics
4. general anesthetics
5. echoencephalography
6. cryosurgery
7. myelography
8. cerebral angiography
9. CSF analysis
10. electromyography
11. analgesics
12. PET
13. tractotomy
14. hypnotics
15. trephination

## MEDICAL RECORD ACTIVITY 14–1

### Subarachnoid hemorrhage

1. In what part of the head did the patient feel pain?
   *Occipital, the back part of the head*
2. What imaging tests were performed, and what was the finding in each test?
   *CT scan showed blood in the cisterna subarachnoidalis and mild acute hydrocephalus. Cerebral angiogram and MRI showed no aneurysm.*
3. How does meningismus differ from meningitis?
   *Meningismus is irritation of the brain and spinal cord with symptoms simulating meningitis but without actual inflammation. Meningitis is an inflammation of the membranes of the spinal cord or brain.*
4. Did the lumbar puncture rule out or confirm a second subarachnoid hemorrhage?
   *It confirmed subarachnoid hemorrhage.*

## MEDICAL RECORD ACTIVITY 14–2

### Consultation report: Acute onset paraplegia

1. What was the original cause of the patient's current problems and what treatments were provided?
   *Fall at work about 15–20 years ago, and she had four subsequent lumbar surgeries*
2. Why was the patient admitted to the hospital?
   *Pain management*
3. What intravenous medications did the patient receive and why was each given?
   *Clonidine for hypertension and methadone for pain*
4. What was the cause of bladder retention?
   *Administration of clonidine*
5. What occurred after the catheter was removed?
   *Subacute onset of paresis, paresthesias, and pain in the legs approximately $2\frac{1}{2}$ to 3 hours later*
6. What three disorders were listed in the differential diagnosis?
   *Subarachnoid hemorrhage, epidural abscess, and transverse myelitis*

# CHAPTER 15 — Special Senses

## LEARNING ACTIVITY 15–3

### Building medical words

1. ophthalmoplegia, ophthalmoparalysis
2. ophthalmology
3. pupilloscopy
4. keratomalacia
5. keratometer
6. scleritis
7. scleromalacia
8. iridoplegia, iridoparalysis
9. iridocele
10. retinopathy
11. retinitis
12. blepharoplegia
13. blepharoptosis
14. otopyorrhea
15. audiometer
16. myringotome
17. amblyopia
18. hyperopia
19. anacusis
20. hyperacusis
21. stapedectomy
22. labyrinthotomy
23. mastoidectomy
24. myringoplasty, tympanoplasty
25. keratotomy

## LEARNING ACTIVITY 15–4

### Matching pathological, diagnostic, symptomatic, and related terms

1. cataract
2. achromatopsia
3. nyctalopia
4. gonioscopy
5. anacusis
6. otitis externa
7. diopter
8. tonometer
9. visual field
10. epiphora
11. strabismus
12. Ménière disease
13. neovascular
14. vertigo
15. exotropia
16. enucleation
17. chalazion
18. amblyopia
19. retinoblastoma
20. tinnitus

## LEARNING ACTIVITY 15–5

### Matching procedures, pharmacology, and abbreviations

1. caloric stimulation test
2. ophthalmoscopy
3. cochlear implant
4. fluorescein angiography
5. otoplasty
6. mydriatics
7. tonometry
8. visual acuity test
9. evisceration
10. beta blockers
11. wax emulsifiers
12. enucleation
13. ST
14. ophthalmic decongestants
15. XT
16. gonioscopy
17. otoscopy
18. audiometry
19. radial keratotomy
20. otic analgesics

## MEDICAL RECORD ACTIVITY 15–1

### Retained foreign bodies

1. Did the patient's surgery involve one or both ears?
   *Bilateral, it involved both ears.*
2. What was the nature of the foreign body in the patient's ears?
   *Retained tympanostomy tubes*
3. What ear structure was involved?
   *Eardrum, or tympanum*
4. What instrument was used to locate the tubes?
   *Operating microscope*
5. What was the material in which the tubes were embedded?
   *Earwax, or cerumen*

## MEDICAL RECORD ACTIVITY 15–2

### Phacoemulsification and lens implant

1. What technique was used to destroy the cataract?
   *Phacoemulsification, an ultrasound technique*
2. In what portion of the eye was the implant placed?
   *Posterior chamber*
3. What anesthetics were used for surgery?
   *Intravenous and retrobulbar block*
4. What was the function of the blepharostat?
   *To separate the eyelids during surgery*
5. What was the function of the keratome?
   *A knife used to incise the cornea*
6. Where was the implant inserted?
   *In the capsular bag*

# Appendix

# B

# Abbreviations

| Abbreviation | Meaning | Abbreviation | Meaning |
|---|---|---|---|
| AAA | abdominal aortic aneurysm | AST | angiotensin sensitivity test; aspartate aminotransferase (cardiac enzyme, formerly called *SGOT*) |
| AB, ab | abortion, antibodies | | |
| ABC | aspiration biopsy cytology | | |
| ABG | arterial blood gas | | |
| ABO | blood groups A, AB, B, and O | Ast | astigmatism |
| | | ATN | acute tubular necrosis |
| ac | before meals | *AU | both ears |
| AC | air conduction | AV | atrioventricular, arteriovenous |
| Acc | accommodation | | |
| ACL | anterior cruciate ligament | Ba | barium |
| ACTH | adrenocorticotropic hormone | BaE | barium enema |
| | | baso | basophil (type of white blood cell) |
| AD | Alzheimer disease | | |
| *AD | right ear | BBB | bundle branch block |
| ADH | antidiuretic hormone (vasopressin) | BC | bone conduction |
| | | BCC | basal cell carcinoma |
| AE | above the elbow | BE | below the elbow |
| AF | atrial fibrillation | BEAM | brain electrical activity mapping |
| AFB | acid-fast bacillus (TB organism) | | |
| | | bid | twice a day |
| AGN | acute glomerulonephritis | BK | below the knee |
| AI | artificial insemination | BM | bowel movement |
| AIDS | acquired immunodeficiency syndrome | BMR | basal metabolic rate |
| | | BNO | bladder neck obstruction |
| AK | above the knee | BP | blood pressure |
| alk phos | alkaline phosphatase | BPH | benign prostatic hyperplasia; benign prostatic hypertrophy |
| ALL | acute lymphocytic leukemia | | |
| ALS | amyotrophic lateral sclerosis; also called *Lou Gehrig disease* | BSE | breast self-examination |
| | | BUN | blood urea nitrogen |
| | | Bx, bx | biopsy |
| ALT | alanine aminotransferase (elevated in liver and heart disease); formerly *SGPT* | C&S | culture and sensitivity |
| | | C1, C2, and so on | first cervical vertebra, second cervical vertebra, and so on |
| AML | acute myelogenous leukemia | CA | cancer; chronological age; cardiac arrest |
| ANS | autonomic nervous system | Ca | calcium; cancer |
| ant | anterior | CABG | coronary artery bypass graft |
| AP | anteroposterior | | |
| APTT | activated partial thromboplastin time | CAD | coronary artery disease |
| | | cath | catheterization; catheter |
| ARDS | acute respiratory distress syndrome | CBC | complete blood count |
| | | CC | cardiac catheterization |
| ARF | acute renal failure | CCU | coronary care unit |
| ARMD, AMD | age-related macular degeneration | CDH | congenital dislocation of the hip |
| AS | aortic stenosis | CHD | coronary heart disease |
| *AS | left ear | CHF | congestive heart failure |
| ASD | atrial septal defect | Chol | cholesterol |
| ASHD | arteriosclerotic heart disease | CK | creatine kinase (cardiac enzyme) |

| Abbreviation | Meaning | Abbreviation | Meaning |
|---|---|---|---|
| CLL | chronic lymphocytic leukemia | ED | erectile dysfunction; emergency department |
| cm | centimeter | EEG | electroencephalogram; electroencephalography |
| CML | chronic myelogenous leukemia | EGD | esophagogastroduo-denoscopy |
| CNS | central nervous system | | |
| $CO_2$ | carbon dioxide | Em | emmetropia |
| COPD | chronic obstructive pulmonary disease | EMG | electromyography |
| | | ENT | ears, nose, and throat |
| CP | cerebral palsy | EOM | extraocular movement |
| CPD | cephalopelvic disproportion | eos | eosinophil (type of white blood cell) |
| CPR | cardiopulmonary resuscitation | ERCP | endoscopic retrograde cholangiopancreatography |
| CS, C-section | cesarean section | | |
| CSF | cerebrospinal fluid | ESR, sed rate | erythrocyte sedimentation rate; sedimentation rate |
| CT | computed tomography | | |
| CT scan, CAT scan | computed tomography scan | ESRD | end-stage renal disease |
| | | ESWL | extracorporeal shockwave lithotripsy |
| CTS | carpal tunnel syndrome | | |
| CV | cardiovascular | EU | excretory urography; also called *intravenous pyelography (IVP)* or *intravenous urography (IVU)* |
| CVA | cerebrovascular accident | | |
| CVS | chorionic villus sampling | | |
| CWP | childbirth without pain | | |
| CXR | chest x-ray, chest radi-ograph | FECG; FEKG | fetal electrocardiogram |
| | | FHR | fetal heart rate |
| cysto | cystoscopy | FHT | fetal heart tone |
| D | diopter (lens strength) | FS | frozen section |
| D&C | dilatation (dilation) and curettage | FSH | follicle-stimulating hormone |
| | | FTND | full-term normal delivery |
| *DC | discharge | FVC | forced vital capacity |
| decub | decubitus (ulcer); bedsore | Fx | fracture |
| derm | dermatology | G | gravida (pregnant) |
| DI | diabetes insipidus; diagnostic imaging | GB | gallbladder |
| | | GBS | gallbladder series |
| diff | differential count (white blood cells) | GC | gonorrhea |
| | | GER | gastroesophageal reflux |
| DJD | degenerative joint disease | GERD | gastroesophageal reflux disease |
| DKA | diabetic ketoacidosis | | |
| DM | diabetes mellitus | GH | growth hormone |
| DOE | dyspnea on exertion | GI | gastrointestinal |
| DRE | digital rectal examination | GU | genitourinary |
| DSA | digital subtraction angiography | GVHR | graft-versus-host reaction |
| | | GYN | gynecology |
| DUB | dysfunctional uterine bleeding | HAV | hepatitis A virus |
| | | Hb, Hgb | hemoglobin |
| DVT | deep vein thrombosis | HBV | hepatitis B virus |
| Dx | diagnosis | HCT, Hct | hematocrit |
| EBV | Epstein-Barr virus | HCV | hepatitis C virus |
| ECG, EKG | electrocardiogram | HD | hemodialysis; hip disarticulation; hearing distance |
| ECHO | echocardiogram; echoencephalogram | | |

| Abbreviation | Meaning | Abbreviation | Meaning |
|---|---|---|---|
| HDL | high-density lipoprotein | K | potassium (an electrolyte) |
| HDN | hemolytic disease of the newborn | KD | knee disarticulation |
| | | KUB | kidney, ureter, bladder |
| HDV | hepatitis D virus | L1, L2, | first lumbar vertebra, second |
| HEV | hepatitis E virus | and so on | lumbar vertebra, and so |
| HF | heart failure | | on |
| HIV | human immunodeficiency virus | LAT, lat | lateral |
| | | LBW | low birth weight |
| HMD | hyaline membrane disease | LD | lactate dehydrogenase; lactic |
| HNP | herniated nucleus pulposus (herniated disk) | | acid dehydrogenase (cardiac enzyme) |
| HP | hemipelvectomy | LDL | low-density lipoprotein |
| HRT | hormone replacement therapy | LH | luteinizing hormone |
| | | LLQ | left lower quadrant |
| *hs | at bedtime | LMP | last menstrual period |
| HSG | hysterosalpingography | LOC | loss of consciousness |
| HSV | herpes simplex virus | LP | lumbar puncture |
| I&D | incision and drainage | LSO | left salpingo-oophorectomy |
| IBS | irritable bowel syndrome | lt | left |
| ICP | intracranial pressure | LUQ | left upper quadrant |
| ID | intradermal | lymphos | lymphocytes |
| IDDM | insulin-dependent diabetes mellitus | MCH | mean corpuscular hemoglobin; mean cell |
| Igs | immunoglobulins | | hemoglobin (average |
| I.M., IM | intramuscular; infectious mononucleosis | | amount of hemoglobin per cell) |
| IMP | impression (synonymous with *diagnosis*) | MCHC | mean cell hemoglobin concentration (average concentration of |
| IOL | intraocular lens | | hemoglobin in a single |
| IOP | intraocular pressure | | red cell) |
| IPPB | intermittent positive-pressure breathing | MCV | mean cell volume (average volume or size of a single |
| IRDS | infant respiratory distress syndrome | | red blood cell; high MCV = macrocytic cells; |
| IS | intracostal space | | low MCV = microcytic |
| ITP | idiopathic thrombocytopenia purpura | | cells) |
| IUD | intrauterine device | MEG | magnetoencephalog- raphy |
| IUGR | intrauterine growth rate; intrauterine growth retardation | MG | myasthenia gravis |
| | | MI | myocardial infarction |
| I.V., IV | intravenous | mix astig | mixed astigmatism |
| IVF-ET | in vitro fertilization and embryo transfer | mL, ml | milliliters |
| | | MRA | magnetic resonance angiogram; magnetic |
| IVP | intravenous pyelography; also called *excretory urography (EU)* or *intravenous urography (IVU)* | | resonance angiography |
| | | MRI | magnetic resonance imaging |
| | | MRI scan | magnetic resonance imaging scan |
| IVU | intravenous urography (IVU); also called *excretory urography (EU)* or *intravenous pyelography (IVP)* | MS | musculoskeletal; multiple sclerosis; mental status; mitral stenosis |

| Abbreviation | Meaning | Abbreviation | Meaning |
|---|---|---|---|
| MSH | melanocyte-stimulating hormone | pH | symbol for degree of acidity or alkalinity |
| MVP | mitral valve prolapse | PID | pelvic inflammatory disease |
| Myop | myopia | PMP | previous menstrual period |
| Na+ | sodium (an electrolyte) | PMS | premenstrual syndrome |
| NB | newborn | PND | paroxysmal nocturnal dyspnea |
| NCV | nerve conduction velocity | | |
| NG | nasogastric | po | by mouth (per os) |
| NIDDM | non-insulin-dependent diabetes mellitus | $Po_2$ | partial pressure of oxygen |
| | | poly, PMN, PMNL | polymorphonuclear leukocyte |
| NIHL | noise-induced hearing loss | | |
| NMTs | nebulized mist treatments | post | posterior |
| NPH | neutral protamine Hagedorn (insulin) | PRL | prolactin |
| | | prn | as required |
| npo | nothing by mouth | PSA | prostate-specific antigen |
| NSAIDs | nonsteroidal anti-inflammatory drugs | PT | prothrombin time, physical therapy |
| $O_2$ | oxygen | PTCA | percutaneous transluminal coronary angioplasty |
| OB | obstetrics | | |
| OCPs | oral contraceptive pills | PTH | parathyroid hormone; also called *parathormone* |
| *OD | right eye | | |
| OD | Doctor of Optometry | PTT | partial thromboplastin time |
| ORTH, ortho | orthopedics | PUD | peptic ulcer disease |
| *OS | left eye | PVC | premature ventricular contraction |
| *OU | both eyes together | | |
| P | phosphorous; pulse | q2h | every 2 hours |
| PA | posteroanterior; pernicious anemia | qam, qm | every morning |
| | | *qd | every day |
| PAC | premature atrial contraction | qh | every hour |
| Pap | Papanicolaou smear | qid | four times a day |
| para 1, 2, 3 | unipara, bipara, tripara (number of viable births) | *qod | every other day |
| | | qpm, qn | every night |
| | | R/O | rule out |
| PAT | paroxysmal atrial tachycardia | RA | rheumatoid arthritis |
| pc, pp | after meals (postprandial) | RAI | radioactive iodine |
| PCL | posterior cruciate ligament | RAIU | radioactive iodine uptake |
| PCNL | percutaneous nephrolithotomy | RBC, rbc | red blood cell, red blood count |
| $Pco_2$ | partial pressure of carbon dioxide | RD | respiratory distress |
| | | RDS | respiratory distress syndrome |
| PCP | *Pneumocystis carinii* pneumonia | RF | rheumatoid factor |
| | | RK | radial keratotomy |
| PCV | packed cell volume | RLQ | right lower quadrant |
| PE tube | pressure-equalizing tube (placed in the eardrum) | ROM | range of motion |
| | | RP | retrograde pyelography |
| PERRLA | pupils equal, round, and reactive to light and accommodation | RSO | right salpingo-oophorectomy |
| | | rt | right |
| | | RUQ | right upper quadrant |
| PET | positron emission tomography | RV | residual volume; right ventricle |
| PFT | pulmonary function tests | SA | sinoatrial |
| PGH | pituitary growth hormone | $Sao_2$ | arterial oxygen saturation |

| Abbreviation | Meaning | Abbreviation | Meaning |
|---|---|---|---|
| SD | shoulder disarticulation | TIA | transient ischemic attack |
| segs | segmented neutrophils | *tid | three times a day |
| SICS | small incision cataract surgery | TKA | total knee arthroplasty |
| | | TKR | total knee replacement |
| SIDS | sudden infant death syndrome | TPR | temperature, pulse, and respiration |
| SLE | systemic lupus erythematosus | TSE | testicular self-examination |
| SNS | sympathetic nervous system | TSH | thyroid-stimulating |
| SOB | shortness of breath | hormone | |
| sono | sonogram | TURP | transurethral resection of |
| sp. gr. | specific gravity | | the prostate (for |
| SPECT | single photon emission computed tomography | | prostatectomy) |
| | | TVH | total vaginal hysterectomy |
| ST | esotropia | Tx | treatment |
| stat | immediately | U&L, U/L | upper and lower |
| STD | sexually transmitted disease | UA | urinalysis |
| | | UC | uterine contractions |
| Sub-Q, subQ | subcutaneous (injection) | ung | ointment |
| Sx | symptom | URI | upper respiratory infection |
| T&A | tonsillectomy and adenoidectomy | US | ultrasound |
| | | VA | visual acuity |
| T$_3$ | triiodothyronine (thyroid hormone) | VC | vital capacity |
| | | VCUG | voiding cystourethrography |
| T$_4$ | thyroxine (thyroid hormone) | VD | venereal disease |
| | | VF | visual field |
| TAH | total abdominal hysterectomy | VSD | ventricular septal defect |
| | | VT | ventricular tachycardia |
| TB | tuberculosis | WBC, wbc | white blood cell, white blood count |
| TFT | thyroid function test | | |
| THA | total hip arthroplasty | XP, XDP | xeroderma pigmentosum |
| THR | total hip replacement | XT | exotropia |

*Although these abbreviations are currently found in medical records and clinical notes, the Joint Commission on Accreditation of Healthcare Organizations (JCAHO) requires their discontinuance. Instead, write out the meanings.

# C

# Glossary of Medical Word Elements

# Medical Word Elements

| Medical Word Element | Meaning |
|---|---|
| **A** | |
| a- | without, not |
| ab- | from, away from |
| abdomin/o | abdomen |
| abort/o | to miscarry |
| -ac | pertaining to, relating to |
| acous/o | hearing |
| acr/o | extremity |
| acromi/o | acromion (projection of scapula) |
| -acusis | hearing |
| -ad | toward |
| ad- | toward |
| aden/o | gland |
| adenoid/o | adenoids |
| adip/o | fat |
| adren/o | adrenal glands |
| adrenal/o | adrenal glands |
| aer/o | air |
| af- | toward |
| agglutin/o | clumping, gluing |
| agora- | marketplace |
| -al | pertaining to, relating to |
| albin/o | white |
| albumin/o | albumin (protein) |
| -algesia | pain |
| -algia | pain |
| allo- | other, differing from the normal |
| alveol/o | alveolus (plural, alveoli) |
| ambly/o | dull, dim |
| amni/o | amnion (amniotic sac) |
| an- | without, not |
| an/o | anus |
| ana- | against; up; back |
| andr/o | male |
| aneurysm/o | a widening, a widened blood vessel |
| angi/o | vessel (usually blood or lymph) |
| aniso- | unequal, dissimilar |
| ankyl/o | stiffness; bent, crooked |
| ante- | before, in front of |

| Medical Word Element | Meaning |
|---|---|
| anter/o | anterior, front |
| anthrac/o | black, coal |
| anti- | against |
| aort/o | aorta |
| append/o | appendix |
| appendic/o | appendix |
| aque/o | water |
| -ar | pertaining to, relating to |
| -arche | beginning |
| arteri/o | artery |
| arteriol/o | arteriole |
| arthr/o | joint |
| -ary | pertaining to, relating to |
| asbest/o | asbestos |
| -asthenia | weakness, debility |
| astr/o | star |
| -ate | having the form of, possessing |
| atel/o | incomplete; imperfect |
| ather/o | fatty plaque |
| -ation | process (of) |
| atri/o | atrium |
| audi/o | hearing |
| audit/o | hearing |
| aur/o | ear |
| auricul/o | ear |
| auto- | self, own |
| ax/o | axis, axon |
| azot/o | nitrogenous compounds |
| **B** | |
| bacteri/o | bacteria |
| balan/o | glans penis |
| bas/o | base (alkaline, opposite of acid) |
| bi- | two |
| bi/o | life |
| -blast | embryonic cell |
| blast/o | embryonic cell |
| blephar/o | eyelid |
| brachi/o | arm |
| brady- | slow |
| bronch/o | bronchus (plural, bronchi) |
| bronchi/o | bronchus (plural, bronchi) |

| Medical Word Element | Meaning |
|---|---|
| bronchiol/o | bronchiole |
| bucc/o | cheek |

## C

| Medical Word Element | Meaning |
|---|---|
| calc/o | calcium |
| calcane/o | calcaneum (heel bone) |
| -capnia | carbon dioxide ($CO_2$) |
| carcin/o | cancer |
| cardi/o | heart |
| -cardia | heart condition |
| carp/o | carpus (wrist bones) |
| cata- | down |
| caud/o | tail |
| cauter/o | heat, burn |
| -cele | hernia, swelling |
| -centesis | surgical puncture |
| cephal/o | head |
| -ception | conceiving |
| cerebell/o | cerebellum |
| cerebr/o | cerebrum |
| cervic/o | neck; cervix uteri (neck of uterus) |
| chalic/o | limestone |
| cheil/o | lip |
| chem/o | chemical; drug |
| chlor/o | green |
| chol/e | bile, gall |
| cholangi/o | bile vessel |
| cholecyst/o | gallbladder |
| choledoch/o | bile duct |
| chondr/o | cartilage |
| chori/o | chorion |
| choroid/o | choroid |
| chrom/o | color |
| chromat/o | color |
| -cide | killing |
| cine- | movement |
| cinemat/o | things that move |
| circum- | around |
| cirrh/o | yellow |
| -cision | a cutting |
| -clasia | to break; surgical fracture |
| -clasis | to break; surgical fracture |

| Medical Word Element | Meaning |
|---|---|
| -clast | to break; surgical fracture |
| clavicul/o | clavicle (collar bone) |
| -cleisis | closure |
| clon/o | clonus (turmoil) |
| -clysis | irrigation, washing |
| coccyg/o | coccyx (tailbone) |
| cochle/o | cochlea |
| col/o | colon |
| colon/o | colon |
| colp/o | vagina |
| condyl/o | condyle |
| coni/o | dust |
| conjunctiv/o | conjunctiva |
| -continence | to hold back |
| contra- | against, opposite |
| core/o | pupil |
| corne/o | cornea |
| cor/o | pupil |
| corp/o | body |
| corpor/o | body |
| cortic/o | cortex |
| cost/o | ribs |
| crani/o | cranium (skull) |
| crin/o | secrete |
| -crine | secrete |
| cruci/o | cross |
| cry/o | cold |
| crypt/o | hidden |
| culd/o | cul-de-sac |
| -cusia | hearing |
| -cusis | hearing |
| cutane/o | skin |
| cyan/o | blue |
| cycl/o | ciliary body of eye; circular, cycle |
| -cyesis | pregnancy |
| cyst/o | bladder |
| cyt/o | cell |
| -cyte | cell |

## D

| Medical Word Element | Meaning |
|---|---|
| dacry/o | tear; lacrimal apparatus (duct, sac, or gland) |
| dacryocyst/o | lacrimal sac |

| Medical Word Element | Meaning |
|---|---|
| dactyl/o | fingers; toes |
| de- | cessation |
| dendr/o | tree |
| dent/o | teeth |
| derm/o | skin |
| -derma | skin |
| dermat/o | skin |
| -desis | binding, fixation (of a bone or joint) |
| di- | double |
| dia- | through, across |
| dipl- | double |
| dipl/o | double |
| dips/o | thirst |
| -dipsia | thirst |
| dist/o | far, farthest |
| dors/o | back (of body) |
| duct/o | to lead; carry |
| -duction | act of leading, bringing, conducting |
| duoden/o | duodenum (first part of small intestine) |
| dur/o | dura mater; hard |
| -dynia | pain |
| dys- | bad; painful; difficult |

## E

| Medical Word Element | Meaning |
|---|---|
| -eal | pertaining to, relating to |
| ec- | out, out from |
| echo- | a repeated sound |
| -ectasis | dilation, expansion |
| ecto- | outside, outward |
| -ectomy | excision, removal |
| -edema | swelling |
| ef- | away from |
| electr/o | electricity |
| -ema | state of; condition |
| embol/o | plug |
| -emesis | vomiting |
| -emia | blood condition |
| emphys/o | to inflate |
| end- | in, within |

| Medical Word Element | Meaning |
|---|---|
| encephal/o | brain |
| end- | within |
| endo- | in, within |
| enter/o | intestine (usually small intestine) |
| eosin/o | dawn (rose-colored) |
| epi- | above, upon |
| epididym/o | epididymis |
| epiglott/o | epiglottis |
| episi/o | vulva |
| erythem/o | red |
| erythemat/o | red |
| erythr/o | red |
| eschar/o | scab |
| -esis | condition |
| eso- | inward |
| esophag/o | esophagus |
| esthes/o | feeling |
| -esthesia | feeling |
| eti/o | cause |
| eu- | good, normal |
| ex- | out, out from |
| exo- | outside, outward |
| extra- | outside |

## F

| Medical Word Element | Meaning |
|---|---|
| faci/o | face |
| fasci/o | band, fascia (fibrous membrane supporting and separating muscles) |
| femor/o | femur (thigh bone) |
| -ferent | to carry |
| fibr/o | fiber, fibrous tissue |
| fibul/o | fibula (smaller bone of lower leg) |
| fluor/o | luminous, fluorescence |
| frotteur/o | to rub |

## G

| Medical Word Element | Meaning |
|---|---|
| galact/o | milk |
| gangli/o | ganglion (knot or knotlike mass) |

| Medical Word Element | Meaning |
|---|---|
| gastr/o | stomach |
| -gen | forming, producing, origin |
| gen/o | forming, producing, origin |
| -genesis | forming, producing, origin |
| gingiv/o | gum(s) |
| glauc/o | gray |
| gli/o | glue; neuroglial tissue |
| -glia | glue; neuroglial tissue |
| -globin | protein |
| glomerul/o | glomerulus |
| gloss/o | tongue |
| glott/o | glottis |
| gluc/o | sugar, sweetness |
| glucos/o | sugar, sweetness |
| glyc/o | sugar, sweetness |
| -gnosis | knowing |
| gonad/o | gonads, sex glands |
| goni/o | angle |
| -graft | transplantation |
| -gram | record, writing |
| granul/o | granule |
| -graph | instrument for recording |
| -graphy | process of recording |
| -gravida | pregnant woman |
| gyn/o | woman, female |
| gynec/o | woman, female |

## H

| Medical Word Element | Meaning |
|---|---|
| hallucin/o | hallucination |
| hedon/o | pleasure |
| hem/o | blood |
| hemangi/o | blood vessel |
| hemat/o | blood |
| hemi- | one half |
| hepat/o | liver |
| hetero- | different |
| hidr/o | sweat |
| hist/o | tissue |
| histi/o | tissue |
| homeo- | same, alike |
| homo- | same |

| Medical Word Element | Meaning |
|---|---|
| humer/o | humerus (upper arm bone) |
| hydr/o | water |
| hyper- | excessive, above normal |
| hypn/o | sleep |
| hypo- | under, below, deficient |
| hyster/o | uterus (womb) |

## I

| Medical Word Element | Meaning |
|---|---|
| -ia | condition |
| -iac | pertaining to, relating to |
| -iasis | abnormal condition (produced by something specified) |
| iatr/o | physician; medicine; treatment |
| -iatry | medicine; treatment |
| -ic | pertaining to, relating to |
| -ical | pertaining to, relating to |
| -ice | noun ending |
| ichthy/o | dry, scaly |
| -ician | specialist |
| -icle | small, minute |
| -icterus | jaundice |
| idi/o | unknown, peculiar |
| -ile | pertaining to, relating to |
| ile/o | ileum (third part of small intestine) |
| ili/o | ilium (lateral, flaring portion of hip bone) |
| im- | not |
| immun/o | immune, immunity, safe |
| in- | in, not |
| -ine | pertaining to, relating to |
| infer/o | lower, below |
| infra- | under, below |
| inguin/o | groin |
| insulin/o | insulin |
| inter- | between |
| intra- | in, within |
| -ion | the act of |
| -ior | pertaining to, relating to |
| irid/o | iris |
| -is | noun ending |

| Medical Word Element | Meaning | Medical Word Element | Meaning |
|---|---|---|---|
| isch/o | to hold back | later/o | side, to one side |
| ischi/o | ischium (lower portion of hip bone) | lei/o | smooth |
| -ism | condition | leiomy/o | smooth muscle (visceral) |
| iso- | same, equal | -lepsy | seizure |
| -ist | specialist | lept/o | thin, slender |
| -isy | state of; condition | leuk/o | white |
| -itic | pertaining to, relating to | lex/o | word, phrase |
| -itis | inflammation | lingu/o | tongue |
| -ive | pertaining to, relating to | lip/o | fat |
| -ization | process (of) | lipid/o | fat |
| | | -lith | stone, calculus |
| | | lith/o | stone, calculus |
| | | lob/o | lobe |
| | | log/o | study of |
| | | -logist | specialist in study of |
| | | -logy | study of |
| | | lord/o | curve, swayback |
| | | -lucent | to shine; clear |
| | | lumb/o | loins (lower back) |
| | | lymph/o | lymph |
| | | lymphaden/o | lymph gland (node) |
| | | lymphangi/o | lymph vessel |
| | | -lysis | separation; destruction; loosening |

## J

| jaund/o | yellow |
|---|---|
| jejun/o | jejunum (second part of small intestine) |

## K

| kal/i | potassium (an electrolyte) |
|---|---|
| kary/o | nucleus |
| kerat/o | horny tissue; hard; cornea |
| kern/o | kernel (nucleus) |
| ket/o | ketone bodies (acids and acetones) |
| keton/o | ketone bodies (acids and acetones) |
| kinesi/o | movement |
| -kinesia | movement |
| kinet/o | movement |
| klept/o | to steal |
| kyph/o | hill, mountain |

## L

| labi/o | lip |
|---|---|
| labyrinth/o | labyrinth (inner ear) |
| lacrim/o | tear; lacrimal apparatus (duct, sac, or gland) |
| lact/o | milk |
| -lalia | speech, babble |
| lamin/o | lamina (part of vertebral arch) |
| lapar/o | abdomen |
| laryng/o | larynx (voice box) |

## M

| macro- | large |
|---|---|
| mal- | bad |
| -malacia | softening |
| mamm/o | breast |
| -mania | state of mental disorder, frenzy |
| mast/o | breast |
| mastoid/o | mastoid process |
| maxill/o | maxilla (upper jaw bone) |
| meat/o | opening, meatus |
| medi- | middle |
| medi/o | middle |
| medull/o | medulla |
| mega- | enlargement |
| megal/o | enlargement |
| -megaly | enlargement |

| Medical Word Element | Meaning | Medical Word Element | Meaning |
|---|---|---|---|
| melan/o | black | neur/o | nerve |
| men/o | menses, menstruation | neutr/o | neutral; neither |
| mening/o | meninges (membranes covering brain and spinal cord) | nid/o | nest |
| | | noct/o | night |
| | | nucle/o | nucleus |
| meningi/o | meninges (membranes covering brain and spinal cord) | nulli- | none |
| | | nyctal/o | night |

**O**

| Medical Word Element | Meaning | Medical Word Element | Meaning |
|---|---|---|---|
| ment/o | mind | obstetr/o | midwife |
| meso- | middle | ocul/o | eye |
| meta- | change, beyond | odont/o | teeth |
| metacarp/o | metacarpus (hand bones) | -oid | resembling |
| metatars/o | metatarsus (foot bones) | -ole | small, minute |
| -meter | instrument for measuring | olig/o | scanty |
| metr/o | uterus (womb); measure | -oma | tumor |
| metri/o | uterus (womb) | omphal/o | navel (umbilicus) |
| -metry | act of measuring | onc/o | tumor |
| mi/o | smaller, less | onych/o | nail |
| micr/o | small | oophor/o | ovary |
| micro- | small | -opaque | obscure |
| mono- | one | ophthalm/o | eye |
| morph/o | form, shape, structure | -opia | vision |
| muc/o | mucus | -opsia | vision |
| multi- | many, much | -opsy | view of |
| muscul/o | muscle | opt/o | eye, vision |
| mut/a | genetic change | optic/o | eye, vision |
| my/o | muscle | or/o | mouth |
| myc/o | fungus | orch/o | testis (plural, testes) |
| mydr/o | widen, enlarge | orchi/o | testis (plural, testes) |
| myel/o | bone marrow; spinal cord | orchid/o | testis (plural, testes) |
| myos/o | muscle | -orexia | appetite |
| myring/o | tympanic membrane (eardrum) | orth/o | straight |
| | | -ory | pertaining to, relating to |
| myx/o | mucus | -osis | abnormal condition; increase (used primarily with blood cells) |

**N**

| Medical Word Element | Meaning | Medical Word Element | Meaning |
|---|---|---|---|
| narc/o | stupor; numbness; sleep | -osmia | smell |
| nas/o | nose | oste/o | bone |
| nat/o | birth | ot/o | ear |
| natr/o | sodium (an electrolyte) | -ous | pertaining to, relating to |
| necr/o | death, necrosis | ovari/o | ovary |
| neo- | new | | |
| nephr/o | kidney | | |

| Medical Word Element | Meaning |
|---|---|
| ox/i | oxygen |
| -oxia | oxygen |
| ox/o | oxygen |
| oxy- | quick, sharp |

## P

| Medical Word Element | Meaning |
|---|---|
| pachy- | thick |
| palat/o | palate (roof of mouth) |
| pan- | all |
| pancreat/o | pancreas |
| -para | to bear (offspring) |
| para- | near, beside; beyond |
| parathyroid/o | parathyroid glands |
| -paresis | partial paralysis |
| patell/o | patella (kneecap) |
| path/o | disease |
| -pathy | disease |
| pector/o | chest |
| ped/i | foot; child |
| ped/o | foot; child |
| pedicul/o | a louse |
| pelv/i | pelvis |
| pelv/o | pelvis |
| pen/o | penis |
| -penia | decrease, deficiency |
| -pepsia | digestion |
| per- | through |
| peri- | around |
| perine/o | perineum |
| peritone/o | peritoneum |
| -pexy | fixation (of an organ) |
| phac/o | lens |
| phag/o | swallowing, eating |
| -phage | swallowing, eating |
| -phagia | swallowing, eating |
| phalang/o | phalanges (bones of fingers and toes) |
| pharmaceutic/o | drug, medicine |
| pharyng/o | pharynx (throat) |
| -phasia | speech |
| phe/o | dusky, dark |
| -phil | attraction for |

| Medical Word Element | Meaning |
|---|---|
| phil/o | attraction for |
| -philia | attraction for |
| phim/o | muzzle |
| phleb/o | vein |
| -phobia | fear |
| phon/o | voice, sound |
| -phonia | voice, sound |
| -phoresis | carrying, transmission |
| -phoria | feeling (mental state) |
| phot/o | light |
| phren/o | diaphragm; mind |
| -phylaxis | protection |
| -physis | growth |
| pil/o | hair |
| pituitar/o | pituitary gland |
| -plakia | plaque |
| plas/o | formation, growth |
| -plasia | formation, growth |
| -plasm | formation, growth |
| -plasty | surgical repair |
| -plegia | paralysis |
| pleur/o | pleura |
| -plexy | stroke |
| -pnea | breathing |
| pneum/o | air; lung |
| pneumon/o | air; lung |
| pod/o | foot |
| -poiesis | formation, production |
| poikil/o | varied, irregular |
| poli/o | gray; gray matter (of brain or spinal cord) |
| poly- | many, much |
| polyp/o | small growth |
| -porosis | porous |
| post- | after, behind |
| poster/o | back (of body), behind, posterior |
| -potence | power |
| -prandial | meal |
| pre- | before, in front of |
| presby/o | old age |
| primi- | first |

| Medical Word Element | Meaning |
| --- | --- |
| pro- | before, in front of |
| proct/o | anus, rectum |
| prostat/o | prostate gland |
| proxim/o | near, nearest |
| pseudo- | false |
| psych/o | mind |
| ptyal/o | saliva |
| -ptosis | prolapse, downward displacement |
| -ptysis | spitting |
| pub/o | pelvis bone (anterior part of pelvic bone) |
| pulmon/o | lung |
| pupill/o | pupil |
| py/o | pus |
| pyel/o | renal pelvis |
| pylor/o | pylorus |
| pyr/o | fire |

## Q

| | |
| --- | --- |
| quadri- | four |

## R

| | |
| --- | --- |
| rachi/o | spine |
| radi/o | radiation, x-ray; radius (lower arm bone on thumb side) |
| radicul/o | nerve root |
| rect/o | rectum |
| ren/o | kidney |
| reticul/o | net, mesh |
| retin/o | retina |
| retro- | backward, behind |
| rhabd/o | rod-shaped (striated) |
| rhabdomy/o | striated (skeletal) muscle |
| rhin/o | nose |
| rhytid/o | wrinkle |
| roentgen/o | x-rays |
| -rrhage | bursting forth (of) |
| -rrhagia | bursting forth (of) |
| -rrhaphy | suture |
| -rrhea | discharge, flow |

| Medical Word Element | Meaning |
| --- | --- |
| -rrhexis | rupture |
| rube/o | red |

## S

| | |
| --- | --- |
| sacr/o | sacrum |
| salping/o | tube (usually fallopian or eustachian [auditory] tubes) |
| -salpinx | tube (usually fallopian or eustachian [auditory] tubes) |
| sarc/o | flesh (connective tissue) |
| scapul/o | scapula (shoulder blade) |
| -sarcoma | malignant tumor of connective tissue |
| -schisis | a splitting |
| schiz/o | split |
| scler/o | hardening; sclera (white of eye) |
| scoli/o | crooked, bent |
| -scope | instrument for examining |
| -scopy | visual examination |
| scot/o | darkness |
| seb/o | sebum, sebaceous |
| semi- | one half |
| sept/o | septum |
| sequestr/o | a separation |
| ser/o | serum |
| sial/o | saliva, salivary gland |
| sider/o | iron |
| sigmoid/o | sigmoid colon |
| silic/o | flint |
| sin/o | sinus, cavity |
| sinus/o | sinus, cavity |
| -sis | state of; condition |
| -social | society |
| somat/o | body |
| somn/o | sleep |
| son/o | sound |
| -spadias | slit, fissure |
| -spasm | involuntary contraction, twitching |
| sperm/o | spermatozoa, sperm cells |

| Medical Word Element | Meaning |
|---|---|
| spermat/o | spermatozoa, sperm cells |
| sphygm/o | pulse |
| -sphyxia | pulse |
| spin/o | spine |
| spir/o | breathe |
| splen/o | spleen |
| spondyl/o | vertebrae (backbone) |
| squam/o | scale |
| staped/o | stapes |
| -stasis | standing still |
| steat/o | fat |
| sten/o | narrowing, stricture |
| -stenosis | narrowing, stricture |
| stern/o | sternum (breastbone) |
| steth/o | chest |
| sthen/o | strength |
| stigmat/o | a point |
| stomat/o | mouth |
| -stomy | forming an opening (mouth) |
| sub- | under, below |
| sudor/o | sweat |
| super- | upper, above |
| supra- | above; excessive; superior |
| sym- | union, together, joined |
| syn- | union, together, joined |
| synapt/o | synapsis, point of contact |
| synov/o | synovial membrane, synovial fluid |

### T

| Medical Word Element | Meaning |
|---|---|
| tachy- | rapid |
| tax/o | order, coordination |
| -taxia | order, coordination |
| ten/o | tendon |
| tend/o | tendon |
| tendin/o | tendon |
| -tension | to stretch |
| test/o | testis (plural, testes) |
| thalam/o | thalamus |
| thalass/o | sea |
| thec/o | sheath (usually refers to meninges) |
| thel/o | nipple |

| Medical Word Element | Meaning |
|---|---|
| therapeut/o | treatment |
| -therapy | treatment |
| therm/o | heat |
| thorac/o | chest |
| -thorax | chest |
| thromb/o | blood clot |
| thym/o | thymus gland |
| -thymia | mind; emotion |
| thyr/o | thyroid gland |
| thyroid/o | thyroid gland |
| tibi/o | tibia (larger bone of lower leg) |
| -tic | pertaining to, relating to |
| till/o | to pull |
| -tocia | childbirth, labor |
| tom/o | to cut |
| -tome | instrument to cut |
| -tomy | incision |
| ton/o | tension |
| tonsill/o | tonsils |
| tox/o | poison |
| -toxic | poison |
| toxic/o | poison |
| trabecul/o | trabecula (supporting bundles of fibers) |
| trache/o | trachea (windpipe) |
| trans- | through, across |
| tri- | three |
| trich/o | hair |
| trigon/o | trigone (triangular region at base of bladder) |
| -tripsy | crushing |
| -trophy | development, nourishment |
| -tropia | turning |
| -tropin | stimulate |
| tubercul/o | a little swelling |
| tympan/o | tympanic membrane (eardrum) |

### U

| Medical Word Element | Meaning |
|---|---|
| -ula | small, minute |
| -ule | small, minute |
| uln/o | ulna (lower arm bone on opposite side of thumb) |

| Medical Word Element | Meaning | Medical Word Element | Meaning |
|---|---|---|---|
| ultra- | excess, beyond | ventricul/o | ventricle (of heart or brain) |
| -um | structure, thing | -version | turning |
| umbilic/o | umbilicus, navel | vertebr/o | vertebrae (backbone) |
| ungu/o | nail | vesic/o | bladder |
| uni- | one | vesicul/o | seminal vesicle |
| ur/o | urine | vest/o | clothes |
| ureter/o | ureter | viscer/o | internal organs |
| urethr/o | urethra | vitr/o | vitreous body (of eye) |
| -uria | urine | vitre/o | glassy |
| urin/o | urine | vol/o | volume |
| -us | condition; structure | voyeur/o | to see |
| uter/o | uterus (womb) | vulv/o | vulva |
| uvul/o | uvula | | |

## V

| | | | |
|---|---|---|---|
| vagin/o | vagina | | |
| valv/o | valve | | |
| varic/o | dilated vein | | |
| vas/o | vessel; vas deferens; duct | | |
| vascul/o | vessel | | |
| ven/o | vein | | |
| ventr/o | belly, belly side | | |

## X

| | |
|---|---|
| xanth/o | yellow |
| xen/o | foreign, strange |
| xer/o | dry |
| xiph/o | sword |

## Y

| | |
|---|---|
| -y | condition; process |

# Appendix

D

# Index of Genetic Disorders

# Appendix

# E

# Index of Diagnostic Imaging Procedures

# Index of Pharmacology

# G

# Index of
# Oncological Terms

# Index